Psychopathology and Function

Second Edition

Psychopathology and Function

Second Edition

Bette R. Bonder, PhD, OTR/L, FAOTA
Professor and Director,
Center for Health Sciences and Human Services
Cleveland State University
Cleveland, Ohio

SLACK Incorporated, 6900 Grove Road, Thorofare, NJ 08086-9447

Note to the Reader

As new scientific information becomes available through basic and clinical research, recommended treatments and drug therapies undergo changes. The editor and publisher have done everything possible to make this book accurate, up-to-date, and in accord with accepted standards at the time of publication. The authors, editor, and publisher cannot accept responsibility for errors or exclusions or for the outcome of the application of material presented herein. There is no expressed or implied warranty of this book or information imparted by it. Any practice described in this book should be applied by the reader to the unique circumstances that may apply in each situation. The reader is advised to always review the provided product literature and use caution when using new or infrequently ordered drugs.

Any review or mention of specific companies or products is not intended as an endorsement by the author or by the publisher.

Publisher: John H. Bond
Acquisitions Editor: Amy E. Drummond
Production Editor: Debra L. Clarke
Art Director: Linda Baker

Bonder, Bette.
Psychopathology and Function/Bette R. Bonder.—2nd ed.
p. cm.
Includes bibliographical references and index.
ISBN 1-55642-270-9
1. Psychology, Pathological. I. Title.
RC454.B5765 1995
616.89—dc20   95-10428

Printed in the United States of America
Published by: SLACK Incorporated
             6900 Grove Road
             Thorofare, NJ 08086-9447

Last digit is print number: 10 9 8 7 6 5 4 3 2

Dedication

For Pat, Aaron and Jordan

Contents

Acknowledgments

This book required the active efforts of many individuals. Gary Kielhofner first asked me to consider writing it, and provided considerable input to the first edition, as did a number of students from the University of Illinois at Chicago. The second edition was brought to completion with the support of Debra Clarke and Amy Drummond at SLACK, and Karen Bradley and Tamara Phillips at Cleveland State University. Many students at Cleveland State University offered helpful suggestions based on their use of the first edition. I am most appreciative of the assistance provided by these individuals. As always, my husband, Pat Bray, and my sons Aaron and Jordan Bray, were supportive and encouraging. They have my profound thanks.

Preface

Any health care provider working in mental health recognizes the importance of psychiatric diagnosis. Many decisions in the mental health system are based on the label which the patient carries. However, most mental health professionals are also aware of the limitations of this label. Most important for occupational therapists, it provides relatively little information about what the individual needs to accomplish in order to survive, or the activities the individual wants to be able to do in order to maintain a high level of life satisfaction. In addition, it does not inform the therapist about the individual's ability to perform those activities.

While occupational therapists must function within the system, their perspective about clients may be markedly different than that of other team members. This is desirable, since optimal well-being is comprised of many factors: physical health, functional abilities, attitudes and so on. All these must be considered in providing the most effective intervention. However, professionals must be able to communicate with each other and for better or for worse, the diagnostic system is the way in which the communication occurs.

This text integrates the perspectives of medicine and occupational therapy, enabling the occupational therapist to convey information in ways the physician (usually psychiatrist) and other team members will understand. It also enables the occupational therapist to interpret what team members are saying about the client in terms of the goals of therapy. While this understanding is crucial, it is also important for occupational therapists to maintain their unique perspective and to make their vital contribution to effective intervention. It is only through this interaction of views that the best possible outcome can be assured for the service recipient.

Introduction to the Second Edition

In the 5 years since the first edition of *Psychopathology and Function,* much has changed in mental health care. Some of the changes were anticipated, most notably the publication of the *Diagnostic and Statistical Manual of Mental Disorders-Fourth Edition* (DSM-IV) (American Psychiatric Association, 1994). This revision of the diagnostic guidelines for mental health practitioners was planned before the ink was dry on DSM-III-R (APA, 1987), and is the result of vast amounts of research and discussion.

Among the unanticipated changes is the massive upheaval in service delivery. As this book goes to press, there is much debate about how health care can best be delivered, how to control costs, and how to assure access for all individuals in the United States. In mental health care, this debate has already resulted in substantial changes in care. Inpatient care for mental disorders is now infrequent, with length of stay reduced to its absolute minimum (Sleek, 1994). Twenty-four hour stays are now common; a week is unusual. Cost control efforts have led to examination of roles of various providers, with exploration of alternatives to physician care being actively sought. Even the availability of care for mental disorders is being questioned, with some movement toward elimination of broad access to mental health services.

In this atmosphere, diagnosis takes on added importance. Demonstrating the validity and reliability of identifiable entities is essential to assuring care for individuals struggling with various mental problems. Thus, the degree to which the development of DSM-IV has been guided by empirical evidence of disorder is a critical factor in its eventual acceptance. As you will see, this is a subject of much debate.

For occupational therapists, and for other providers of care for individuals with psychiatric symptoms, diagnosis continues to be one of several factors guiding intervention. This edition of *Psychopathology and Function* expands its exploration of the ways in which occupational therapists interact with the diagnostic system in providing care. It also examines the role of all health care providers in attending to symptoms of mental disorder in individuals receiving care for other problems. Although the debate rages about care for psychiatric disorders, the reality is that every health care provider in every setting is likely to encounter individuals who display signs of these problems. This reality has significant impact on all care provided.

This book is designed to guide occupational therapists in three areas: 1) understanding their clients, 2) communicating with other professionals, and 3) providing care to real people in real life, assuring that quality of life is maintained or enhanced for those being served. The text is not intended to provide comprehensive coverage of the occupational therapy process in mental health. Many other books discuss that subject from a variety of perspectives. This text is designed as an overview of the kinds of clients with whom occupational therapists and other health care providers are likely to work, and to give therapists an understanding of the ways in which other mental health professionals view these individuals. By understanding the context for service, occupational therapists can enhance their intervention and define their unique contribution to mental health.

References

American Psychiatric Association (1987). *Diagnostic and Statistical Manual of Mental Disorders* (3rd ed. rev.) Washington, DC: Author.

American Psychiatric Association (1994). *Diagnostic and Statistical Manual of Mental Disorders* (4th ed.) Washington, DC: Author.

Sleek, S. (July, 1994). Merits of long, short therapy debated. *American Psychological Association Monitor,* 40-41.

Introduction to the First Edition

The field of mental health has undergone vast changes in the last 25 years. Experimentally validated information about both etiology and treatment of psychiatric disorders has grown enormously, allowing for increasingly effective intervention and, in many instances, more positive prognosis. New information has changed the face of mental health treatment for the individual and, at the same time, altered the systems in which intervention is offered.

In spite of the increase in knowledge, much remains to be learned. The etiology of some syndromes remains a mystery, while heated debate continues as to whether other syndromes are the result of biology, environment, learning, or some combination of these. Treatment is, in some instances, still a matter of trial and error, with providers making educated guesses about which of the existing interventions might make a difference. Even when a specific therapy is generally accepted as the treatment of choice, the reasons for its efficacy may be poorly understood.

At the same time, health care in general has become increasingly complex, both in terms of treatment and the systems in which care is delivered. Patients, their families and employers, third party payers, and health care providers, all struggle with issues about quality of care, cost, and the rights of the various interested parties. Occupational therapists, like other health care providers, have had to adapt to these increasing complexities in order to continue to provide high quality care.

Occupational therapy as a profession originated in mental health (Bruce & Borg, 1987). The earliest therapists provided activities which were thought "useful," and "healthful," in order to divert individuals from their problems, as "moral treatment" emerged as a theory for intervention. Meyer (1977) for example, believed mental illness to be a "problem of living," and felt that a balance of work, leisure, and rest would restore health.

The emerging beliefs of occupational therapy fit within the two primary forms of treatment employed by physicians and other mental health care providers at that time. For individuals who were psychotic (severely disturbed and out of contact with reality), removal from the environment and placement in an institution was the norm. It was felt that these disorders were largely intractable, and little could be done except to relieve the families of the burden of caring for their bizarre relatives. There was some suspicion that these illnesses had a physical component, which resulted in the employment of insulin shock, psychosurgery, and, later, electroshock treatments. For those who were "neurotic" (emotionally disturbed but in contact with reality), psychoanalysis or other verbal therapies were implemented, usually while the patient continued to reside at home. This form of treatment often meant years of intensive verbal therapy focused on discussion of experiences which might have molded maladaptive emotional reactions.

The most striking change in mental health care was the discovery of a variety of psychopharmacological agents in the middle of this century. These drugs made it possible to control many psychotic symptoms, as well as depression and anxiety. At the same time, a variety of new theories about behavior increased the range of therapies from which treatment choices were made. Behavior therapy, cognitive therapy, and family therapies are among the alternatives which have emerged. These theories have been investigated with a variety of research methodologies, so that effectiveness can be more clearly established.

Many of the new therapies are brief. While earlier types of interventions may have continued for years, many of the newer types of treatment are designed to reach maximum effectiveness within a few weeks or months. In addition, many are provided outside of institutional settings, in community mental health centers, day treatment centers, or other community-based facilities.

In addition to (and perhaps in response to) the rapid growth of knowledge about psychiatric disorders, there has been a proliferation of mental health professions. Early in the century, psychiatrists, psychologists, social workers, and nurses were the primary providers of care. Added to the list now, in addition to occupational therapists among many others, are vocational counselors, as well as recreation, art, music, and dance therapists. The roles of these professionals may be blurred, with overlap among them. To function effectively together, each must bring a strong sense of professional identity, and a clear picture of what he or she may contribute to the well-being of the client.

There is now one more interested party in mental health care: the entity that funds treatment. It was not uncommon earlier in the century for the individual or the family to pay directly for services received. The norm now is for an employer, an insurance company, or the government to support care. As costs have soared, these organizations have become increasingly involved in decision making about the kinds of care to be provided, the circumstances under which they will be provided, and the duration. There is constant review of the efficacy of treatment, and the payers demand that the effectiveness of each intervention be demonstrated by observable changes in behavior or symptoms.

All these factors have made service provision in mental health a complex proposition. The well-being of the individual is now frequently weighed against the interests of the various parties involved in each situation. It is in this complex system that occupational therapists must now operate, and strive to provide quality services to individuals and families with mental health problems.

In order to function effectively, occupational therapists must have a clear understanding of the needs of the individual, of the system in which they are providing care, of the roles of other professionals, and of their own contributions to care. There are several factors which must be considered. First, when occupational therapists offer treatment in mental health, they generally do so as part of a treatment team. This team is usually headed by a psychiatrist, a physician with specialized training in mental illness. The medical background of the team leader is significant, because it contributes to the importance of diagnosis as a starting place for treatment. While this delineation of authority is less prominent in some types of community treatment environments, diagnosis may still be emphasized.

As noted above, payment for services is almost always provided, at least in part, by someone other than the identified patient. In most cases, the other is an insurance company or the government. Increasingly, employers are providing their own insurance for employees and are acting as the third party payers. As these others pay, they are involved in decisions about care. Their interests may be somewhat different than those of the patient, with cost containment an important factor. They are interested in service which is effective, but is within reasonable cost limits. One of the ways in which they control costs is by reviewing diagnoses and prognoses and paying only for treatments that have been demonstrated through research and practice to be effective for the specific disorder. Thus diagnosis assumes importance in terms of the kinds of treatment which are likely to be reimbursed.

In focusing on the individual's ability to perform those tasks required in daily life, occupational therapists respond to both the needs of the patient and the wishes of third party payers. Enhancing function may serve to make individuals less dependent, enable them to live without support from the environment, or to minimize the need for such support. Thus occupational therapists provide a vital service with the potential to increase function and quality of life and decrease costs.

However, occupational therapists must work within the existing treatment milieu. This presents several difficulties. First, and most importantly, psychiatric diagnosis does not always predict functional performance. As Williams (1988) indicates "(Diagnosis) does not imply that all people with a particular mental disorder are alike; on the contrary they may differ in many important ways that can affect treatment and outcome" (p. 203). Individuals labeled as schizophrenic may function in very different ways, some able to live reasonably independently, others almost totally dependent. Second, it may be difficult for occupational therapists to articulate their goals in a system where diagnosis and symptoms generally reflect psychological rather than functional characteristics. For example, people with schizophrenia may be described in terms of cognitive and sensory distortions, rather than in terms of the ways in which those distortions affect their ability to work or care for themselves.

The purpose of this book is to describe for therapists the diagnostic system currently used in the United States and to discuss the role of occupational therapy within that system. The emergence of the current classification system will be reviewed, and the relationship of psychiatric diagnosis to the occupational therapy process considered. Then major classification categories will be described with regard to incidence of the disorders, symptomatology, etiology, and prognosis. Most importantly, functional performance will be examined for the various categories, in terms of both skills (motor, cognitive, sensory, etc.) and activities (work, leisure, activities of daily living, etc.). Discussion of the implications of performance for occupational therapy intervention will be included. The final chapter deals with psychotropic medications. Medication has emerged as a primary form of treatment by psychiatrists, regardless of orientation. All mental health professionals should understand the effects of these agents as well as the potential side effects. Occupational therapy treatment must often be planned with these effects in mind. For this reason, medication as a form of intervention will be considered in some detail.

By developing a clear understanding of psychopathology and psychiatric diagnosis, and the role of occupational therapy within that context, occupational therapists can be best equipped to provide optimal service to clients.

References

American Psychiatric Association, Task Force on Nomenclature (1994). *Diagnostic and Statistical Manual of Mental Disorders (4th ed.)*. Washington, D.C..

Bruce, M. A., & Borg, B. (1987). *Frames of reference in psychosocial occupational therapy.* Thorofare, NJ: SLACK.

Meyer, A. (1977). The philosophy of occupation therapy. *American Journal of Occupational Therapy, 31,* 639-642.

Williams, J. B. W. (1988). Psychiatric classification. In J. A. Talbott, R. E. Hales, & S. C. Yudofsky (Eds.), *The American Psychiatric Press Textbook of Psychiatry* (pp.201-223). Washington, DC: American Psychiatric Press.

Chapter 1
Psychiatric Diagnosis and the Classification System

There are numerous theories about psychiatric disorders with widely varying implications for intervention. Medical, behavioral, analytical, and neuropsychological approaches differ greatly in terms of their postulates about the origins of psychiatric disorder and methods for intervening. This creates a dilemma for service providers. Without a common ground for understanding, communication among professionals becomes impossible. The resolution of the dilemma has been the development of a common system of classification, the *Diagnostic and Statistical Manual.* Since its appearance in 1952, it has undergone several revisions, the current version being the *Diagnostic and Statistical Manual of Mental Disorders, Fourth Edition* (DSM-IV) (American Psychiatric Association [APA], 1994). Mental health professionals can converse through DSM-IV regardless of theoretical orientation. As has been noted, "mental health professionals need a common language with which to communicate about the types of psychological problems for which they assume professional responsibility. A diagnosis is simply a way of summarizing a large amount of information into a shorthand term" (Spitzer, Skodal, Gibbon, & Williams, 1983, p. xvi).

Communication is a vital function of a classification system, but there are others. According to Williams (1988), such a system provides a guide to cause, and by extension, assessment and treatment of disorders. For example, "physical" disorders must be differentiated from psychiatric syndromes, as treatment relates to such distinctions (Hall, Gardner, Stickney, LeCann, & Popkin, 1980). In addition, description of the characteristics of each disorder is vital to efforts to improve diagnostic reliability and to distinguish among disorders. Finally, classification assists in research to further examine causes and treatment of mental disturbance. Without a shared system for identification of distinct disorders, such research is almost impossible. For example, diagnostic criteria assist in distinguishing specific groups of individuals to be studied, behaviors to be examined, and outcomes which are of interest to the researcher.

Emergence of the DSM

In 1840, the United States had a one-category classification system for mental illness, that category being "Idiocy" (Williams, 1988). By 1880 the system had increased to eight categories. Over time, as understanding and awareness increased, the classification system was refined, eventually being formalized as a chapter in the International Classification of Diseases (ICD) now in its 10th edition (World Health Organization [WHO], 1990), and as the DSM.

The DSM later to be known as DSM-I, was published in 1952 by the (APA). It was a major breakthrough for the field of mental health, as it provided the first comprehensive volume describing the range of mental disorders. The descriptions were quite general, however, making diagnosis unreliable. As psychiatric knowledge grew, it became clear that a revision was needed.

DSM-II appeared in 1968, following 3 years of work by the APA. It coincided with the eighth revision of the ICD. The differences between DSM-I and DSM-II were minor, with some changes in the names of syndromes and minor changes in descriptive language. Like DSM-I, though, descriptions were general and often vague. A major criticism of both DSM-I and DSM-II was the poor reliability of diagnosis. Professionals were often unable to consistently identify the same disorder in a specific patient (Klerman, 1988), or the diagnosis might change over time even if nothing had happened to change the behavior or symptoms of the individual.

DSM-III represented a major change in the nature of the diagnostic process. As with DSM-II, its development coincided with a revision of the ICD. American psychiatrists were concerned that the ICD-9 lacked many specific diagnoses which were well accepted in the United States on the basis of research data. There was also concern that the glossary was inadequate in the area of mental health (Williams, 1988).

Furthermore, in the 1960s and 1970s, there was heated debate about the nature of mental illness, and even its existence. Szasz (1974) argued that mental illness was a cultural phenomenon, rather than a disease. He suggested that mental illness was used as a label to explain deviant, and therefore socially unacceptable, behavior, and that the purpose of the label was to provide an excuse to control such behavior. Supporting this argument was the poor reliability of diagnoses. If two professionals were unlikely to make the same diagnosis of a patient, Szasz argued, perhaps it was because they were responding to cultural imperatives rather than to any real problem with the individual's behavior.

The 1970s saw several advances which contributed to the discussion. Foremost among these was the vastly increased knowledge about psychopharmacology and biology. For the first time, biological factors in mental disturbance could be identified, both in terms of genetic and biochemical characteristics. At the same time, research capabilities were enhanced through development of new research methodologies, and through development of clinical instruments which were found to be reliable (Klerman, 1988). This meant that professionals were consistent in their views of specific patients, and that diagnosis was stable over time if the patient did not change. Among the instruments which emerged at that time was the *Research Diagnostic Criteria* (RDC) (Spitzer, Endicott, & Robins, 1975). The emergence of such measures demonstrated that it was possible to provide clear, consistent guidelines which allowed for discrimination among symptom constellations.

Thus, in 1974, the APA appointed a committee to begin development of DSM-III, a task which ultimately took 6 years. Both the process of development and the product were novel, representing a significant departure from DSM-II. The process involved not only a great deal of committee work to develop descriptions and diagnostic criteria, but also a major research effort to validate diagnoses and determine reliability in a systematic fashion. During the research phase, more than 12,000 individuals were evaluated (Spitzer, Forman, & Nee, 1979). Clinicians from across the United States completed reports and commented on any difficulties using the system.

The interrater reliability studies involved 796 patients, each of whom was evaluated by two clinicians. All five newly developed axes (component diagnostic subgroups) were studied. Because these were field studies, some variables were poorly controlled, but even so the new classification system had reliability coefficients in the range of .7 (Axis I) to .6 (Axis II) (Williams, 1985). This means, roughly, that professionals agreed 60% to 70% of the time. The attempt to confirm reliability was, itself, novel. It should be noted that some later studies have found lower reliability, especially for Axis II (Mellsop, Varhgese, Joshua, & Hicks, 1982).

The product was notably different from DSM-II. First of all, the number of diagnoses was expanded to more than 150. In addition, descriptions were designed to be as specific as possible, with criteria about constellations of symptoms, onset of the disorder, duration, and probable course. This specificity was an important factor in assuring reliability, and represented the first classification to provide operational criteria (Klerman, 1988). Operational criteria are specific, observable characteristics that describe a particular syndrome or disorder. It is also noteworthy that DSM-II provided descriptive psychopathology rather than inferred etiology. In other words, the guide described what patient behavior the clinician saw, not what caused it. In addition, descriptions were largely atheoretical, that is, without reference to particular theories or points of view, making the product an effective mechanism for communication among therapists subscribing to divergent treatment philosophies (Williams, 1988).

DSM-III also acknowledged that diagnosis alone might not provide sufficient data to implement treatment. As a result, several new categories were developed to provide additional information, making it the first multiaxial classification system (Klerman, 1988). These axes made it possible not only to name a syndrome, but also to identify: 1) the type of personality of the individual in whom the problem was occurring, (AXIS II) 2) accompanying medical conditions of significance to treatment and prognosis, (AXIS III) 3) levels of stress encountered by the individual, (AXIS IV) and 4) recent levels of function (AXIS I).

Inclusion of this last axis is of particular importance to occupational therapists, as it represents an acknowledgment that diagnosis alone does not adequately describe function. It is also noteworthy that Axis V appears to be the most reliable of the axes with a correlation coefficient somewhere between .7 and .8 (Williams, 1988).

In DSM-III, categories were hierarchical, based on the assumption that disorders higher on the hierarchy had symptoms found in those lower, but not the opposite. Later research challenged this assumption (Boyd, Burke, Grundberg, Holzer, & Rae, 1984), one of the many findings that led to the almost immediate effort to revise DSM-III. DSM-III-R (revised) was published in 1987 and reflected advances in scientific knowledge. One change was the deletion of the assumption of hierarchies (Williams, 1988). While changes were minor, they reflected an effort to resolve problems with DSM-III and an effort to disseminate new knowledge as quickly as possible. Before DSM-III-R was completed, discussion had turned to the development of DSM-IV (APA, 1994). As with other editions of DSM, this revision was timed to coincide with a revision of the ICD (Kendall, 1991). The 10th edition of that volume appeared in 1990, by which time DSM-IV was nearing completion.

The process by which DSM-IV (APA, 1994) was developed was intended to be a careful, thoughtful, largely empirical one. Task groups of experts for each existing and proposed diagnostic category began by undertaking massive reviews of research literature (Widiger, Frances, Pincus, & Davis, 1990). These reviews were to serve as metaanalyses to guide the working groups about whether or not to include each diagnosis, and what criteria would be listed.

A series of field trials of the proposed criteria was also undertaken (APA, 1994). Twelve trials including more than 6,000 subjects were designed to examine the reliability and clinical utility of the proposed categories.

Decisions were ultimately guided by a set of standards. Criteria for addition of a new category or exclusion of an existing category were to be more stringent than criteria for retaining what existed (APA, 1994). This was done to avoid unnecessary changes which would confuse practitioners and reduce researchers' ability to track long-term consequences of mental disorder and treatment. In addition, an effort was made, where possible, to conform categories to those in IDC-10 (WHO, 1990), which was close to completion prior to publication of DSM-IV (Kendall, 1991).

Efforts were made to conform to the best possible scientific evidence in developing criteria (Francis, Widiger et al., 1991). Issues of reliability, validity, and utility were considered with an eye to assuring the highest possible standards.

Several new factors were included in DSM-IV. Among them were recognition of cultural differences in psychiatric constructs (Fabrega, 1992). DSM-IV includes an appendix listing terms that are applied to mental disorders in other cultures which might be encountered by practitioners in the United States. So, for example, "nervios" and "zar" are briefly explained in their cultural context. Another factor is recognition of the relationship between spiritual difficulties and mental disorders (APA, 1994).

The development of DSM-IV was a political as well as a scientific process, with numerous and sometimes heated arguments about inclusion and exclusion of categories (Caplan, 1991). One dispute, for example, relates to the inclusion of a diagnosis of "self-defeating personality disorder" (SDPD) which had been included in the appendices of DSM-III-R (APA, 1987) as a potential diagnosis requiring more study. Feminists argued that this validated the tendency of the legal system to "blame the victim" for crimes committed against him or her (e.g., that battered wives brought their problems upon themselves). A proposal to add a category for "delusional dominating personality disorder" (Caplan, 1991) to be applied to the batterer to counterbalance SDPD was rejected by the task force examining the issue, to the anger of those proposing it. Among other potential diagnoses considered were caffeine abuse (Hughes, Oliveto, Helzer, Higgins, & Bickel, 1992) and psychotic major depression (Schatzberg & Rothschild, 1992); both were rejected. Those involved in the development of DSM-IV themselves indicate that while scientific criteria should be primary and the burden of proof higher for change in categories, the issue of potential for stigmatizing the individual (or alternatively, excusing behavior because of psychiatric disorder) was important to consider in decision making (Pincus, Francis, Davis, First, & Widiger, 1992).

Some disputes raged around criteria for existing categories. For example, the committee on gender identity disorders expressed concern that criteria could not be applied equally to males and females because of cultural differences in acceptability of behaviors (Bradley et al., 1991). King and Strain (1992) indicated that there were significant problems in the category of somatoform pain disorder because of the difficulties in clearly differentiating between normal and abnormal reactions to pain. In fact, the whole issue of whether pain was organic versus nonorganic (that is, the result of a known "physical" agent like a bacterium or the result of some unknown "nonphysical" agent) was a heated one (Spitzer, Williams, First, & Kendler, 1989).

Another dispute was based in theory. DSM-IV purports to be atheoretical, but there has been some concern that this led to elimination of important constructs. Psychoanalysts and other dynamically oriented therapists wanted to see defense mechanisms added as a sixth axis (Skodol & Perry, 1993). This conflict was resolved by the inclusion of these terms in an extensive glossary. Issues about how many axes and what dimensions they should reflect were numerous (Schacht, 1993). For example, family therapists believed that because so many problems center around family interactions, a new axis should be added to reflect family circumstances (Lange, Schaap, & von Widenfelt, 1993).

Concern was also expressed that the committees developing DSM-IV (APA, 1994) were comprised almost entirely of physicians, resulting in a tilt in the content toward a medical model (DeAngelis, 1991). Pressure from psychologists, social workers, and other mental health professionals resulted in their inclusion in the process, but physicians still dominated the deliberations.

One argument was that the development of DSM-IV was premature (Zimmerman, Jampala, Sierles, & Taylor, 1991). Among the concerns expressed was the fact that although they were gaining acceptance, DSM-III and III-R were not yet fully implemented in clinical settings (Maser, Kaelber, & Weise, 1991) and that change would be resisted (Morey & Ochoa, 1989; Smith & Kraft, 1989). Another worry was that rapid change in diagnostic categories would reduce researchers' ability to follow outcomes longitudinally, or to compare research results for a specific disorder.

The working groups for DSM-IV fully recognized such dilemmas (Frances, First et al., 1991), noting that

> *The Task Force has not resolved fully, nor indeed expects to resolve fully, any of these issues. Instead, the Task Force is attempting to find balanced, if imperfect solutions to reflect the best available knowledge* (p. 407).

Thus, the development of the classification system can be seen as a complex scientific and political process, which has involved physicians, psychologists, social workers, and some political or special interest groups. While final decisions made about DSM-IV are based primarily on the consensus of authorities (Spitzer, 1991), and while it remains an imperfect system, DSM-IV is, for better or worse, the system by which professionals now communicate.

Format of DSM-IV

As noted, DSM-IV is a multiaxial classification system comprised of five axes (Figure 1-1). Axis I represents psychiatric diagnosis; Axis II, personality disorders and mental retardation; Axis III, significant accompanying medical conditions; Axis IV, degree of stress within the 12 months preceding diagnosis; and Axis V, level of function. On this last axis, two numbers can be listed: 1) current level of function and 2) highest level of function within the past 12 months. Diagnosis on all five axes is designed to provide

Figure 1-1. Axes in DSM-IV.

Axis I:	Clinical Disorders Other conditions that may be a focus of clinical attention
Axis II:	Mental Retardation Personality Disorders
Axis III:	General Medical Conditions
Axis IV:	Psychosocial and Environmental Problems
Axis V:	Global Assessment of Functioning

American Psychiatric Association (1994).
The Diagnostic and Statistical Manual of Mental Disorders (4th ed, pg. 25). Washington, DC: Author.

maximum information about the individual's condition.

Appendix A of this text contains the summary pages from DSM-IV. The categories listed there are discussed in detail in the body of the text, with clarifying examples of behavior and specific symptoms which must be present to support a given diagnosis. This description includes considerations such as duration of symptoms and course of the disorder.

Axis I includes diagnoses of specific psychiatric syndromes or disorders. Each category includes a description of major features of the disorder, the symptoms that must be present to warrant the diagnosis, and a discussion of accompanying features which may or may not be present. Age of onset and course of the disorder are described, as are predisposing factors, prevalence, and familial pattern. A section on impairment briefly discusses the social and occupational implications of the disorder. Complications which may occur are included, and finally, a discussion of differential diagnosis provides a summary of the characteristics which distinguish the disorder from others and a list of other diagnoses to consider if criteria do not fit the presenting picture.

Axis II includes mental retardation and personality disorders, which are defined as long-standing patterns of adaptation. Individuals may have psychiatric diagnoses without personality disorders, or vice versa, but they often accompany each other. A distinguishing characteristic of a personality disorder is its usually negative effect on those around the individual (Klerman, 1988), frequently resulting in a disordered social system. Mental retardation is included on this axis, because like the personality disorders, it is considered a condition which emerges early and continues throughout life, sometimes underlying or accompanying an Axis I condition. This definition of Axis II is somewhat different from DSM-III-R, in which other conditions were included on this dimension. There has been controversy about making Axis I/Axis II distinctions (Widiger & Shea, 1991), but given the decision criteria for change in the DSM, the Axis remains for now.

Axis III allows for diagnosis of coexisting medical conditions, coded according to the ICD-10 (WHO, 1990) categories. Medical conditions which might affect the course of the psychiatric disorder or the types of treatments to be implemented are noted on this axis, as are those which might have an impact on overall function.

Axis IV describes psychosocial and environmental problems. Among the factors might be noted on this axis are educational and housing difficulties, and problems with access to health care. This represents a change from DSM-III-R (APA, 1987), in which Axis IV was for noting level and source of stress. This change was due to dissatisfaction of clinicians using the axis, as well as disappointing results from the limited research data about its reliability (Skodol, 1991).

Axis V reflects the individual's highest level of function within the 12 months preceding diagnosis, as well as current level of function. Psychological, social, and vocational functioning are rated on a 0 to 90 point scale, with general descriptions of each 10-point range to provide guidance in making an assessment. This is, at present, the most subjective of the axes, as specific behaviors are not included. However, a moderate correlation has been noted between severity of symptoms and function (Klerman, 1988), i.e., there is a moderate relationship between the degree of psychological impairment and performance. This axis was included in an attempt to acknowledge strengths of the client, as well as deficits (thus *highest* level of function rather than average level of function). In spite of its relative subjectivity, this is the most reliable of the axes (Axis III has not been subjected to any reliability studies) (Bonder, 1990). In general, clinicians reported being satisfied with Axis V (Skodol, 1991). Further, no better measures of function were found (Goldman, Skodol, & Lave, 1992), so the axis remains unchanged from earlier versions of DSM.

Not all axes are used by all clinicians. It is most typical that diagnoses will be made on Axes I and II, and often Axis III diagnoses are included when there is a significant medical condition. However, Axes IV and V are often omitted, a problem for occupational and other therapists who may be greatly concerned with function.

Figure 1-2 below provides the description of one common diagnosis, dysthymic disorder, as it appeared in DSM-I, DSM-II, DSM-III, DSM-III-R, and as it is now seen in DSM-IV. Among the obvious differences is the change in name from depressive neurosis. Increasing specificity can be noted in each revision, increasing the probability of reliable diagnosis, and thus the clarity of therapeutic choice.

What follows in this text is discussion of the relationship of diagnosis to

Figure 1-2. Changes in the Diagnosis of Depression: DSM-I to DSM-IV.

DSM-I	000-X06 Depressive Reaction
	The anxiety in this reaction is allayed, and hence partially relieved, by depression and self-deprecation. The reaction is precipitated by a current situation, frequently by some loss sustained by the patient, and is often associated with a feeling of guilt for past failures or deeds. The degree of the reaction in such cases is dependent upon the intensity of the patient's ambivalent feeling toward his loss (love, possession) as well as upon the realistic circumstances of the loss.
	The term is synonymous with "reactive depression" and is to be differentiated from the corresponding psychotic reaction. In this differentiation, points to be considered are (1) life history of patient, with special reference to mood swings (suggestive of psychotic reaction), to the personality structure (neurotic or cyclothymic) and to precipitating environmental factors and (2) absence of malignant symptoms (hypochondriacal preoccupation, agitation, delusions, particularly somatic, hallucinations, severe guilt feelings, intractable insomnia, suicidal ruminations, severe psychomotor retardation, profound retardation of thought, stupor).
DSM-II	300.4 Depressive Neurosis
	This disorder is manifested by an excessive reaction of depression due to an internal conflict or to an identifiable event such as the loss of a love object or cherished possession. It is to be distinguished from *Involutional melancholia (q.v.)* and *Manic-depressive illness (q.v.). Reactive depressions or Depressive reactions* are to be classified here.

Figure 1-2. Changes in the Diagnosis of Depression: DSM-I to DSM-IV (continued).

DSM-III	Diagnostic Criteria for Dysthymic Disorder
	A. During the past 2 years (or 1 year for children and adolescents) the individual has been bothered most or all of the time by symptoms characteristic of the depressive syndrome but that are not of sufficient severity and duration to meet the criteria for a major depressive episode (although a major depressive episode may be superimposed on Dystheymic Disorder).
	B. The manifestations of the depressive syndrome may be relatively persistent or separated by periods of normal mood lasting a few days to a few weeks, but no more than a few months at a time.
	C. During the depressive periods there is either prominent depressed mood (e.g., sad, blue, down in the dumps, low) or marked loss of interest or pleasure in all, or almost all, usual activities and pastimes.
	D. During the depressive period at least three of the following symptoms are present: (1) insomnia or hypersomnia (2) low energy level or chronic tiredness (3) feelings of inadequacy, loss of self-esteem, or self-deprecation (4) decreased effectiveness or productivity at school, work, or home (5) decreased attention, concentration, or ability to think clearly (6) social withdrawal (7) loss of interest in or enjoyment of pleasurable activities (8) irritability or excessive anger (in children, expressed toward parents or caretakers) (9) inability to respond with apparent pleasure to praise or rewards (10) less active or talkative than usual, or feels slowed down or restless (11) pessimistic attitude toward the future, brooding about past events, or feeling sorry for self (12) tearfulness or crying (13) recurrent thoughts of death or suicide
	E. Absence of psychotic features, such as delusions, hallucinations, or incoherence, or loosening of associations.
	F. If the disturbance is superimposed on a pre-existing mental disorder, such as Obsessive Compulsive Disorder or Alcohol Dependence, the depressed mood, by virtue of its intensity or effect on functioning, can be clearly distinguished from the individual's usual mood.

Figure 1-2. Changes in the Diagnosis of Depression: DSM-I to DSM-IV (continued).

DSM III-R	Diagnostic Criteria for 300.4 Dysthymic Disorder

	A. Depressed mood for most of the day, for more days than not, as indicated either by subjective account or observation by others, for at least 2 years. **Note:** In children and adolescents, mood can be irritable and duration must be at least 1 year.
	
	B. Presence, while depressed, of two (or more) of the following:
	    (1) poor appetite or overeating
	    (2) insomnia or hypersomnia
	    (3) low energy or fatigue
	    (4) low self-esteem
	    (5) poor concentration or difficulty making decisions
	    (6) feelings of hopelessness
	
	C. During the 2-year period (1 year for children or adolescents) of the disturbance, the person has never been without the symptoms in Criteria A and B for more than 2 months at a time.
	
	D. No Major Depressive Episode (see p. 327) has been present during the first 2 years of the disturbance (1 year for children and adolescence); i.e., the disturbance is not better accounted for by chronic Major Depressive Disorder, or Major Depressive Disorder, In Partial Remission.
	
	Note: There may have been a previous Major Depressive Episode provided there was a full remission (no significant signs or symptoms for 2 months) before development of the Dysthymic Disorder. In addition, after the initial 2 years (1 year in children or adolescents) of Dysthymic Disorder, there may be superimposed episodes of Major Depressive Disorder, in which case both diagnoses may be given when the criteria are met for a Major Depressive Episode.
	
	E. There has never been a Manic Episode (see p. 332), a Mixed Episode (see p. 335), or a Hypomanic Episode (see p. 338), and criteria have never been met for Cyclothymic Disorder.
	
	F. The disturbance does not occur exclusively during the course of a chronic Psychotic Disorder, such as Schizophrenia or Delusional Disorder.
	
	G. The symptoms are not due to the direct physiological effects of a substance (e.g., a drug of abuse, a medication) or a general medical condition (e.g., hypothyroidism).
	
	H. The symptoms cause clinically significant distress or impairment in social, occupational, or other important areas of functioning.
	
	Specify if: Early Onset: if onset is before age 21 years
	Late Onset: if onset is age 21 years or older
	
	Specify (for most recent 2 years of Dysthymic Disorder):
	With Atypical Features (see p. 384)

**Figure 1-2. Changes in the Diagnosis of Depression:
DSM-I to DSM-IV (continued).**

DSM IV	Diagnostic Criteria for 300.4 Dysthymic Disorder

	A. Depressed mood for most of the day, for more days than not, as indicated either by subjective account or observation by others, for at least 2 years. **Note:** In children and adolescents, mood can be irritable and duration must be at least 1 year.
	
	B. Presence, while depressed, of two (or more) of the following:
	
	    (1) poor appetite or overeating
	    (2) insomnia or hypersomnia
	    (3) low energy or fatigue
	    (4) low self-esteem
	    (5) poor concentration or difficulty making decisions
	    (6) feelings of hopelessness
	
	C. During the 2-year period (1 year for children or adolescents) of the disturbance, the person has never been without the symptoms in Criteria A and B for more than 2 months at a time.
	
	D. No Major Depressive Episode (see p. 327) has been present during the first 2 years of the disturbance (1 year for children and adolescence); i.e., the disturbance is not better accounted for by chronic Major Depressive Disorder, or Major Depressive Disorder, In Partial Remission.
	
	Note: There may have been a previous Major Depressive Episode provided there was a full remission (no significant signs or symptoms for 2 months) before development of the Dysthymic Disorder. In addition, after the initial 2 years (1 year in children or adolescents) of Dysthymic Disorder, there may be superimposed episodes of Major Depressive Disorder, in which case both diagnoses may be given when the criteria are met for a Major Depressive Episode.
	
	E. There has never been a Manic Episode (see p. 332), a Mixed Episode (see p. 335), or a Hypomanic Episode (see p. 338), and criteria have never been met for Cyclothymic Disorder.
	
	F. The disturbance does not occur exclusively during the course of a chronic Psychotic Disorder, such as Schizophrenia or Delusional Disorder.
	
	G. The symptoms are not due to the direct physiological effects of a substance (e.g., a drug of abuse, a medication) or a general medical condition (e.g., hypothyroidism).
	
	H. The symptoms cause clinically significant distress or impairment in social, occupational, or other important areas of functioning.
	
	Specify if: Early Onset: if onset is before age 21 years
	Late Onset: if onset is age 21 years or older
	
	Specify (for most recent 2 years of Dysthymic Disorder):
	With Atypical Features (see p. 384)

occupational therapy and consideration of major diagnostic categories, with emphasis on what is known or theorized about etiology and course of the disorders, the types of treatments currently being employed and the efficacy of those treatments. That information is linked to probable effects on the occupational performance of the individual, and recommendations made about potential interventions for occupational therapy.

References

American Psychiatric Association Task Force on Nomenclature (1952). *The Diagnostic and Statistical Manual of Mental Disorders* (1st ed.). Washington, DC: Author.

American Psychiatric Association Task Force on Nomenclature (1968). *The Diagnostic and Statistical Manual of Mental Disorders* (2nd ed.). Washington, DC: Author.

American Psychiatric Association Task Force on Nomenclature (1980). *The Diagnostic and Statistical Manual of Mental Disorders* (3rd ed.). Washington, DC: Author.

American Psychiatric Association Task Force on Nomenclature (1987). *The Diagnostic and Statistical Manual of Mental Disorders* (3rd ed. rev.). Washington, DC: Author.

American Psychiatric Association Task Force on Nomenclature (1994). *The Diagnostic and Statistical Manual of Mental Disorders* (4th ed.). Washington, DC: Author.

Bonder, B. R. (1990). Occupational therapy update: Disease and dysfunction: The value of axis V. *Hospital and Community Psychiatry, 41,* 959-960, 964.

Boyd, J. H., Burke, J. D., Grundberg, E., Holzer, C. E., & Rae, D. S. (1984). Exclusion criteria of DSM-III: A study of co-occurrence of hierarchy-free syndromes. *Archives of General Psychiatry, 41,* 983-989.

Bradley, S. J., Blanchard, R., Coates, S., Green, R., Levine, S. B., Meyer-Bahlburg, H. F. L., Pauly, I. B., & Zucker, K. J. (1991). Interim report of the DSM-IV subcommittee on gender identity disorders. *Archives of Sexual Behavior, 20,* 333-343.

Caplan, P. J. (1991). How *do* they decide who is normal? The bizarre, but true, tale of the DSM process. *Canadian Psychology, 32,* 162-170.

DeAngelis, T. (June, 1991). DSM being revised, but problems remain. *American Psychological Association Monitor,* 12-13.

Fabrega, H. (1992). Diagnosis interminable: Toward a culturally sensitive DSM-IV. *Journal of Nervous and Mental Disease, 180,* 5-7.

Frances, A. J., First, M. B., Widiger, T. A., Miele, G. M., Tilly, S. M., Davis, W. W., & Pincus, H. A. (1991). An A to Z guide to DSM-IV conundrums. *Journal of Abnormal Psychology, 100,* 407-412.

Frances, A., Widiger, T. A., First, M. B., Pincus, H. A., Tilly, S. M., Miele, G. M., & Davis, W. W. (1991). DSM-IV: Toward a more empirical diagnostic system. *Canadian Psychology, 32,* 171-173.

Goldman, H. H., Skodol, A. E., & Lave, T. R. (1992). Revising axis V for DSM-IV: A review of measures of social functioning. *American Journal of Psychiatry, 149,* 1148-1156.

Hall, R. C. W., Gardner, E. R., Stickney, S. K., LeCann, A. G., & Popkin, M. K. (1980). Physical illness manifesting as psychiatric disease. *Archives of General Psychiatry, 37,* 989-995.

Hughes, J. R., Oliveto, A. H., Helzer, J. E., Higgins, S. T., & Bickel, W. K. (1992). Should caffeine abuse, dependence, or withdrawal be added to DSM-IV and ICD-10? *American Journal of Psychiatry, 149,* 33-40.

Kendall, R. E. (1991). Relationship between the DSM-IV and the ICD-10. *Journal of Abnormal Psychology, 100,* 297-301.

King, S. A., & Strain, J. J. (1992). Revising the category of somatoform pain disorder. *Hospital and Community Psychiatry, 43,* 217-219.

Klerman, G. L. (1988). Classification and DSM-III-R. In A. M. Nicholi (Ed.), *The new Harvard guide to psychiatry* (pp. 70-87). Cambridge, MA: Belknap Press.

Lange, A., Schaap, C., & von Widenfelt, B. (1993). Family therapy and psychopathology:

Developments in research and approaches to treatment. *Journal of Family Therapy, 15,* 113-146.

Maser, J. D., Kaelber, C., & Weise, R. E. (1991). International use and attitudes toward DSM-III and DSM-III-R: Growing consensus in psychiatric classification. *Journal of Abnormal Psychology, 100,* 271-279.

Mellsop, G., Varghese, F., Joshua, S., & Hicks, A. (1982). The reliability of Axis II of DSM-III. *American Journal of Psychiatry, 139,* 1360-1361.

Morey, L., & Ochoa, F. (1989). An investigation of adherence to diagnostic criteria: Clinical diagnosis of the DSM-III personality disorders. *Journal of Personality Disorders, 3,* 180-192.

Pincus, H. A., Frances, A., Davis, W. W., First, M. B., & Widiger, T. A. (1992). DSM-IV and new diagnostic categories: Holding the line on proliferation. *American Journal of Psychiatry, 149,* 112-117.

Schacht, T. E. (1993). How do I diagnose thee? Let me count the dimensions. *Psychological Inquiry, 4,* 115-118.

Schatzberg, A. F., & Rothschild, A. J. (1992). Psychotic (delusional) major depression: Should it be included as a distinct syndrome in DSM-IV? *American Journal of Psychiatry, 149,* 733-745.

Skodol, A. E. (1991). Axis IV: A reliable and valid measure of psychosocial stressors? *Comprehensive Psychiatry, 32,* 503-515.

Skodol, A. E., & Perry, J. C. (1993). Should an axis for defense mechanisms be included in DSM-IV? *Comprehensive Psychiatry, 34,* 108-119.

Smith, D., & Kraft, W. (1989). Attitudes of psychiatrists toward diagnostic options and issues. *Psychiatry, 52,* 66-77.

Spitzer, R. L. (1991). An outsider-insider's views about revising the DSMs. *Journal of Abnormal Psychology, 100,* 294-296.

Spitzer, R. L., Endicott, J., & Robins, R. C. (1975). Research diagnostic criteria (RDC). *Psychopharmacology Bulletin, 11,* 22-24.

Spitzer, R. L., Forman, J. B. W., & Nee, J. (1979). DSM-III field trials I: Initial interrater diagnostic reliability. *American Journal of Psychiatry, 136,* 818-820.

Spitzer, R. L., Skodol, A. E., Gibbon, M., & Williams, J. B. W. (1983). *Psychopathology: A case book.* New York: McGraw-Hill.

Spitzer, R. L., Williams, J. B. W., First, M., & Kendler, K. (1989). A proposal for DSM-IV: Solving the "organic/nonorganic" problem. *Journal of Neuropsychiatry, 1,* 126-127.

Szasz, T. (1974). *The myth of mental illness.* (2nd ed.). New York: Harper & Row.

Widiger, T. A., Frances, A. J., Pincus, H. A., & Davis, W. W. (1990). DSM-IV literature reviews: Rationale, process, and limitations. *Journal of Psychopathology and Behavioral Assessment, 12,* 189-202.

Widiger, T. A., & Shea, T. (1991). Differentiation of axis I and axis II disorders. *Journal of Abnormal Psychology, 100,* 399-406.

Williams, J. B. W. (1985). The multiaxial system of DSM-III: Where did it come from and where should it go? *Archives of General Psychiatry, 42,* 181-186.

Williams, J. B. W. (1988). Psychiatric classification. In J. A. Talbott, R. E. Hales, & S. C. Yudofsky (Eds.), *The American Psychiatric Press textbook of psychiatry.* Washington, DC: American Psychiatric Press, 201-223.

World Health Organization (1990). *International Classification of Diseases* (10th Ed.). Geneva: Author.

Zimmerman, M., Jampala, C., Sierles, F. S., & Taylor, M. A. (1991). DSM-IV: A nosology sold before its time? *American Journal of Psychiatry, 148,* 463-467.

Chapter 2
DSM-IV and Occupational Therapy

Before proceeding to a discussion of the various diagnostic categories, it is important to consider the relationship of psychiatric diagnosis to the occupational therapy process. Occupational therapists work within a system in which diagnosis is important, but their view of disorder differs from that of other mental health professionals. The difference revolves around the importance of function in everyday activities, the causes of dysfunction, goals of treatment, and methods for intervening. This chapter provides only a general overview, and readers should refer to texts which deal with the occupational therapy process in mental health. However, in order to understand how occupational therapy fits in the mental health system, some discussion of the differing views of dysfunction is necessary.

It is important to recognize that what constitutes psychiatric disturbance is not fixed or absolute. Porter (1987) noted that "what is mental and what is physical, what is mad and what is bad, are not fixed points but culture relative (p.10)." Ideas have changed through the centuries about what constitutes mental illness and what interventions are appropriate. Shifts from acceptance of deviant behavior in the community to institutionalization and back to community centered care, from so-called "rational" to "moral" to medical treatment, from optimism to pessimism about the probability that individuals can "get better" have all been influenced by and have influenced ideas about the origins and treatments of mental disorders.

Some theorists have speculated that deviance emerges from early childhood experiences (the analytic view), while others suspect that the problem is faulty learning (behaviorists) (Cuvo, 1992), or a skewed set of interpretations about events (cognitive therapies). Other theories emphasize neurobiological explanations for behavior (Jaeger & Douglas, 1992), or interactional models (Lange, Schaap, & von Widenfelt, 1993). Szasz (1974) felt that psychiatric disorder did not exist, but was, instead, a reflection of lack of acceptance of behavior which was outside the norm.

DSM-IV purports to be atheoretical, to apply regardless of one's view of the origins of psychiatric disturbance. However, the diagnostic process in itself reflects the medical model (DeAngelis, 1991). It implies that there are specific syndromes or disorders which constitute discrete and distinguishable entities identified on the basis of constellations of symptoms, including psychological characteristics, behaviors, and physical findings. Thus the model can be thought of as a disease model (Rogers, 1982). The purpose of intervention in this model is to cure disease.

This model presents certain problems in psychiatric practice (Antonosky, 1972). Not all psychological theories fit neatly into the medical model. For example, behaviorists attempt to remediate problematic behaviors, and cognitive therapists attempt to alter the ways in which clients view the world and their own situations. Neither of these approaches focuses on curing disease. Even so, the importance of the medical model to psychiatry continues to be evident in the centrality of the diagnostic process.

There are a number of reasons why diagnosis may be so important. Several of these have been noted in the previous chapter. Communication among professionals is facilitated by the common language provided by diagnosis (Spitzer, Skodal, Gibbon, & Williams, 1988). Decisions of third party payers are simplified by the process of attaching a label to a set of symptoms, and outcomes can be better evaluated based on change in that set of symptoms. For these reasons, it is unlikely that the diagnostic system will disappear any time in the near future.

Psychiatrists have acknowledged that diagnosis is only loosely related to function. It was for this reason that Axis V was developed. And it is clear that Axis V correlates with severity of disorder, rather than with specific diagnosis (Klerman, 1988). Individuals who are diagnosed as schizophrenic may present with widely varying functional abilities, some able to hold jobs, for instance, while others may require the constant attention of an inpatient psychiatric facility. (It is also true that individuals diagnosed with a particular disorder may vary as related to other symptoms as well. Not all schizophrenics are alike [APA, 1994].) First and his colleagues (1992) suggests that behaviors may be more helpful than abstract constructs in making diagnoses. Further, there is acknowledgement that once the "disease" has been ameliorated, residual dysfunction may remain to be addressed (Jaeger & Douglas, 1992).

Occupational Therapy View of Mental Disorder

Occupational therapists focus on function, both in explaining psychiatric disorder and in intervening (Rogers, 1982). While physicians focus on disease, occupational therapists focus on performance. It is quite possible to have a disease which results in no functional deficit, or at least not one which requires intervention. An individual who has a head cold has a disease, but may carry on with normal activities.

On the other hand, some individuals who have no diagnoseable disease, either physical or psychological, have deficits in performance. Children from socioeconomically deprived backgrounds may have difficulty adapting to the expectations in a school setting; adults from isolated rural settings might show performance deficits when they move to the city to take factory jobs. These do not constitute diseases in the medical sense, but occupational therapists would be concerned about remediating the performance deficits.

This view of the individual is a consistent tenet of occupational therapy regardless of the theoretical orientation of the individual. Thus, individuals who adhere to Kielhofner's (1985) Model of Human Occupation, a general systems model, or Allen's (1985) cognitive approach, a neurobiological model, would all focus on function as the central concern of assessment and intervention. The specific problems identified on the basis of these theories would differ, as would the interventions, but the long term goal is to enhance function.

This perspective is reflected in the Uniform Terminology Checklist (AOTA, 1994). This is a summary of the skills and performance which are the focus of occupational therapy (see Appendix B). Major performance areas, activities of daily living, work, and play or leisure, have been identified. For successful performance in each of these areas, a wide range of skills are needed, including sensorimotor, cognitive, and psychosocial skills. These performance areas and skills are the focus of occupational therapy. Kielhofner (1992) identifies three central assumptions of occupational therapy:

1. Human beings have an occupational nature.
2. Human beings may experience occupational dysfunction.
3. Occupation can be used as a therapeutic agent (p.49).

From those three assumptions, several goals for therapy emerge:

1. Evaluate human behavior and function in terms of occupational performance, the components of that performance and the required adaptive behavior.
2. Support the optimum health of each person based on the individual's needs and the community demands for occupational performance.
3. Develop, improve, reestablish, promote or maintain normal occupational function and performance throughout the human life span.
4. Prevent, remediate, or minimize dysfunctional occupational performance and adaptive behavior throughout the human life span (Reed & Sanderson, 1980, p.11-12).

Thus the occupational therapist examines the abilities of the individual in the identified performance areas, considers which skills are deficient, preventing maximum performance, and sets about remediating those deficits, or, in the case of the individual at risk, preventing them.

Within these broad parameters, therapists develop interventions based on a set of theoretical beliefs about human performance and its enhancement. A number of models assist in understanding behavior. Among these are the cognitive disabilities model,(Allen, 1985) the model of human occupation (see Kielhofner, 1992 for a discussion of these models), the rehabilitation model (Anthony, 1979), and the occupational adaptation model (Schkade & Schultz, 1992; Schultz & Schkade, 1992). Figure 2-1 provides a brief summary of the beliefs of these models. While not an exhaustive list, this group includes several theories which are in common use, and which hold promise for future development.

Figure 2-1. Some Theories of Occupational Therapy Practice in Mental Health.

THEORY	BELIEFS ABOUT DYSFUNCTION	INTERVENTION	OUTCOMES
Model of Human Occupation (Kiehlhofner & Burke, 1980)	Maladaptive cycles of input, output, feedback; does not meet need for exploration and mastery	*Assessment* Evaluation of subsystems, environment, feedback. *Intervention* facilitate age appropriate occupation	Adaptive cycles; Age appropriate subsystems
Rehabilitation (Anthony, 1977)	Psychiatric disability: deficits in skilled performance	*Assessment* Present and needed skills. *Intervention* Step organized program includes physical fitness, vocational activities	Increased repertoire of skilled behavior: physical, emotional, intellectual
Cognitive Model (Allen, 1985)	Cognitive impairment	*Assessment* Allen Cognitive Levels test *Intervention* Monitoring changes based on medical intervention; environmental modification	Supported performance based on reduced environmental demand
Occupational Adaptation (Schultz & Schkade, 1992; Schkade & Schultz, 1992)	Ineffective adaptive response; ineffective occupational response	*Assessment* Information about occupational role expectations, person systems, occupational adaptation. *Intervention* Focuses on enhanced occupational adaptation	Effective occupational performance; effective occupational adaptation

The occupational therapy process in mental health is similar to that in other kinds of intervention. The first step is assessment to determine strengths and weaknesses. Extensive discussion of existing mechanisms for assessment can be found in Christiansen and Baum (1991). It is imperative that occupational therapists focus their assessment on appropriate concerns for their discipline, ie. on performance (Bonder, 1993).

Treatment goals are based on the individual's strengths and deficits, the activities the individual needs and wants to perform, and the social, economic, and environmental resources available to the individual. In psychiatry, intervention falls into three primary categories: 1) enhancing skills and performance; 2) altering attitudes about skills and performance; and 3) altering the environment to maximize skills and performance.

The first category includes teaching, training, and skill enhancement through practice. The occupational therapist might provide cooking classes, classes on job seeking (Richert, 1990), etc. Another approach is to provide practice. A client might be assigned a job in the clinic through which work related skills can be learned. This category also includes interventions which remediate underlying skills. A child who is retarded might be provided with intense kinesthetic and proprioceptive input through swinging and spinning (Humphries, Snider, & McDougall, 1993). According to sensory integration theory, this might better organize the central nervous system, thus enhancing higher level skills (Ayres, 1972). Another example, based on developmental theory, would be providing the same child with practice on lower level skills, balance on a balance beam, for instance, to assist the child in gradually achieving higher order skills in a step by step fashion (Bruce & Borg, 1987).

The second major type of intervention relates to the individual's attitudes and beliefs. Individuals who have been diagnosed with various psychiatric disorders often have inaccurate or skewed views of themselves. Inaccurate self-concept and lowered self-esteem are common among these individuals, regardless of specific diagnosis; both may lead to ineffective performance. Such individuals may not know that they can do particular activities, or may feel a chronic sense of failure. They may need practice simply expressing themselves (Gibson & Richert, 1993). Providing opportunities for success may bolster sagging self-esteem, and review of performance of a variety of activities may allow for more accurate self-assessment. The model of human occupation (Kielhofner, 1985) suggests that clients need to have and be aware of their own valued goals in order to perform effectively.

The third form which intervention typically takes is environmental modification. It has been theorized that some individuals do not have great capacity to modify their own performance, but that they may benefit from modifications in the environment which reduce demand (Allen, 1985). Another way of viewing this set of interventions is that many individuals do not know how to construct for themselves the most supportive environments, and that they can benefit from learning how to do so. Since setting can influence the performance of the individual, modification of the setting, whether by the therapist or the individual, will maximize function (Rogers, 1982).

The passage of the Americans with Disabilities Act (Crist & Stoffel, 1992) has increased the importance of this last form of intervention. The act specifies that employers must make reasonable accommodations in the workplace for individuals with disabilities, including those with mental disorders. The occupational therapist has valuable expertise to lend to this effort. Specifically, the therapist should help the individual identify the components or characteristics of the job which are problematic, then work with the individual and the employer to identify reasonable accommodations which can be made. More frequent breaks, a less stimulating environment, more specific instructions, and frequent feedback are all examples of modifications which may help an individual with a mental disorder cope with a job.

In recent years there has been a movement away from inpatient treatment which has altered occupational therapy practice in mental health in significant ways (Gusich & Silverman, 1991; Wilberding, 1991). First, therapists now identify a role in crisis intervention and prevention of mental disorder (Miller & Robertson, 1991). Perhaps even more central to practice is the understanding that distinctions between physical and psychological disorder are always arbitrary to some extent. Therapists increasingly recognize that their clients in other settings may well have psychiatric disorders (Mayou, Hawton, Feldman, & Ardern, 1991; Stoudemire, 1991). For example, it is well established that depression is common in individuals who have had cerebrovascular accidents (Allman, 1991). Thus, therapists in rehabilitation settings must be sensitive to the issues of motivation, self-esteem, guilt, and sadness which may accompany this disorder.

Therapists must also be aware of cultural considerations related to mental disorders (Dillard et al., 1992). As is explicit in DSM-IV (APA, 1994), cultures differ in their perspectives on psychiatric disorders. Therapists must select culturally relevant activities which will be meaningful and motivating to the individual client in the context of his or her environment.

The primary modality employed by occupational therapists in all areas of practice is activity. This includes all the kinds of activities in which individuals normally engage: routine daily activities such as cooking, cleaning, and self-care; work activities, including studying and volunteer activities (Lang & Cara, 1989); leisure and play, including sports, crafts, and expressive activities such as art, writing, and dance. The belief is that a balance of these activities promotes the best possible quality of life for the individual (Meyer, 1977). Figure 2-2 lists the primary areas of occupational therapy focus and some of the specific goals and modalities which might be used to intervene.

Figure 2-2. Objectives of Occupational Therapy Treatment.

Objective	Sample Treatment Goals	Sample Approaches
Enhance skills and performance	1. Improve ADL skills: grooming hygiene	Education (teach skill or performance)
	2. Improvement in IADL skills in budgeting and money manage-housekeeping etc.	Practice: (provide experience)
	3. Enhance work related skills: job seeking, interviewing, relating to co-workers	Reinforcement–used alone or in connection with education
	4. Improve orientation	Reality orientation
		Sensory stimulation
Improve self-image and self expression	1. Increase self-esteem	Provide activities with high probability of successful outcome
	2. Encourage accurate self-assessment	Provide feedback on outcomes
	3. Increase ability to recognize	Use of art activities: drawing, painting, writing, dance
Modify environment to maximize function	1. Reduce stress of environment	Move to smaller community, more structured living space
	2. Provide performance cues	Reduce clutter, label cabinets
	3. Encourage environmental support	Link community services, church group

A psychiatrist might look at a client who presents with depressed mood and lethargy and say, "Here is someone who has a dysthymic disorder. Let us treat the client with antidepressant medication and with verbal therapy to allow him to ventilate his feelings."

The occupational therapist might look at the same client and say, "Here is someone who has a pervasive sense of failure and no clear goals in life. Let us provide him with activities which will affirm his strengths and help him identify some goals which will give his life meaning."

The two approaches are clearly different. In the best possible situation, they are complimentary, each providing the client with something which will enhance his satisfaction with life, as well as his ability to contribute to society.

Therapists must be aware that individuals with mental disorders are likely to present in all areas of practice. Treatment in rehabilitation, acute care, long term care, industrial settings, and schools will be affected by the co-existing mental disorders of clients. For example, instructions may be misunderstood by someone with a psychotic disorder, motivation may be affected by presence of depression, and so on.

In working with clients with mental disorders in settings not designated specifically to manage such problems, therapists ashould keep in mind the principles described here and in more extensive texts on psychiatirc treatment. Instructions may need to be given more clearly or repeatedly, and goals related to self-concept or self-esteem included. Referral to appropriate health care professionals can also be quite helpful. Many individuals do not realize themselves that they have a condition which can be treated.

Therapists increasingly provide this care in facilities which may or may not be labeled as mental health institutions (Richert & Gibson, 1993). Treatment may be in quarter or half-way houses, community centers, sheltered living facilities, schools, and in clients' homes.

As these changes occur, there is much "role blurring" among disciplines (Gibson & Richert, 1993). In addition to occupational therapists, the client may be treated by a psychiatric nurse, social worker, psychologist, art, music, dance, or recreation therapist, vocational counselor, and psychiatrist.

The nurse is responsible primarily for nursing care, medical management, and, in inpatient settings, promoting the therapeutic milieu (Gibson & Richert, 1993). Social workers deal with family issues, and with discharge planning. Psychologists typically complete psychological assessments, and in some settings provide individual and group psychotherapy. Art, music, and dance therapists offer opportunities for expression through non-verbal means using the expressive arts as their media. Vocational counselors focus on work related skills and abilities, while recreation therapists focus on leisure abilities and interests. The psychiatrist provides medical care and prescribes medications, including psychotropic medications and may also provide psychotherapy.

Occupational therapists focus on assessment and remediation of perform- ance of work, leisure, and self-care and the underlying skills required to accomplish those activities. Their holistic view of activity helps them integrate the perspectives of art, music, dance, recreation therapists, and vocational counselors. They emphasize sensory, neuromotor, cognitive and psychological skills required for performance (Christiansen & Baum, 1991).

Ideally, these professionals work together to provide the best care for the client. In reality, however, roles sometimes overlap. Further, as cost containment becomes an issue, efforts may be made to reduce the number of different therapists involved with each client. Occupational therapists have a broad perspective, and can focus on issues vital to the client; they also have an obligation to recognize their limitations and call on others as appropriate.

The following chapters describe the diagnostic categories in DSM-IV (APA, 1994), including diagnostic criteria, etiology, symptoms, and prognosis. They then describe the functional consequences of the disorder, and typical treatment. Those which are most likely to require occupational therapy services are emphasized, others described briefly. In reading them, you will see that individuals with a variety of disorders may benefit from similar occupational therapy interventions. This is due to the differences between concepts relevant to medical diagnosis and occupational diagnosis. It is important to keep in mind the limitations of the diagnostic system, as well as the central goal of occupational therapy, the enhancement of performance.

References

Allen, C. (1985). *Occupational therapy for psychiatric diseases: Measurement and management of cognitive disabilities.* Boston: Little Brown & Co.

Allman, P. (1991). Depressive disorders and emotionalism following stroke. *International Journal of Geriatric Psychiatry, 6,* 377-383.

American Occupational Therapy Association (1994). *Uniform Terminology Checklist* (3rd ed.). Rockville, MD: Author.

American Psychiatric Association (1994). *Diagnostic and Statistical Manual of Mental Disorders* (4th ed.). Washington, DC: Author.

Anthony, W. A. (1979). *The principles of psychiatric rehabilitation.* Amherst, MA: Human Resource Development Press.

Antonosky, A. (1972). Breakdown: A needed fourth step in the conceptual armamentarium of modern medicine. *Social Science and Medicine, 6,* 537-544.

Ayres, A. J. (1972). *Sensory integration and learning disorders.* Los Angeles: Western Psychiatric Services.

Bonder, B. R. (1993). Issues in assessment of psychosocial components of function. *American Journal of Occupational Therapy, 47,* 211-216.

Bruce, M. A., & Borg, B. (1987). *Psychosocial occupational therapy: Frames of reference for intervention.* Thorofare, NJ: SLACK Incorporated.

Christiansen, C., & Baum, C. (1991). *Occupational therapy: Overcoming human performance deficits.* Thorofare, NJ: SLACK Incorporated.

Crist, P. A. H., & Stoffel, V. C. (1992). The Americans with Disabilities Act of 1990 and employees with mental impairments: Personal efficacy and the environment. *American Journal of Occupational Therapy, 46,* 434-443.

Cuvo, A. J. (1992). Gentle teaching: On the one hand...but on the other hand. *Journal of Applied Behavior Analysis, 25,* 873-877.

DeAngelis, T. (June, 1991). DSM being revised, but problems remain. *American Psychological Association Monitor,* 12-13.

Dillard, M., Andonian, L., Flores, O., Lai, L., MacRae, A., & Shakir, M. (1992). Culturally competent occupational therapy in a diversely populated mental health setting. *American Journal of Occupational Therapy, 46,* 721-726.

First, M. B., Frances, A., Widiger, T. A., Pincus, H. A., & Davis, W. W. (1992). *Behavioral Assessment, 14,* 297-306.

Gibson, D., & Richert, G. Z. (1993). The therapeutic process. In H. L. Hopkins & H. D. Smith (Eds.), *Occupational therapy* (8th ed., pp. 557-566). Philadelphia: J. B. Lippincott.

Gusich, R. L., & Silverman, A. L. (1991). Basava day clinic: The model of human occupation as applied to psychiatric day hospitalization. *Occupational Therapy in Mental Health, 11,* 113-134.

Humphries, T. W., Snider, L., & McDougall, B. (1993). Clinical evaluation of the effectiveness of sensory integrative and perceptual motor therapy in improving sensory integrative function in children with learning disabilities. *Occupational Therapy Journal of Research, 13,* 163-182.

Jaeger, J., & Douglas, E. (1992). Neuropsychiatric rehabilitation for persistent mental illness. *Psychiatric Quarterly, 63,* 71-94.

Kielhofner, G. (Ed.) (1985). *A model of human occupation: Theory and application.* Baltimore: Williams and Wilkins.

Kielhofner, G. (1992). *Conceptual foundations of occupational therapy.* Philadelphia: F. A. Davis.

Klerman, G. L. (1988). Classification and DSM-III-R. In A. M. Nicholi (Ed.), *The new Harvard guide to psychiatry* (pp. 70-87). Cambridge MA: Belknap Press.

Lang, S. K., & Cara, E. (1989). Vocational integration for the psychiatrically disabled. *Hospital and Community Psychiatry, 40,* 890-892.

Lange, A., Schaap, C., & von Widenfelt, B. (1993). Family therapy and psychopathology: Developments in research and approaches to treatment. *Journal of Family Therapy, 15,* 113-146.

Mayou, R., Hawton, K., Feldman, E., & Ardern, M. (1991). Psychiatric problems among medical admissions. *International Journal of Psychiatry in Medicine 21,* 71-84.

Meyer, A. (1977). The philosophy of occupational therapy. *American Journal of Occupational Therapy, 31,* 639-642.

Miller, V., & Robertson, S. (1991). A role for occupational therapy in crisis intervention and prevention. *Australian Occupational Therapy Journal, 38,* 143-146.

Porter, R. (1987). *A Social history of madness.* New York: Weidenfeld & Nicolson.

Reed, K., & Sanderson, S. R. (1980). *Concepts of occupational therapy.* Baltimore: Williams & Wilkins.

Richert, G. Z. (1990). Vocational transition in acute care psychiatry. *Occupational Therapy in Mental Health, 10,* 43-62.

Richert, G. Z., & Gibson, D. (1993). Practice settings. In H. L. Hopkins & H. D. Smith (Eds.), *Occupational therapy* (8th ed., pp. 546-551). Philadelphia: J. B. Lippincott.

Rogers, J. C. (1982). Order and disorder in medicine and occupational therapy. *American Journal of Occupational Therapy, 36,* 29-35.

Schkade, J. K., & Schultz, S. (1992). Occupational adaptation: Toward a holistic approach for contemporary practice, part 1. *American Journal of Occupational Therapy, 46,* 829-838.

Schultz, S., & Schkade, J. K. (1992). Occupational adaptation: Toward a holistic approach for contemporary practice, part 2. *American Journal of Occupational Therapy, 46,* 917-926.

Spitzer, R. L., Skodal, A. E., Gibbon, M., & Williams, J. B. W. (1988). *Psychopathology: A casebook.* New York: McGraw-Hill.

Stoudemire, A. (1991). Psychological factors affecting physical condition and DSM-IV. *Psychosomatics, 34,* 8-11.

Szasz, T. (1974). *The myth of mental illness* (2nd ed.). New York: Harper & Row.

Wilberding, D. (1991). The quarterway house: More than an alternative of care. *Occupational Therapy in Mental Health, 11*, 65-92.

Recommended Reading

Allen, C. (1985). *Occupational therapy for psychiatric diseases: Measurement and management of cognitive disabilities.* Boston: Little Brown & Co.

Barris, R., Kielhofner, G., & Watts, J. H. (1988). *Occupational therapy in psychosocial practice.* Thorofare, NJ: SLACK Incorporated.

Bruce, M. A., & Borg, B. (1988) *Psychosocial occupational therapy: Frames of reference for intervention.* Thorofare, NJ: SLACK Incorporated.

Christiansen, C., & Baum, C. (1991). *Occupational therapy: overcoming human performance deficits.* Thorofare, NJ: SLACK Incorporated.

Kielhofner, G. (1992). *Conceptual foundations of occupational therapy.* Philadelphia: F. A. Davis.

Chapter 3
Disorders of Infancy, Childhood, and Adolescence

These disorders are characterized by onset in the early years of life. While they appear early, many of them are lifelong problems, making their functional implications substantial. The disorders may be present at birth, as in the case of some types of mental retardation, or may appear in adolescence, as in the case of some anxiety disorders (Figure 3-1).

Figure 3-1. Disorders of Infancy, Childhood, and Adolescence.

- Mental retardation
- Learning disorders (Academic skills disorders)
- Motor skills disorders
- Communications disorder
- Pervasive developmental disorders:
    Autism
    Other
- Disruptive behavior disorders:
    Attention deficit hyperactivity disorder
    Conduct disorder
    Oppositional defiant disorder
- Separation anxiety disorder

Diagnoses listed in other categories and covered in later chapters (e.g., mood disorders) may also be applied to children or adolescents. These are disorders that typically emerge during adulthood, but may occur earlier. Their manifestation in children may differ, but symptoms are similar to those seen in adults. Thus while age of onset is an important factor in differential diagnosis, it is one of many which must be considered.

Childhood and adolescence are characterized by numerous stresses which may lead to disorders not specifically listed in this section. Depression, suicidal ideation or action, substance abuse, adjustment disorders, and sexual acting out are not uncommon. Some theorists suggest that these difficulties may be part of normal development, particularly during adolescence (Freud, 1958). This view is supported by those who feel that modern society presents more difficult dilemmas than existed in earlier times, among these parental divorce, early placement in day care, and availability of and peer pressure to use drugs and alcohol (Nicholi, 1988).

This view has been disputed, however. Some researchers have found adolescents to be largely well adjusted (Offer, Marcus, & Offer, 1970). The evidence is unclear. It appears, for example, that approximately 10% to 20% of children with divorced families develop long-term functional problems (Jellinek & Herzog, 1988) while others appear to do as well as their peers. Disputes about what constitutes "normal" childhood and adolescence and what reflects dysfunction await resolution through further research.

The issue of what is normal and what represents dysfunction severe enough to warrant diagnosis must be considered in examining disorders of infancy, childhood, and adolescence. DSM-IV (APA, 1994) has attempted to be quite specific about the symptoms that must be present in order for diagnosis to be made, but there remains an element of subjectivity, which some practitioners suggest is particularly problematic where the young are concerned.

As with all psychiatric diagnoses, those of childhood and adolescence may occur independently, or in conjunction with other problems. The concept of dual diagnosis is a frequent theme in the literature, referring to someone who has two concurrent diagnoses, for example, retardation and depression (Reiss & Rojahn, 1993) or any of a number of other psychiatric disorders (Bregman, 1991). Dual diagnosis complicates both the diagnostic process and treatment, requiring integration of treatment approaches (Mulcahy, 1992). The issue of dual diagnosis is discussed in greater detail in Chapter 5.

This chapter reviews the diagnoses of infancy, childhood, and adolescence most likely to be seen by occupational therapists.

Mental Retardation

Three characteristics must be present for this diagnosis: 1) subaverage intelligence, 2) deficits in adaptive functioning in at least two areas, and 3) the appearance of both prior to age 18 (Figure 3-2). Intelligence (IQ) is usually measured on any of the standard intelligence tests such as the Stanford-Binet or Weschler Intelligence Scale for Children (Zimmerman & Woo-Sam, 1984), with 70 being the score used to define retardation. This cut-off is arbitrary, and IQ tests typically have standard errors of roughly $\pm$ 4 points. Thus, the diagnosis must be made cautiously.

Figure 3-2. Disorders of Childhood: Symptoms and Deficits.

Disorder	Symptoms	Functional Deficits
Mental Retardation	1. Subaverage intelligence	Global ADL/IADL, work, leisure
	2. Deficits in adaptive function	Global motor, sensory motor, social, cognitive
	3. Appears before age 18	Range from mild to severe
Autistic Disorder	1. Impaired social interaction	Global ADL/IADL, work, leisure
	2. Impaired communication	Global motor, sensory motor, sensory, cognitive, psychological, social
	3. Restricted activity repertoire	Usually severe
	4. Onset during infancy or childhood	
Attention Deficit Hyperactive Disorder (ADHD)	1. Restlessness, distractability	Social, school, leisure
	2. Excessive activity	Mild to severe
	3. Impulsivity	Usually improve during adolescence
	4. Onset before age 7	
Conduct Disorder	1. Has engaged in at least three antisocial acts within past twelve months	Social, leisure, school
Separation Anxiety Disorder	1. Excessive anxiety	School, social, leisure

Etiology and Incidence

The etiology of retardation is well-established in some cases, but not in others. Some genetic disorders, trisomy 21 (Down syndrome) or fragile X syndrome (Hodapp et al., 1992), for example, cause retardation, as will some prenatal problems such as prenatal malnutrition or fetal alcohol syndrome (Phelps & Grabowski, 1992). A variety of physical problems during early childhood may also lead to retardation (Reber, 1992), including exposure to toxic substances such as lead, diseases such as meningitis, and injury, especially head trauma.

Environmental factors may also contribute to retardation. Absence of adequate stimulation or parental deprivation may lead to slowed development and low IQ. Early malnutrition is also a factor (Galler, Ramsey, Solimano, & Lowell, 1983). Bijou (1992) identifies a number of categories of causes, including biomedical pathology, cultural-familial conditions, and restricted development. At least 30% of cases, however, have no identifiable cause (Reber, 1992).

It appears that mental retardation is present in approximately 1% of the population (Reber, 1992).

Prognosis

To some extent, prognosis is dependent on cause. In some instances, retardation may be reversed when the cause of the retardation is removed. Absence of environmental stimulation, for example, may result in developmental lag (Reber, 1992). If parents can be taught to make the environment more stimulating, the retardation may be remediated and the child may achieve normal function. Some government programs, such as Project Head Start, appear to have positive effects on IQ for many children who are somewhat delayed developmentally (these programs were not designed for children who are mentally retarded, however).

Similarly, where a biological cause can be established, medical treatment of the underlying problem may prevent retardation from worsening, although generally speaking the existing damage will be permanent. For example, if retardation is the result of lead toxicity, agents may be introduced that remove lead from the system. This treatment will prevent further damage, but will generally not reverse damage that has already occurred (Galler et al., 1983). Prompt treatment of diseases such as meningitis, when such treatment exists, may also minimize the probability of retardation or limit damage.

In most cases, however, individuals with mental retardation remain delayed throughout life (Zigman, Schupf, Silverman, & Sterling, 1989). Functional ability can be enhanced, and most interventions with individuals who are mentally retarded focus on some form of education or training. These may include behavior modification (Reber, 1992), or any of a variety of educational approaches. Depending on degree of retardation, the individual may be taught to cook simple meals, to dress and maintain personal hygiene, and to perform simple vocational tasks, making some individuals relatively independent and self-sufficient. While function may be remediated, individuals who are retarded by definition do not achieve the same level as their peers who are not retarded.

Education may extend to the family, both for purposes of prevention (educating pregnant women about the need for good nutrition, for example) and for management of the retarded child. This may reduce some of the stress that has been noted in families with children who have mental retardation (Baker, Landen, & Kashima, 1991; Cullen, MacLeod, Williams, & Williams, 1991).

Depending on the degree of impairment, institutionalization may be necessary. Individuals who are profoundly retarded may be unable to learn the skills that would enable them to live even in sheltered environments in the community. For many less severely impaired individuals, however, many types of sheltered environments, special schools, and later, independent living, may provide alternatives to institutionalization.

Implications for Function and Treatment

Retardation is classified as mild (IQ 55 to 70), moderate (IQ 40 to 55), severe (IQ 25 to 40), or profound (IQ below 25). These are approximate ranges, but provide a rough guide to expected function. While IQ and functional ability are correlated, a variety of factors may impact on the functional picture presented by individuals with similar IQ scores. There has been much discussion, for example, about the possibility of cultural bias of IQ tests (Zimmerman & Woo-Sam, 1984), which might cause a low score in someone who otherwise has a reasonable level of function. In fact there has been much controversy around this point, with some researchers feeling that IQ tests should not be used to identify retardation. As an example, some children from deprived backgrounds may know a great deal of street jargon, but have limited vocabularies for English words used in the larger society. Furthermore, the concept of environmental press (Murray, 1938) suggests that the environment can be structured to minimize demands on the individual, thus supporting existing abilities.

Generally speaking, individuals who have low IQs show performance deficits in most areas of function. These may present as delays in the development of specific abilities, the absence of some abilities, or deficits in the skill with which activities are performed. For example, a child who is mentally retarded might sit relatively late, might not sit at all, or might sit with poor control and posture. A individual with profound retardation may never acquire speech or learn to feed him- or herself, while an individual who is only mildly retarded may learn to read and do simple arithmetic problems. In general, individuals with mild to moderate mental retardation tend to be concrete in their thinking, and require simple, repeated instructions in order to learn tasks.

Except where there are obvious physical signs of retardation at birth, in the case of trisomy 21, for example, functional delays observed by parents are most likely to result in the identification of individuals with mental retardation. Parents typically become concerned when a child does not sit, walk, or talk at the expected time.

Functional deficits tend to be pervasive, though as with all children, some areas may be more delayed than others. Functional decrements also are related to types of retardation (Bregman & Hodapp, 1991). For example, activities of daily living (ADL) are a relative strength for individuals with fragile X syndrome as compared with individuals with trisomy 21 (Zigler & Hodapp, 1991). A child with mental retardation is likely to have motor, social, cognitive, sensory, and psychological deficits, though he or she may have relatively less motor delay than cognitive delay, or less social delay than motor delay. For example, some children who are retarded may be quite sociable, but have difficulty with academic skills. Deficits are also roughly correlated with IQ, so that a profoundly retarded child is likely to have severely impaired function in all areas.

Deficits occur in all performance areas: play, social interaction, ADL, and education. These translate into later deficits in work, play, leisure, and ADL/Instrumental Activities of Daily Living (IADL). Hellendoorn and Hoekman (1992) found that play was age appropriate for mental rather than chronological age.

Intervention is generally medical and educational/behavioral. Medical treatment focuses on reversing treatable conditions and maximizing health to preserve intact function. Provision of adequate nutrition and exercise, and monitoring of health in individuals unable to report symptoms is vital to optimal functioning.

Medication may be used for individuals who have accompanying behavioral problems or are self-injurious (Aman, 1991). While the value of medication as an adjunct to intervention is not clear, it is considered worth pursuing since about 25% of individuals with mental retardation have such behaviors (Meador & Osborn, 1992).

For children, educational approaches are most often employed. For those with mild impairment, "mainstreaming," inclusion to the greatest degree possible in the regular school system, is the intervention of choice. They may have special classes during the course of the day, and attend regular classes when possible. Those more severely impaired will attend special schools.

Behavioral interventions can be valuable for both children and adults (Carr & Carlson, 1993; Repp & Karsh, 1992). Enhanced social and vocational function can be obtained by carefully outlining the steps involved in each task, and then providing reinforcement as the individual accomplishes each step. The approach, called "self-management," encourages the individual to verbalize and rehearse steps in specific activities (Ferretti, Cavalier, Murphy, & Murphy, 1993). Less attention has been paid to leisure performance, but there is every reason to believe that this, too, can be enhanced through behavioral and educational approaches. Community based instruction (McDonnell, Hardman, Hightower, Keifer-O'Donnell, & Drew, 1993) and job training (Simmons & Flexer, 1992) with emphasis on repeated practice is successful in enhancing adaptive skills. Similarly, functional communication training (Durand & Carr, 1992) can yield long-term improvements in ability.

Residential intervention may be necessary for some individuals (Bruininks, Chen, Lakin, & McGrew, 1992). In these settings, interaction with staff can lead to more independent functioning (Fleming & Reile, 1993). Fleming and Reile (1993) found that 80% of studies of such programs reported positive or mixed results.

It is important to note, however, that while many types of treatment appear to promote optimal function, none completely reverses retardation, except cases where it is medically possible to do so. On the other hand, recent evidence suggests that some types of retardation (trisomy 21, for instance) have better prognoses than assumed in the past. Some of these individuals achieve quite good function, and report very positive levels of life satisfaction.

Implications for Occupational Therapy

For individuals who are retarded, the goal of treatment is most often habilitation (enabling) rather than rehabilitation, since they must acquire skills they never had, rather than regain those lost. Since function is not consistently poor (Bregman & Hodapp, 1991), it is important to understand the cause of retardation for the individual, as well as his or her own particular strengths.

In general, goals of occupational therapy focus on enabling maximal performance. This requires careful assessment of both deficits and strengths. Individuals who are retarded often wish to do the same activities as their peers (Edgerton, 1976) and are able to accomplish many developmental milestones, albeit more slowly than others. Although recognition of strengths is important in working with any client, it is particularly vital with these individuals as their strengths are often overlooked.

At the same time, realistic appraisal is necessary. It is essential to understand what constitutes the starting point for a particular individual, and the duration of the learning process for a particular skill may place limits on eventual achievement.

Individuals who are profoundly retarded are unlikely to acquire more than extremely minimal skills. Early intervention may need to focus on eating and on movement to facilitate dressing in much the same way as a therapist might approach a child with severe cerebral palsy (Carrasco & Powell, 1989). Sensory integration and sensory stimulation may be of value (Reisman, 1993).

With children who are less severely retarded, training and education may prove quite valuable, particularly when practice is built in. For example, body awareness may facilitate dressing skills. In one school, children aged 6 to 10 years old spent several weeks playing "Simon Says," pointing to body parts on dolls, doing the Hokey Pokey ("you put your left foot in . . ."), and so on. Two months later they were ready to begin putting legs into pant legs and arms into sleeves. It should be noted that sensory stimulation is also a component of these activities.

Identifying leisure activities at which they can succeed is also important for these children. Many have siblings they would like to emulate, but Little League may be beyond them unless leagues are specially organized. Not only must the individual identify leisure interests, but he or she must also have the mobility skills to get to those activities (McInerney & McInerney, 1992). Training and practice in use of public transportation is an essential factor in addressing all performance areas.

As these children age, vocational training and training in independent living skills become increasingly important. This includes training in social skills (Margalit & Ronen, 1993) and sex education (Rhodes, 1993). Although individuals who are retarded may desire the same activities as their peers who are not retarded, they tend to conceptualize at a concrete level. Since many will live independently or in semi-sheltered environments, they need to understand the accompanying responsibilities. One young woman, for example, expressed a wish for a child until she sat through an independent living group while a baby-doll cried in the background. Another young man planned to go to the movies every day until the therapist had him put his pay from the sheltered workshop in piles to represent rent, food, transportation, etc.

Technological devices can provide some assistance (Sandknop, Schuster, Wolery, & Cross, 1992) as a means of structuring the environment to reduce demand. Devices must be carefully evaluated and training should be provided until the individual is comfortable with their use. It is important to choose wisely since some devices add to rather than reduce complexity of tasks.

In general, for both children and adults, sensory stimulation can be helpful in focusing attention. Presenting tasks in small steps allows for practice in sequence (Martin, 1989). An additional focus must be on self-esteem, since these individuals often compare themselves negatively to others, and must deal with pejorative comments by others. Mainstreamed children, for example, must contend with schoolmates who call them "moron" or "dummy."

As can be inferred from this discussion, treatment may occur in a variety of sites, including the home, a special school, a regular school, an institution, a sheltered workshop, or a supervised living facility (Martin, 1989). Each requires sensitivity on the part of the therapist to the needs of the client in that setting, and the possibility of movement from setting to setting (e.g., into a supervised apartment when custodial parents die). Children nearing the end of the educational process may need intensive work on vocational skills.

Learning Disorders (Academic Skills Disorders)

The learning disorders section of DSM-IV (APA, 1994) has been greatly expanded and clarified. It now identifies a number of different conditions, including reading disorder, mathematics disorder, and disorder of written expression. The expansion of this section is of particular importance to occupational therapists because of the frequency with which they treat children with these problems. For each diagnosis, characteristics which must be present include achievement substantially below age appropriate expectations and difficulties in daily life and/or academic performance because of the deficit.

Etiology and Incidence

Taken together, the learning disabilities are found in somewhere between 2% and 10% of schoolchildren (APA, 1994). Data for individual disorders are not available because most studies group them together.

Etiology is not well-established, although most literature supports a biological/neurological component. Family studies indicate a genetic factor, as well (Gilger, Pennington, & Defries, 1991; Smith, 1992).

Treatment and Prognosis

Some children grow out of their learning difficulties over time. For these children, the disorder may represent a developmental lag rather than a chronic disorder. Other children, however, experience long-term negative consequences. Behavior problems are common (McGrath & Grant, 1993), possibly because children with this disorder may have trouble keeping up in class and become frustrated. Similarly, self-esteem may suffer as the child recognizes he or she is not able to do what others can. Best outcomes seem to be in families where adequate support networks are available (McGrath & Grant, 1993). When teachers and parents work together in planning and implementing treatment, outcomes seem better than when only the school or parent provides intervention (Shukla, 1989).

Identification of the difficulty is a particular concern. Often these disorders are not noted until the child is in school, sometimes well along in school (Chesson, McKay, & Stephenson, 1991). Because many of these children have normal or above average intelligence, they may be able to compensate for their difficulties until schoolwork becomes complex (Stephenson, McKay, & Chesson, 1990). Late identification causes difficulty because the child may already have developed a sense of low self-esteem or behavioral problems.

Treatment must begin with careful assessment to determine the exact nature of the difficulty (Farrell, Dunning, & Foley, 1989). Following assessment, plans can be made to remediate deficits, often through occupational therapy. In addition, teachers can develop instructional plans which make use of alternate pathways available to the child. For example, a child with auditory learning difficulties may be able to make use of visual substitutes and vice versa. These adaptive mechanisms can be extremely helpful, but must be individual. For example, one child with a disorder of written expression had great difficulty writing, but was able to use a computer with ease.

Implications for Occupational Therapy

There is a vast body of literature about occupational therapy for children with learning disabilities. Treatment of such children is a primary role for therapists in school systems. Screening is a particularly important role (Chesson et al., 1991) since parents and teachers may not know what to look for. Informing parents and teachers about signs of learning disorders can be quite valuable.

Further, occupational therapists assist teachers and parents in managing the difficulties, and in providing direct treatment to the child. Sensory-integration is among the interventions which appear to be of value (Humphries, Snider, & McDougall, 1993; Kinnealey & Miller, 1993). For elaboration on the role of occupational therapy with children with learning disorders, Pratt and Allen (1989) is a useful reference.

Motor Skills Disorder

This disorder, which is labeled developmental coordination disorder, is characterized by incoordination, clumsiness, or delays in meeting developmental motor milestones for sitting, walking, etc. These symptoms must have an impact on performance, and must not be the result of a physical disorder such as cerebral palsy.

Etiology and Incidence

In children aged 5 to 11, incidence is estimated at about 6% (APA, 1994). Etiology is not clear, although a biological component is suspected.

Prognosis and Treatment

As with learning disorders, some children simply grow out of their difficulties. However, in about half these children, difficulties persist beyond age 12 (Geuze & Borger, 1993). In those for whom the disorder is more chronic, teachers report behavioral and learning difficulties. Treatment is similar to that for learning disorders.

Implications for Occupational Therapy

Occupational therapists are very involved in treatment of this disorder. In addition to screening, assessment, and consultation with teachers and parents, therapists provide direct treatment (Kinnealey & Miller, 1993).

Communication Disorders

Included in this category are expressive language disorder, mixed expressive-receptive language disorder, phonological disorder, and stuttering. Expressive language disorder is characterized by difficulty producing sounds in an age appropriate fashion, as well as difficulty with vocabulary, sentence structure, and grammar. It is very common among young children. By age 17, incidence drops to about half a percent (APA, 1994). Expressive-receptive language disorder has these characteristics along with receptive difficulties such as problems understanding others' language. Phonological disorder is typified by pronunciation difficulties without the accompanying problems with language usage.

Stuttering is an impairment of speech fluency. It may be an inability to produce specific sounds, or an inability to control repetitions of sounds or words. As the disorder becomes established, anxiety about speaking appears, exacerbating the problem. Delay in language development and articulation problems are common among children who stutter (Homzie, Lindsay, Simpson, & Hasenstab, 1988).

In these disorders, functional impairment depends on the severity of the disorder, the individual's determination, and the understanding of others. Leisure and academic pursuits may be more difficult (Black, 1987) because of these communication difficulties. Treatment is most often provided by speech therapists, but occupational therapists may be involved if there is any accompanying learning disability, or damage to self-esteem that might be remedied through success with activities.

Pervasive Developmental Disorders

Autism

Although this is a rare condition, it has received considerable notice possibly because of the extreme nature of the deficits with which it is associated. A number of popular books (c.f. Greenfield, 1986) have brought it to the attention of the general public. In order for the diagnosis to be made, social interaction, communication, and activity must be impaired. Children with autism have severe social deficits, lack speech or have peculiar speech patterns, and have unusual stereotyped movements like hand flapping. Infants with autism have been noted to be hypoactive, to avoid gaze, and to have reduced emotional expression (Adrien et al., 1993). Children with autism may sit without making eye contact or speaking, while engaging in some self-stimulating behavior, possibly spinning their bodies or twirling their hair for hours on end. They show poor cognitive flexibility, verbal reasoning, complex memory, and complex language association (Minshew, Goldstein, Muenz, & Payton, 1992), but less deficit in associative memory and rule learning in abstract thinking.

Autism often occurs in the presence of other disorders, particularly mental retardation. It must be distinguished from schizophrenia and other psychotic disorders (Phelps & Grabowski, 1991). Differential diagnosis is done based on the severe language deficits which occur in autism, as well as the probable low IQ. Autism is distinct from pure mental retardation because of the variability of IQ in different areas which occurs in autism (Siegel, 1991).

Etiology and Incidence

The etiology of autism is increasingly well understood. At one point it was considered a problem of inadequate parenting, believed to be associated with maternal coldness, absence, or rejection (Weininger, 1993). This idea has been largely discredited, and current hypotheses center on the possibility of some sort of neurological dysfunction. It is known, for example, that autistic children have poor receptive language and symbol use (Atlas, 1987) supporting the notion of CNS deficits. There is a growing body of evidence that autism is a neurological disorder, probably of prenatal origin (Phelps & Grabowski, 1991).

Incidence is roughly 4 to 5 per 10,000 population (Verheij & van Loon, 1992). The disorder is much more common in males.

Prognosis

Prognosis is poor for at least two thirds of individuals with autism (Gillberg, 1991). While some individuals may show unpredictable improvements, the majority continue to be fairly impaired throughout life and some may deteriorate in adolescence. In particular, social impairment and behavioral and psychiatric symptoms have been found to persist (Rumsey, Rapoport, & Scheery, 1985). Factors which help predict long-term outcomes include IQ and speech abilities at age 5.

Some studies have shown gradual improvement in symptoms. However, Rumsey and colleagues (1985) studied 14 autistic individuals, 9 of whom were considered high functioning, and found that all had ongoing social and occupational impairment. Skill and performance are globally and chronically affected although improvement may occur. Kanner (1992) reported on a long-term follow-up of 11 individuals diagnosed as autistic in 1943. He found that only two were significantly improved.

Implications for Function and Treatment

Autistic individuals show extreme impairments in social functioning, ability to communicate, and in performance of most activities. These impairments are often characterized by peculiarities in performance, as well as absence of performance. For example, an autistic individual may be able to speak, but may put words together in ways which are not meaningful to others. Similarly, he or she may be able to perform specific fine motor tasks, but unable to put them together into a meaningful sequence of activities to accomplish a specific task.

The deficits in function are quite severe, usually precluding most forms of normal goal-oriented occupation. Autistic individuals are usually unable to perform ADL and IADL, have disturbed patterns of play, and are unable to study and, later, to work. Communication skills are particularly poor (Atlas, 1987).

Because the etiology is as yet unclear, treatment is not well-established. Most interventions currently employed are behavioral, with a focus on speech development, increasing behaviors such as ADL skills, or decreasing undesirable behaviors such as peculiar movements (McEachin, Smith, & Lovaas, 1993). More and more autistic children are in public schools, often in special classes, although the majority of programs are still provided at special schools or inpatient settings, as they are usually designed to provide high levels of input throughout the day.

Behavior modification has been employed for specific deficits. One study focused on affectionate behavior (McEvoy et al., 1985), reporting on an effort to teach autistic children to express positive emotion to those around them. The authors reported that some very limited improvement occurred. Because of the severity of dysfunction, behavioral programs usually focus on small components of performance, making global improvement an extremely long-term goal. Environmental enrichment with sensory stimulation has been employed with some success, in an effort to provide more general intervention (Ward, 1985). McEachin and colleagues (1993) reported that behavioral treatment may have long-term positive effects.

Medical intervention focuses on drug treatment to ameliorate symptoms. Clomipramine and pimozide are among the drugs used with some evidence of positive outcome (Ernst et al., 1992; Gordon, State, Nelson, Hamburger, & Rapoport, 1993).

Implications for Occupational Therapy

Because autistic children are so severely impaired, observation must often substitute for formal assessment, and treatment goals must be sensitive to the probability that change will occur in very small steps.

Ideally, adaptive behavior, cognitive, motor, and perceptual skills should be evaluated (Nelson, 1981), but this often proves difficult because of the profound communication deficits characteristic of these children. A wide range of assessment and intervention strategies is essential because of the severe and comprehensive dysfunction found in children who are autistic (Huebner, 1992).

Many of the intervention strategies used with children who are severely or profoundly retarded, including sensory stimulation and sensory integration, may be attempted (Herman, 1980). There is evidence that these interventions may help focus attention and reduce self-stimulating behavior (Toigo, 1992). In general, focus is on basic self-care and communication. Motivation and attention are key issues. Behavioral techniques may be helpful both in enhancing attention and in training autistic children to perform sequences of activities related to self-care.

There is some evidence that play behavior can be enhanced using self-management intervention (Stahmer & Schriebman, 1992). This involves demonstration of appropriate toy use, followed by reinforcement of appropriate play. Similar interventions in a highly structured milieu seem somewhat helpful in other performance areas (Rogers & Lewis, 1989).

Other Pervasive Developmental Disorders

DSM-IV (APA, 1994) includes several other pervasive developmental disorders distinct from autistic disorder. These other diagnoses are arrived at based on differences in symptoms (Gillberg, 1992). For example, a child with Rett syndrome is more likely to show extreme social aloofness than are those with fragile X syndrome (Gillberg, 1992). Subtle differences in symptoms have implications for choice of therapy (Verheij & van Loon, 1992). Verheij and van Loon (1992) recommend careful assessment of sensory, sensorimotor, attention, cognitive, emotional, and speech development, and the impact of these on play. Their recommendation is that treatment focus on 1) reducing anxiety, 2) eliminating impeding behavior, and 3) stimulating growth and development, largely through education and behavior modification.

Disruptive Behavior Disorders

These disorders are reflected in behavior which may initially be more disturbing to others than to the individual. However, the presence of these disorders may have long-term effects on self-esteem and social participation, as the individual is likely to receive considerable social censure and rejection as a result of his or her behavior. In addition, manifested behaviors may interfere with learning, causing long term academic problems.

Attention Deficit Hyperactivity Disorder (ADHD)

This disorder is characterized by excessive inattention, impulsiveness, and hyperactivity. Typically, the child has difficulty attending to others, and is extremely active physically. Problematic behaviors, including at least six specific symptoms of inattention, impulsiveness, or hyperactivity must be present for at least 6 months for the diagnosis to be made. The behaviors must be judged to be more severe than in normal children, a criterion which presents significant diagnostic difficulties, as noted below. In addition, the behaviors must interfere with social, academic, or vocational performance. The problem behaviors must appear prior to age 7 to be diagnosed as ADHD. The diagnosis is problematic, as individual adult tolerance for activity in children varies. What is labeled "youthful exuberance" in some families may be intolerable to other parents. In some children, the diagnosis is not made until the school years, when ADHD may interfere with ability to complete school work. In other instances the diagnosis may be made on the basis of the adult's difficulty accepting the behavior, rather than on clearly disturbed behavior on the part of the child. For the most part, however, these children are easily recognizable. They respond to the slightest distraction, running to chase dust, sunlight, and every small sound, rather than focusing on tasks for periods of time. Their level of activity is often exhausting just to watch.

The diagnosis of Attention Deficit Disorder without hyperactivity is even more difficult (Goodyear & Hynd, 1992) because inattention may be misunderstood as disinterest, daydreaming, or inability.

Etiology and Incidence

Etiology of ADHD is not clearly established, although it is suspected that it may occur in the presence of neurological damage or a disordered central nervous system. First described by Hoffman in 1926, it was originally called Minimal Brain Damage. Later it was known as hyperkinesis, then hyperactivity (Rutter & Taylor, 1978). Current theories suggest that the problem is one of CNS organization (Jellinek & Herzog, 1988). Children with ADHD have been found to be more field dependent than others (Stoner & Glynn, 1987). This means that they have difficulty separating figures from the background in pictures, a difficulty that would contribute, among other things, to reading difficulties and problems with visual discrimination tasks. This would also contribute to difficulty filtering out normal distractions in the environment. They also have more frequent language disorders than other children (Love & Thompson, 1988), supporting the idea of CNS disturbance. The disorder also seems to be more common in families where other relatives have had the diagnosis, suggesting a familial or genetic component (Biederman, 1991).

This is a common disorder, occurring in 3% to 5% of the population (APA, 1994). It is much more common in males.

Prognosis

Prognosis is good for some children, who seem to "outgrow" the disorder as they get older (Lie, 1991). Many do well, with no evidence of higher rates of alcoholism or criminal behavior. Learning disabilities and motor and perceptual problems may disappear over time, or be compensated for. Some researchers dispute this scenario, however, suggesting that adults often show identical symptoms to children (Bellack, 1992; Lie, 1991).

A potential negative consequence of ADHD is the possibility that the child will become depressed or develop low self-esteem as a result of the social disapproval or academic difficulties which often accompany the disorder. Understandably, the prognosis is less favorable if ADHD is accompanied by retardation or some other behavioral disorder (e.g. conduct disorder) (August, Stewart, & Holmes, 1983; Lie, 1991). Comorbidity of these disorders seems common (Biederman, Newcorn, & Sprich, 1991) and may account for some of the differences in prognosis reported in various research studies. Hechtman, Weiss, and Perlman (1980) found ongoing problems with heterosexual relationships, assertiveness, and self-esteem, and Lie (1991) indicated that ADHD is associated in some studies with lower school and vocational achievement.

Implications for Function and Treatment

Children with ADHD are able to function in many areas. They are usually able to perform age-appropriate ADL and IADL and to play and to interact with peers on some level. Generally speaking, social and academic performance are most impaired. Peers and adults may find the excessive activity and difficulty concentrating annoying, and avoid or chastise the child. In some instances, poor impulse control leads the child to behave in socially inappropriate or antisocial fashion, again leading to disapproval or to legal difficulties.

In the academic sphere, poor concentration and impulse control present significant problems (Lie, 1991). Not only is learning impaired, but teachers find these children difficult to manage. They often do poorly in school and then become anxious about their performance, exacerbating their learning difficulties. Other activities that require concentration or attention may be difficult or impossible for these children, limiting the play and leisure activities in which they are able to participate.

Medication is used frequently to control ADHD (Gomez & Cole, 1991). Amphetamines, Ritalin in particular, are often used. The exact mechanism by which they work is not known but they seem effective in focusing attention. There is some controversy about the use of these drugs, as their long-term effects are not thought to be adequately understood. In addition, some researchers believe that they are used too freely, particularly in cases where the diagnosis may be marginal. Most importantly, effectiveness of the drugs is not clear (Gomez & Cole, 1991). It seems that positive effects result in more manageable behavior rather than improved academic performance. For this reason, there has been concern that the drugs are "abused" in the sense that they provide relief for the adult, while some less intrusive approaches might be equally effective for the child.

Other interventions are both behavioral and environmental (Gomez & Cole, 1991). Behavioral approaches attempt to reinforce efforts to concentrate and control hyperactivity. Environmental approaches are used to design low stimulus environments in which distractions are kept to a minimum. Biofeedback has also been used with some success (Weitman, personal communication, October, 1994). There is evidence that multiple forms of intervention are better than drugs alone (Gomez & Cole, 1991).

Implications for Occupational Therapy

As the name of the disorder implies, attention is an important factor in working with these children (Pratt & Allen, 1989). Several approaches may be useful. Environmental structuring to minimize distraction may help the child focus on the task at hand. Occupational therapy may also provide patterned, sequenced sensory input to attempt to help the child better organize his or her surroundings. Both relaxation (Kwako, 1980) and perceptual motor training (Christ, 1980) have been reported as helpful.

In addition, self-esteem is an important issue for these children. Identification of activities they can do well can be enormously helpful in convincing them, often despite repeated scoldings from exasperated adults, that they do have strengths.

Often, the occupational therapist works with parents and teachers to teach them to manage problematic behaviors. Assisting them to structure the learning or home environment optimally, or to break tasks into chunks, or to provide deep touch to help the child gain control may help the adult cope better, and the child function better.

Conduct Disorder

This diagnosis is made if, within 12 months of diagnosis of ADHD, the individual has engaged in at least three episodes of behavior in which societal norms are violated, such as aggression, destruction of property, lying or theft, or violation of rules. The diagnosis may be made for children or adolescents, or occasionally for adults who do not meet the criteria for antisocial personality.

Etiology and Incidence

Etiology of this disorder is not clearly established, although there is speculation that, like antisocial personality, it may be the result of either inconsistent or overprotective parenting. Behaviorists suggest that the result of these parental styles is poor understanding of the consequences of behavior, while psychodynamic theorists suggest that there is poor development or integration of the superego. In addition, environmental and socioeconomic explanations have been advanced, suggesting that this behavior is the result of social or family disadvantage (Gardner, 1992). It occurs frequently in combination with disorders like ADHD and depression (Ben-Amos, 1992; Wierson, Forehand, & Frame, 1992), and it has been suggested that it may be a consequence of the CNS damage or the negative appraisals of self which occur as a result of ADHD or LD.

This disorder occurs in roughly 6% to 16% of males and 2% to 9% of females (APA, 1994).

Prognosis

Milder forms of the disorder seem to have reasonably good prognoses, while the more severe form predicts later delinquent and adult antisocial behavior (Faretra, 1981; Robins, 1978). As the disorder coexists with others, including enuresis (Faretra, 1981), retardation, ADHD, depression, and substance abuse, if the coexisting condition is remediated, the conduct disorder may also improve. Similarly, if the environment is altered or improved, symptoms may subside. However, when there are coexisting conditions the prognosis is worse (Clarke & Clarke, 1988). For some individuals, the conduct disorder is evident primarily in group situations, and removing the child from the disordered group reduces the problematic behavior (Lahey, Loeber, Quay, Frick, & Grimm, 1992).

In general, about half of all cases are reported to have very poor outcomes (Clarke & Clarke, 1988). However, Wierson and colleagues (1992) provide a comprehensive review of outcome studies, and conclude they are inadequate, in part because of differing definitions of the disorder and unclear inclusion criteria for subjects.

Implications for Function and Treatment

Many of these individuals have difficulty with school/work performance, possibly as the result of cognitive or attention deficits, possibly as a result of attitudinal problems (Wierson et al., 1992). As a rule, ADL and IADL functions are not impaired. Leisure and play tend to focus on socially unacceptable activities, as acting out may take the place of more normal endeavors.

These children are likely to have social difficulties, which may stem from poor ability to detect and understand social cues from others (Dodge, 1983; Dodge, Murphy, & Buchsbaum, 1984). This finding has led to speculation that training in these skills might improve function and reduce symptoms.

Glasser (1975) recommended a type of milieu therapy he labeled reality therapy as a mechanism for making individuals accountable for their behavior. This is one of many milieu treatments which have been attempted, including the behavioral approach of the token economy, with rewards or reinforcements for acceptable behavior. Milieu treatments are those in which the entire environment is carefully structured to have therapeutic impact.

A whole range of treatment options is available, including psychotherapy, behavior therapy, social learning, cognitive therapy, academic intervention, parent training, and recreational programming (Wierson et al., 1992). Pharmacotherapy may also be attempted, including anticonvulsants, antidepressants, and beta blockers (Stewart, Myers, Burket, & Lyles, 1990). The effectiveness of any of these is not well documented.

Implications for Occupational Therapy

Occupational therapists work with children with conduct disorders in several ways. First, energy may be channeled to more appropriate activities, with copious reinforcement for acceptable behavior. Expectations for behavior during such activities must be carefully identified and reasonable positive or negative outcomes systematically provided.

Second, self-esteem of these children must be considered. Experiences of success can be of great value in building a more positive self-concept.

Finally, opportunities for expression must be provided. Many of these children come from disturbed environments. They may be unable to verbally express feelings adequately and may do better through play, art, music, or movement.

At the same time, the possibility of coexisting deficits must be considered. ADHD should be addressed, as should other disorders.

Oppositional Defiant Disorder

A less severe variant of conduct disorder is oppositional defiant disorder. According to DSM-IV (APA, 1994), this disorder is diagnosed based on a pattern of hostile or defiant behavior of at least 6 months' duration, which causes noticeable impairment of function. It is reported to be related to conduct disorder, but diagnostically different enough to be listed separately (Lahey et al., 1992). Risk of problems with the legal system is much lower, and school problems tend to be less severe. Similarly, prognosis is better over the long term. Interventions are similar to those used with individuals with conduct disorder.

Separation Anxiety Disorder

This disorder is typified by anxiety or panic related to threatened separation from familiar caretakers or presence of unfamiliar adults. Onset is prior to age 18, duration is at least 4 weeks, and the disorder causes functional decline. The decline relates to reluctance to go to school or engage in other activities away from the immediate family.

Other anxiety disorders can occur in children and adolescents, including obsessive compulsive disorder (Swedo, Leonard, & Rapoport, 1992; Thomsen, 1992). These are discussed in Chapter 8.

Etiology and Incidence

The etiology of this disorder is not well understood, although it may have a biological basis, as is suspected of some of the adult anxiety disorders. There has also been speculation about premature separation from a primary caregiver as a cause (Bowlby, 1969).

This disorder occurs in 4% of the population and is more common in females (APA, 1994).

Prognosis

In some instances, the disorder disappears spontaneously, sometimes after only one episode. In other cases, it may become severe and disabling, as the individual may develop a social phobia or school phobia, and refuse to leave the home. The child may have a stomachache every morning, or cry and scream when the school bus comes. Remediation is easiest in those situations where there are clear environmental factors, such as excessive pressure to perform well in school, contributing to the problem. Altering the environment may be quite effective in those situations. One child got sick at school every morning before computer class. She improved when she received individual tutoring that convinced her she could handle the work.

Implications for Function and Treatment

As noted, in severe cases, school, social, and leisure activities may be severely compromised. Individuals may become so anxious at the thought of having to perform in one of these spheres that they become physically ill. ADL are usually not affected, nor are IADL which may be performed in the home. However, those activities which require interaction with strangers or leaving familiar environments may be all but impossible. It appears to be performance, i.e., school and leisure activity, rather than motor, social, or other skills which is impaired.

Treatment is not well understood, although some theorists suspect that altering home circumstances to provide a more stable, less pressuring environment may be helpful. Some behavioral techniques are also attempted, although such methods as systematic desensitization, which are helpful with some anxious adults, may be too complex for young children (King & Ollendick, 1989). Flooding has had little systematic evaluation, while reports of cognitive therapies seem promising.

Implications for Occupational Therapy

Relaxation techniques may be helpful to children with anxiety disorders. Using mental imagery to picture success, enjoyment, and relaxation can provide a useful prelude to anxiety-provoking activities.

In addition, activities can in themselves be relaxing, particularly if those that are enjoyable to the child can be identified. Sometimes pairing a pleasant activity with one that evokes anxiety can relieve feelings of distress. The student who felt sick before computer class did well when the task was playing computer games rather than doing schoolwork. The positive association later generalized to other computer activities.

Expressive arts may be beneficial as a way to uncover and explore fears. A child who was afraid to leave his room drew pictures of enormous snakes and spiders. It turned out he had encountered a snake in his basement that had greatly frightened him. It was then possible to address his fear.

Other Disorders of Infancy, Childhood, and Adolescence

There are numerous other disorders that may occur in younger individuals. Some are the same as those which occur in adults, including schizophrenia (Werry & McClellan, 1992), adjustment disorder (Newcorn & Strain, 1992), and mood disorders (Werry & McClellan, 1992). Suicidal behavior has been noted in children as young as preschool, although the reasons for the behavior differ from those of adults (Fasko & Fasko, 1991). The most common cause was expected punishment; others were escape from an unpleasant situation and a desire for reunion with a significant other who had died.

There are also a number of other childhood disorders (APA, 1994). These include several eating, tic, elimination disorders, elective mutism, stereotypic movement disorder, and reactive attachment disorder. These disorders are discussed briefly in Chapter 10.

References

Adrien, J. L., Lenoir, P., Martineau, et al. (1993). Blind ratings of early symptoms of autism based upon family home movies. *Journal of the American Academy of Child and Adolescent Psychiatry, 32,* 3.

Aman, M. G. (1991). Pharmacotherapy in the developmental disabilities: New developments. *Australia and New Zealand Journal of Developmental Disabilities, 17,* 183-199.

American Psychiatric Association (1994). *Diagnostic and Statistical Manual of Mental Disorders* (4th ed.). Washington, DC: Author.

Atlas, J. A. (1987). Symbol use by developmentally disabled children. *Psychological Reports, 61,* 207-214.

August, G. J., Stewart, M. A., & Holmes, C. S. (1983). A four-year follow-up of hyperactive boys with and without conduct disorder. *British Journal of Psychiatry, 143,* 192-198.

Baker, B. L., Landen, S. J., & Kashima, K. J. (1991). Effects of parent training on families of children with mental retardation: Increased burden or generalized benefit? *American Journal of Mental Retardation, 96,* 127-136.

Bellack, L. (1992). Comorbidity of attention deficit hyperactivity disorder and other disorders. *American Journal of Psychiatry, 149,* 147-148.

Ben-Amos, B. (1992). Depression and conduct disorders in children and adolescents: A review of the literature. *Bulletin of the Menninger Clinic, 56,* 188-208.

Biederman, J. (1991). Attention Deficit Hyperactivity Disorder (ADHD). *Annals of Clinical Psychiatry, 31,* 9-22.

Biederman, J., Newcorn, J., & Sprich, S. (1991). Comorbidity of attention deficit hyperactivity disorder with conduct, depressive, anxiety and other disorders. *American Journal of Psychiatry, 148,* 564-577.

Bijou, S. W. (1992). Concepts of mental retardation. *The Psychological Record, 42,* 305-322.

Black, J. A. (1987). A comparative study of the perception of freedom-in-leisure between stuttering and nonstuttering individuals. *Journal of Fluency Disorders, 12,* 291-304.

Bowlby, J. (1969). *Attachment and loss.* New York: Basic Books.

Bregman, J. (1991). current developments in the understanding of mental retardation. Part II: Psychopathology. *Journal of American Academy of Children Adolescent Psychiatry, 30,* 861-872.

Bregman, J., & Hodapp, R. M. (1991). Current developments in the understanding of mental retardation. Part I: Biological and phenomenological perspectives. *Journal of American Children Adolescent Psychiatry, 30,* 5, 707-719.

Bruininks, R. H., Chen, T. H., Lakin, K. C., & McGrew, K. S. (1992). Components of personal competence and community integration for persons with mental retardation in small residential programs. *Research in Developmental Disabilities, 13,* 463-479.

Carr, E. G., & Carlson, J. I. (1993). Reduction of severe behavior problems in the community using a multicomponent treatment approach. *Journal of Applied Behavior Analysis, 26,* 157-172.

Carrasco, R. C., & Powell, N. (1989). Children with cerebral palsy. In P. N. Pratt & A. S. Allen (Eds.), *Occupational therapy for children* (2nd ed., pp. 396-421). St. Louis, C.V. Mosby.

Chesson, R., McKay, C., & Stephenson, E. (1991). The consequences of motor/learning difficulties for school-age children and their teachers: Some parental views. *Support for Learning, 4,* 173-177.

Christ, P. A. H. (1980). Electromyographic biofeedback and perceptual motor training for hyperactivity. *Occupational Therapy in Mental Health, 1,* 47-57.

Clarke, A. M., & Clarke, A. D. B. (1988). The adult outcome of early behavioural abnormalities, *International Journal of Behavioral Development, 11,* 3-19.

Cullen, J. C., MacLeod, J. A., Williams, P. D., & Williams, A. R. (1991). Coping, satisfaction, and the life cycle in families with mentally retarded persons. *Issues in Comprehensive Pediatric Nursing, 14,* 193-207.

Dodge, K. A. (1983). Behavioral antecedents of peer social status. *Child Development, 54,* 1386-1399.

Dodge, K. A., Murphy, R. R., & Buchsbaum K. (1984). The assessment of intention-cue detection skills in children: Implications for developmental psychopathology. *Child Development, 55,* 163-173.

Durand, V. M., & Carr, E. G. (1992). An analysis of maintenance following functional communication training. *Journal of Applied Behavior Analysis, 25,* 777-794.

Edgerton, R., & Bercovici, S. (1976). The cloak of competence years later. *American Journal of Mental Deficiency, 80,* 485-497.

Ernst, M., Magee, H. J., Gonzalez, N. M., Locascio, J. J., Rosenberg, C. R., & Campbell, M. (1992). Pimozide in autistic children. *Psychopharmacology Bulletin, 28,* 187-191.

Faretra, G. (1981). A profile of aggression from adolescence to adulthood: An 18-year-old follow-up of psychiatrically disturbed and violent adolescents. *American Journal of Orthopsychiatry, 51,* 439-453.

Farrell, P., Dunning, T., & Foley, J. (1989). Methods used by educational psychologists to assess children with learning difficulties. *School Psychology International, 10,* 47-55.

Fasko, S. N., & Fasko, D. (1990-91). Suicidal behavior in children. *Psychology: A Journal of Human Behavior, 27-28,* 10-16.

Ferretti, R. P., Cavalier, A. R., Murphy, M. J., & Murphy R. (1993). The self-management of skills by persons with mental retardation. *Research in Developmental Disabilities, 14,* 189-205.

Fleming, R. K., & Reile, P. A. (1993). A descriptive analysis of client outcomes associated with staff interventions in developmental disabilities. *Behavioral Residential Treatment, 8,* 29-43.

Freud, A. (1958). Adolescence. *Psychoanalytic Study of Children, 13,* 255-278.

Galler, J. R., Ramsey, F., Solimano, G., & Lowell, W. E. (1983). The influence of early malnutrition on subsequent behavioral development: II. classroom behavior. *Journal of the American Academy of Child Psychiatry, 22,* 16-22.

Gardner, F. E. M. (1992). Parent-child interaction and conduct disorder. *Educational Psychology Review, 4,* 135-163.

Geuze, R., & Borger, H. (1993). Children who are clumsy: Five years later. *Adapted Physical Activity Quarterly, 10,* 10-21.

Gilger, J. W., Pennington, B. F., & Defries, J. C. (1991). Risk for reading disability as a function of parental history in three family studies. *Reading and Writing: An Interdisciplinary Journal, 3,* 17-29.

Gillberg, C. (1991). Outcome in autism and autistic-like conditions. *Journal of the American Academy of Child and Adolescent Psychiatry, 30,* 375-382.

Gillberg, C. (1992). Subgroups in autism: Are there behavioral phenotypes typical and underlying medical conditions? *Journal of Intellectual Disability Research, 36,* 201-214.

Glasser, W. (1975). *Reality therapy: A new approach to psychiatry.* New York: Perennial Library/Harper & Row.

Gomez, K., & Cole, C. (1991). Attention deficit hyperactivity disorder: A review of treatment alternatives. *Elementary School Guidance & Counseling, 26,* 106-115.

Goodyear, P., & Hynd, G. W. (1992). Attention-deficit disorder with (ADD/H) and without (ADD/WO) hyperactivity: Behavioral and neuropsychological differentiation. *Journal of Clinical Child Psychology, 21,* 273-305.

Gordon, C., State, R. C., Nelson, J. E., Hamburger, S. D., & Rapoport, J. (1993). A double-blind comparison of clomipramine, desipramine, and placebo in the treatment of autistic disorder. *Archives of General Psychiatry, 50,* 441-447.

Greenfield, J. (1986). *A client called Noah.* New York: Henry Holt and Co.

Hechtman, L. Weiss, G., & Perlman, T. (1980). Hyperactives as young adults. *Canadian Journal of Psychiatry, 25,* 478-482.

Hellendoorn, J., & Hoekman, J. (1992). Imaginative play in children with mental retardation. *Mental Retardation, 30,* 255-263.

Herman, B. E. (1980). A sensory-integrative approach to the psychotic child. *Occupational Therapy in Mental Health, 1,* 57-68.

Hodapp, R., Leckman, J. F., Dykens, E. M., Sparrow, S. S., Zelinsky, D. G., & Ort, S. I. (1992). K-ABC profiles in children with fragile X syndrome, Down syndrome, and nonspecific mental retardation. *American Journal of Mental Retardation, 97,* 39-46.

Homzie, M. J., Lindsay, J. S., Simpson, J., & Hasenstab, S. (1988). Concomitant speech, language, and learning problems in adult stutterers and in members of their families. *Journal of Fluency Disorders, 13,* 261-277.

Huebner, R. A. (1992). Autistic disorder: A neuropsychological enigma. *American Journal of Occupational Therapy, 46,* 487-501.

Humphries, T. W., Snider, L., & McDougall, B. (1993). Clinical evaluation of the effectiveness of sensory integrative and perceptual motor therapy in improving sensory integrative function in children with learning disabilities. *Occupational Therapy Journal of Research, 13,* 163-182.

Jellinek, M. S., & Herzog, D. B. (1988). The child. In A. M. Nicholi (Ed.), *The new Harvard guide to psychiatry* (pp. 607-636). Cambridge, MA: Belknap Press.

Kanner, L. (1992). Follow-up study of eleven autistic children originally reported in 1943. *Focus on Autistic Behavior, 7,* 1-11.

Kinnealey, M., & Miller, L. J. (1993). Sensory integration/learning disabilities. In H. L. Hopkins & H. D. Smith (Eds.), *Occupational therapy* (8th ed., pp. 489-494). Philadelphia: J. B. Lippincott.

King, N. J., & Ollendick, T. H. (1989). Children's anxiety and phobic disorders in school settings: Classification, assessment, and intervention issues. *Review of Educational Research, 59,* 431-434.

Kwako, R. (1980). Relaxation as therapy for hyperactive children. *Occupational Therapy in Mental Health, 1,* 29-45.

Lahey, B. B., Loeber, R., Quay, H. C., Frick, P. J., & Grimm, J. (1992). Oppositional defiant and conduct disorders: Issues to be resolved by DSM-IV. *Journal of American Academy Child Adolescent Psychiatry, 31,* 539-546.

Lie, N. (1991, suppl.). Follow-ups of children with attention deficit hyperactivity disorder. *Acta Psychiatria Scandinavia, 85,* 5-40.

Love, A. J., & Thompson, M. G. G. (1988). Language disorders and attention deficit disorders in young children referred for psychiatric services: Analysis of prevalence and a conceptual synthesis. *American Journal of Orthopsychiatry, 58,* 52-64.

Margalit, M., & Ronen, T. (1993). Loneliness and social competence among preadolescents and adolescents with mild mental retardation. *Mental Handicap Research, 6,* 97-111.

Martin, M. J. (1989). Children with mental retardation. In P. N. Pratt, & A. S. Allen (Eds.), *Occupational Therapy for Children* (2nd ed., pp. 422-441.). St. Louis, C.V. Mosby.

McDonnell, J., Hardman, M. L., Hightower, J., Keifer-O'Donnell, R., & Drew, C. (1993). Impact of community-based instruction on the development of adaptive behavior of secondary-level students with mental retardation. *American Journal of Mental Retardation, 97,* 575-584.

McEachin, J. J., Smith, T., & Lovaas, O. I. (1993). Long-term outcome for children with autism who received early intensive behavioral treatment. *American Journal on Mental Retardation, 97,* 359-372.

McEvoy, M. A., Nordqueist, V. M., Twardosz, S., Heckaman, K. A., Wehby, J. H., & Denny, R. K. (1985). Promoting autistic children's peer interaction in an integrated early childhood setting using affection activities. *Journal of Applied Behavioral Analysis, 21,* 193-200.

McGrath, M., & Grant, G. (1993). The life cycle and support networks of families with a person with a learning difficulty. *Disability, Handicap & Society, 8,* 25-41.

McInerney, C. A., & McInerney, M. (1992). A mobility skills training program for adults with developmental disabilities. *American Journal of Occupational Therapy, 46,* 233-239.

Meador, D. M., & Osborn, R. G. (1992). Prevalence of severe behavior disorders in persons with mental retardation and treatment procedures used in community and institutional settings. *Behavioral Residential Treatment, 7,* 299-314.

Minshew, N., Goldstein, G., Muenz, L., & Payton, J. (1992). Neuropsychological functioning in nonmentally retarded autistic individuals. *Journal of Clinical and Experimental Neuropsychology, 14,* 749-761.

Mulcahy, M. (1992). Evaluation of treatment in the psychiatry of mental retardation. *International Journal of Mental Health, 21,* 77-94.

Murray, H. A. (1938) *Explanations in personality.* New York: Oxford Press.

Nelson, D. L. (1981). Evaluating autistic clients. *Occupational Therapy in Mental Health, 1,* 1-22.

Newcorn, J. H., & Strain, J. (1992). Adjustment disorder in children and adolescents. *Journal of the American Academy of Child and Adolescent Psychiatry, 31,* 318-326.

Nicholi, A. M., Jr. (1988). The adolescent. In A. M. Nicholi (Ed.), *The new Harvard guide to psychiatry* (pp. 637-664). Cambridge, MA: Belknap Press.

Offer, D., Marcus, D., & Offer, J. L. (1970). A longitudinal study of normal adolescent boys. *American Journal of Psychiatry, 126,* 917-924.

Phelps, L., & Grabowski, J. (1991). Autism: Etiology, differential diagnosis, and behavioral assessment update. *Journal of Psychopathology and Behavioral Assessment, 13,* 107-125.

Phelps, L., & Grabowski, J. (1992). Fetal alcohol syndrome: Diagnostic features and psychoeducational risk factors. *School Psychology Quarterly, 7,* 112-128.

Pratt, P. N., & Allen, A. S. (1989). *Occupational therapy for children* (2nd ed.). St. Louis: C. V. Mosby.

Reber, M. (1992). Mental retardation. *The Interface of Psychiatry and Neurology, 15,* 511-522.

Reiss, S., & Rojahn, J. (1993). Joint occurrence of depression and aggression in children and adults with mental retardation. *Journal of Intellectual Disability Research, 37,* 287-294.

Reisman, J. (1993). Using a sensory integrative approach to treat self-injurious behavior in an adult with profound mental retardation. *The American Journal of Occupational Therapy, 47,* 403-411.

Repp, A. C., & Karsh, K. G. (1992). An analysis of a group-teaching procedure for persons with developmental disabilities. *Journal of Applied Behavior Analysis, 25,* 701-712.

Rhodes, R. (1993). Mental retardation and sexual expression: An historical perspective. *Sexuality and Disabilities, 8,* 1-27.

Robins, L. N. (1978). Sturdy childhood predictors of adult antisocial behaviors: Replication from longitudinal studies. *Psychology & Medicine, 8,* 611-622.

Rogers, S., & Lewis, H. (1989). An effective day treatment model for young children with pervasive developmental disorders. *Journal of the American Academy of Child and Adolescent Psychiatry, 28,* 207-214.

Rumsey, J. M., Rapoport, J. L., & Scheery, W. R. (1985). Autistic children as adults: Psychiatric, social and behavioral outcomes. *Journal of the American Academy of Child and Adolescent Psychiatry, 24,* 465-473.

Sandknop P., Schuster, J., Wolery, M., & Cross, D. (1992). The use of an adaptive device to teach students with moderate mental retardation to select lower priced grocery items. *Education and Training in Mental Retardation, 27,* 219-229.

Shukla, R. P. (1989). Identification of educationally handicapped children and non-instructional responsibilities of teachers: Concept analysis and suggestions. *Indian Journal of Disability and Rehabilitation, 3,* 73-80.

Siegel, B. (1991). Toward DSM-IV: A developmental approach to autistic disorder. *Pervasive Developmental Disorders, 14,* 53-68.

Simmons, T. J., & Flexer, R. W. (1992). Community based job training for persons with mental retardation: An acquisition and performance replication. *Community-Based Job Training,* 261-272.

Smith, S. (1992). Familial patterns of learning disabilities. *Annals of Dyslexia, 42,* 143-158.

Stahmer, A. C., & Schreibman, L. (1992). Teaching children with autism appropriate play in unsupervised environments using a self-management treatment package. *Journal of Applied Behavior Analysis, 25,* 447-459.

Stephenson, E., McKay, C., & Chesson, R. (1990). An investigative study of early developmental factors in children with motor/learning difficulties. *British Journal of Occupational Therapy, 53,* 4-6.

Stewart, J. T., Myers, W. C., Burket, R. C., & Lyles, W. B. (1990). A review of pharmacotherapy of aggression in children and adolescents. *Journal of the American Academy of Child and Adolescent Psychiatry, 29,* 269-277.

Stoner, S. B., & Glynn, M. A. (1987). Cognitive styles of school-age children showing attention deficit disorders with hyperactivity. *Psychological Reports, 61,* 119-125.

Swedo, S. E., Leonard, H. L., & Rapoport, J. L. (1992). Childhood-onset obsessive compulsive disorder. *Obsessional Disorders, 15,* 767-775.

Thomsen, P. H. (1992). Obsessive-compulsive disorder in adolescence. *Psychopathology, 25,* 301-310.

Toigo, D. (1992). Autism: Integrating a personal perspective with music therapy practice. *Music Therapy Perspectives, 10,* 13-20.

Verheij, F., & van Loon, H. (1992). Pervasive developmental disorders not otherwise specified: A developmental-psychopathological approach for the development of made-to-measure treatment planning. *Acta Paedopsychiatrica, 55,* 235-242.

Ward, A. J. (1978). Early childhood autism and structural therapy: Outcome after 3 years. *Journal of Consulting and Clinical Psychology, 46,* 227-238.

Weinenger, O. (1993). Attachment, affective contact, and autism. *Psychoanalytic Inquiry, 13,* 49-62.

Werry, J. S., & McClellan, J. M. (1992). Predicting outcome in child and adolescent (early onset) schizophrenia and bipolar disorder. *Journal of the American Academy of Child and Adolescent Psychiatry, 31,* 147-150.

Wierson, M., Forehand, R. L., & Frame, C. L. (1992). Epidemiology and treatment of mental health problems in juvenile delinquents. *Advances in Behavioral Research and Therapy, 14,* 93-120.

Zigler, E., & Hodapp, R. M. (1991). Behavioral functioning in individuals with mental retardation. *Annual Review of Psychology, 42,* 29-50.

Zigman, W. B., Schupf, N., Silverman, W. P., & Sterling, R. C. (1989). Changes in adaptive functioning of adults with developmental disabilities. *Australia and New Zealand Journal of Developmental Disabilities, 15,* 277-287.

Zimmerman, I. L., & Woo-Sam, J. M. (1984). Intellectual assessment of children. In G. Goldstein & M. Hersen (Eds.), *Handbook of Psychological Assessment* (pp. 57-76). New York: Pergamon Press.

Chapter 4
Delirium and Dementia

This section of DSM-IV (APA, 1994) includes diagnoses which are associated with biological etiologies, all of which are characterized by cognitive dysfunction. There are three major categories: delirium, which is a disturbance of consciousness and cognition developed over a short time; dementia, with multiple cognitive deficits without change in consciousness; and amnestic disorder, with disturbances in memory without other cognitive impairments. According to Tucker, Caine, Folstein, and colleagues (1992) this is a section of DSM-IV which has been changed substantially from DSM-III-R (APA, 1987).

Delirium

Delirium is characterized by global changes in cognition, with accompanying alteration of consciousness (Figures 4-1 and 4-2). The individual will have diminished awareness of the environment and be disoriented to time, place, and, sometimes, to self as well. In addition to altered consciousness, delirium presents with inability to maintain attention, disorganized thinking, changes in psychomotor activity or sleep, perceptual disturbances, and memory impairment. Onset is generally rapid, and a precipitating event can frequently be identified.

Figure 4-1. Distinguishing Delirium from Dementia.

Delirium	Dementia
Cognitive change Altered consciousness	Cognitive change Full consciousness

Examples:
    Substance intoxication delirium
    Substance withdrawal delirium
	Examples:
	    Dementia of the Alzheimer's type
	    Vascular dementia

Figure 4-2. Delirium and Dementia: Symptoms and Deficits.

Disorder	Symptoms	Functional Deficits
Delirium	1. Reduced attention	Global ADL/IADL, work, leisure
	2. Disorganized thinking	Global sensory, sensory motor, cognitive, social, psychological
	3. Altered consciousness	
	4. Rapid onset	
Dementia	1. Memory impairment	Global ADL/IADL, work, leisure
	2. Cognitive impairness	Global sensory, sensory motor, cognitive, social, psychological
	3. 1 and 2 interfere with function	May be mild to severe
	4. No altered consciousness	

Etiology and Incidence: Treatment and Prognosis

Delirium may accompany a high fever, head trauma, encephalitis, substance abuse, tumors, and many other physical conditions. Differential diagnosis on Axis III is critical, as the cause of delirium defines treatment. Delirium is extremely common, occurring in 10% to 15% of individuals on medical and surgical wards (Lipowski, 1992). It is typically transient, resolving in days or weeks, either through cure of the underlying biological disorder, or through death, which occurs in about 14% of cases (Lipowski, 1992).

Implications for Function: Implications for OccupationalTherapy

Individuals with delirium show marked functional decrements in all spheres as a result of altered consciousness and diminished cognition. They are unable to accomplish activities at the performance level, and skills will show marked deficits. Occupational therapists are only occasionally involved in treatment of individuals with delirium, most often when the delirium persists accompanying a prolonged state of coma. In these instances, the therapist may be asked to provide sensory stimulation to encourage resolution of the coma, and to provide passive range of motion to minimize contractures which might occur as a result of prolonged bedrest and inactivity.

Dementia

Dementia is characterized by memory loss in the presence of full consciousness. Abstract thinking and judgment are impaired. Aphasia, apraxia, and other cognitive and motor dysfunction may be noted, along with personality changes, such as newly developing paranoia. In order for the diagnosis to be made, symptoms must be sufficiently severe to interfere with vocational or social functioning. Changes in consciousness are not noted. Cognitive loss in dementia is far beyond age associated memory impairment (Caine, 1993) the sort of minor memory change which is characteristic of normal aging but is *not* disabling.

Etiology and Incidence

There are a large number of possible causes of dementia. They include Alzheimer's disease, vascular disease (multi-infarct dementia), Huntington's chorea, Pick's disease, Jakob-Creutzfeldt disease, and multiple sclerosis. There are other, reversible causes of dementia, including depression (Riley, 1994) and metabolic and nutritional problems, and there is a group of dementias labeled pseudodementia (e.g., Ganser's syndrome) which are thought to be psychogenic rather than biological in origin (Jeste, Gierz, & Harris, 1990). Differential diagnosis is difficult at present, but vital to effective treatment. By far the most common dementing illness is Dementia of the Alzheimer's Type (DAT) or Alzheimer's disease (AD). It is believed to account for at least half of dementias in the elderly, with a prevalence of three to four million individuals (Selkoe, 1992).

Distinguishing among the dementias is done on the basis of both laboratory findings and the nature of the symptoms. DAT and Pick's are primarily cortical, while Huntington's and Parkinson's diseases are subcortical (Cummings, 1982). Multi-infarct and Jakob-Creutzfeldt are mixed. The subcortical dementias have more extrapyramidal signs, such as ataxia and tremor, while the cortical dementias have more cognitive symptoms such as memory loss, personality change, and visuospatial impairment. Identification of these symptom differences is an important step in diagnosis.

Multi-infarct dementia, a vascular dementia, can be diagnosed by computerized axial tomography (CAT scan), as it is caused by small infarcts or cerebral vascular tears. Symptoms include spotty loss of function, which progresses through rather abrupt changes in performance followed by periods of relative stability. DAT, on the other hand, shows more global loss, and more gradual, continuous progression. These differences may be quite subtle, however.

Pseudodementia (Ganser's syndrome) is characterized by a course which is not deteriorating, and by differences between the subjective reports of the individual about severity and the objective findings. Typically objective signs are less severe than those reported by the individual (Jeste et al., 1990). "Approximate answers" to questions (e.g., $3+3=7$) (Jeste et al., 1990) are also typical. This disorder is not a form of malingering, as there is no conscious attempt to mislead. It may, instead, be a hysterical or psychotic episode. Prevalence is uncertain, but probably about 2% of dementias are pseudodementia.

Depressive dementia is characterized by slowing and poverty of response (Riley, 1994). The individual may not respond to questions at all, or may give very brief responses. Psychomotor slowing is also a sign of this type of dementia, which is responsive to psychotropic medication. A caution for care providers is the possibility that a depressive dementia may be superimposed on another irreversible dementia, causing excess disability. If the depression is treated, symptoms may be reduced, although the course of the underlying dementia will not be altered (Alexopoulos & Abrams, 1991).

Diagnosis of DAT must be made by exclusion. It can be confirmed only through brain biopsy or autopsy. If other causes of dementia, including depression, metabolic disorders, and multi-infarct dementia can be ruled out, a diagnosis of DAT will be made.

The precise etiology of DAT is not known, although autopsy reveals a characteristic pattern of neuritic plaques and tangles (Byrne, Smith, & Arie, 1991) as well as changes in the hippocampus. A variety of etiological factors have been hypothesized. The most prevalent theories at present include a genetic explanation (Rosenberg, 1993) possibly related to defects of chromosomes 21, 14, or 19. The finding that chromosome 21 is involved was related to the observation that individuals with trisomy 21 who live into their 40s almost always show characteristic symptoms and cortical changes associated with Alzheimer's disease. A slow virus (as has been demonstrated in Jakob-Creutzfeldt disease), or some unexplained loss of neurotransmitters have also been proposed as causes. A buildup of a protein known as amyloid has been identified (Rosenberg, 1993), although the cause of this buildup is not established.

It appears that there may be more than one type of DAT (Fenn, Luby, & Yesavage, 1993). A number of researchers have speculated that there is a familial (genetic) form of DAT which differs symptomatically from other forms, as well as having a different etiology (Heston, Mastri, Anderson, & White, 1981; Silverman, Breitner, Mohs, & Davis, 1986). While this type of Alzheimer's disease has been difficult to document because of diagnostic problems and deaths from unrelated causes, an autosomal dominant familial form has been identified.

A distinction has been made between early and late onset dementia (Chui, Teng, Henderson, & Moy, 1985). Early onset dementia is more severe, with worse aphasia (speech difficulty) and presence of agraphia (difficulty writing) early on (Brandt, Mellitz, & Rovner, 1989). Some researchers have speculated that the early onset type is the familial type, but this contention is still open to debate with research both supporting and refuting this supposition.

There has been increasing research about DAT, which has been found to be present in approximately 50% of all nursing home residents (Seltzer, 1988). Since the numbers are likely to increase, considerable attention has been given to the disorder. Other dementias are also increasing. Possibly because of differential life expectancies, the disorders are more common in women.

Prognosis
Prognosis for DAT is always poor. The disease progresses to total incapacity and death. The speed of progress is quite variable, however. Some researchers speculate that early onset DAT is more likely to progress rapidly, to result in greater dysfunction, and to cause death within a few years. By contrast, later onset DAT is thought to progress more slowly, with the possibility of functional plateaus which last for long periods of time. Different course as a result of age of onset is not clearly established, but it is known that DAT will progress over time, and is always fatal.

Prognosis for multi-infarct dementia is variable. Existing damage is irreversible. The progress of the disease may be slow, and may not be progressive. Treatment of coexisting high blood pressure or vascular disease may slow or stop deterioration of function.

The other irreversible dementias also have poor long-term prognoses. The only one with any particularly effective treatment is Parkinson's disease, which can be treated symptomatically with a medication, levodopamine (L-dopa). Otherwise, management rather than treatment is the goal of intervention.

When dementia is caused by depression or is a pseudodementia, prognosis is relatively good (Jeste et al., 1990). The underlying psychological disorder is often treatable, improving cognitive function. It is also important to recognize that individuals with Alzheimer's disease may also be depressed. Treatment of the depression may dramatically improve function for a while. One man reported that when his mother was placed in a cogenial residential facility she regained her ability to play bridge, although many symptoms of her Alzheimer's disease remained.

Implications for Function and Treatment

Dementia has a devastating impact on all areas of function. As it progresses, occupational, social, and ADL/IADL skills disappear, until ultimately, swallowing and even breathing may become difficult. In fact, death often occurs as a result of pneumonia which is the result of inability to clear the lungs (Burns, 1992). As noted above, the progress of the disease is somewhat variable and rather unpredictable. Some residual function may be retained for long periods of time.

DAT has been described as progressing through three stages (Berila, 1994). The first symptom identified is usually memory impairment. The individual may put water on the stove to boil and forget to turn it off, or may go out and forget how to get back home. The memory difficulties may lead to work problems and carelessness in personal grooming. For example, the individual may forget how to do work tasks or forget to bathe. During the second stage, aphasia, apraxia (movement difficulties), disorientation, and restlessness appear. It is common during this phase to see the individual pacing around the house for hours on end, forgetting who people are, even those closest to him or her, and having difficulty finding words. In some individuals, an attempt to deal with the word-finding problem is made by talking around the word. Thus "radio" may be called the machine with a switch that talks.

Personality changes also occur. Temper outbursts are common as the individual finds his or her limitations extremely frustrating. In addition, as ability to understand the environment worsens, the individual becomes fearful and, often, paranoid. When personal items are missing, the individual often assumes that they have been stolen. Finally, memory becomes severely impaired, and total loss of sensory and cognitive abilities occurs. The individual becomes bedridden and incontinent, unable to chew or swallow.

Some specific characteristics of the symptoms are worth noting. First, personality and social behavior may be maintained well into the disease. In fact, some individuals learn to cover their impairment so well that it is not recognized by others until the disease is well along. It is only after listening for awhile that the other person becomes aware that verbalizations, however pleasant, make no sense. The memory and sensory losses also have some specific characteristics. Problems seem to arise in the encoding of information, so the defect is in recent, rather than immediate or remote, memory (LaRue, 1982). This means that the individual will be able to process what is happening at the moment and what happened 50 years ago, but not what happened that morning. In addition, extraneous memories seem to intrude on function, leading to confabulation and perseveration. An individual who is questioned about family members may present a long, rambling description of sisters and brothers, but not remember spouse and children. This is a characteristic which distinguishes DAT from depression, which is more likely to lead to absence of response.

Language, especially word finding, is almost universally impaired. Articulation, however, remains intact until very late in the disease course (Murdoch, Chenery, Wilks, & Boyle, 1987). The individual can say words, but not put them together in a meaningful way. Aphasia is thought to be worse in the familial type, and agraphia is a defining feature of familial DAT. Visuospatial deficits are common, as are visual field losses (Steffes & Thralow, 1987). The individual thus has difficulty with walking and other activities which require spatial discrimination. Temporal distortions are also common (Cummings, 1982), with the person unable to keep track of time, day, or season.

Other dementias are characterized by different functional deficits. Pick's disease, which has an earlier onset than DAT (usually ages 40 to 60), manifests itself first with behavioral and affective changes (Cummings, 1982). Cognitive changes including aphasia occur later. Unlike DAT, motor and sensory changes are rare, and occur later in the disease course. Visuospatial deficits are also rare.

Multi-infarct dementia has less predictable functional consequences, as changes are dependent on the location and extent of cerebral damage (Hachinski, Lassen, & Marshall, 1974). In addition, progress of the disease is inconsistent. There may be long periods of plateau and sudden decrements in performance.

Depressive dementias are a manifestation of depression most likely to appear in the elderly (Riley, 1994). Instead of symptoms of sadness and hopelessness, the depression presents with confusion and memory impairment. Unlike the dementias described above, however, motor slowing and reduced levels of response to the environment are seen. This type of dementia is reversible through drug therapy. Hysterical dementias are those which have no identifiable biological base, and seem to be the result of psychological conflict and stress rather than biology. They are usually identifiable by the course, which is atypical for any of the known dementias, and by the fact that the dementia may come and go, with periods of normal function interspersed with problem behavior. Usual treatment for these dementias is psychotherapy and possibly drug therapy.

There are other causes of dementia, as well, including Korsakoff's, Wernicke's, and syphilitic dementia. Korsakoff's and Wernicke's are both attributable to long-term alcoholism, syphilitic to tertiary syphilis. All are irreversible, although they may stabilize rather than progress. Each has its own particular course and symptoms. Korsakoff's, for example, presents with amnesia for recent events. The individual remembers quite clearly up to a particular point in time, perhaps 10 years ago, and has no memory for anything which occurred from that time to the present.

A new dementia emerging in rapidly growing numbers is that related to human immunodeficiency virus (HIV) (Egan, 1992). Approximately 5% to 10% of the HIV-infected population has signs of dementia, even before development of acquired immunodeficiency syndrome (AIDS).

AIDS dementia complex has many of the features of other dementias, but progresses very rapidly. It is separate from some of the opportunistic infections which cause encephalitis or other CNS diseases. Its manifestations are global cognitive impairment including memory deficits, intellectual impairment, poor concentration, and memory. According to Navia and colleagues (1986), inflicted individuals maintain the ability to do simple ADL, but are not functionally independent. Social, leisure, and vocational performance are severely compromised. Late stage individuals are severely dysfunctional in all spheres. Maintenance doses of AZT may prevent or delay onset of AIDS-associated dementia (Egan, 1992).

Available treatment of individuals with dementing illnesses is minimal, except in those cases where a reversible cause can be identified. In the majority of cases, however, treatment is symptomatic and behavioral. If the individual is wandering at night, for example, a low dose of a sleeping medication may be administered (Schneider & Sobin, 1991). In cases where severe paranoia appears, medication may also be tried. Medical intervention presents problems, though, as drugs may be sedating, making symptoms such as confusion worse. Some symptoms can be reasonably well-managed for some period of time.

Experimentation with new medications is ongoing. One which has received considerable notice is tetrahydroaminoacridine (THA) (Minthon et al., 1992). The drug seems to have modest impact on cognition as measured by neuropsychological tests. However, no improvement on self-care measures has been noted, and only about one third of individuals show any improvement at all.

The most common dementias, however, cannot be cured, nor can the progression be stopped, or in most cases, even slowed. Much intervention focuses on the individual's caregiver, who must learn how to manage the behaviors. The caregiver may be taught how to give simple instructions, how to deal with temper outbursts, and so on (Fisher & Carstensen, 1990).

Implications for Occupational Therapy

Occupational therapists have a vital role to play in the treatment of dementing illnesses. Because of the incurable and usually progressive nature of the disorders, interventions which focus on management and maximizing quality of life are quite valuable. In the early stages of these disorders, efforts can be made to help the individual maintain function and autonomy (Trace & Howell, 1991). This may be done through environmental adaptation, education, and use of assistive devices, particularly memory aids. Van Deusen (1992) recommends teaching compensatory techniques for visuospatial problems and apraxia during the early stages of the disorder.

As the individual's function declines, focus shifts to helping caregivers cope with emerging deficits (Berila, 1994). Again, environmental adaptation can be useful (Josephsson et al., 1993). This includes simplifying the environment, reducing the number of stimuli, and also adding various safety devices, such as automatic turn-off switches for stoves, and door alarms to warn off wandering. The caregiver must be educated about the course of the disease and given information about how to deal with problems. It may be helpful to provide information about how to feed the person, how to modify clothing, and so on.

Other suggestions include careful use of community services to reduce caregiver burden (Baum, 1991), carefully patterned sensory stimulation to minimize the potential for sensory deprivation syndrome (Bryant, 1991), and physical therapy to encourage mobility (Pomeroy, 1993).

For both the individual and the caregiver, quality of life is a major issue. For the individual, activity should be encouraged at whatever level they can perform. Day treatment programs provide structured activities and stimulation at a level which the individual can manage. The caregiver is often overwhelmed and exhausted by the needs of the individual, and must be encouraged to take time for his or her own leisure. At some point, nursing home placement may be necessary, and the occupational therapist may join with others who are involved in care to help the caregiver make this decision.

At all stages of the disorder, psychotherapy and other expressive therapies should be considered (Bonder, 1994). The individual often needs to express emotions, and particularly as the disorder is diagnosed earlier, this becomes increasingly possible through verbal therapies. Where verbal expression is not possible, art, music, and dance may be valuable in assisting the individual to cope. A number of first-person accounts of the disorder are now available (Davis, 1989; McGowin, 1993) and it is clear that such expression makes a significant difference in quality of life.

References

Alexopoulos, M. D., & Abrams, R. C. (1991). Depression in Alzheimer's disease. *The Psychiatric Clinics of North America, 14,* 2, 327-340.

American Psychiatric Association (1987). *Diagnostic and Statistical Manual of Mental Disorders* (3rd ed. rev.). Washington, DC: Author.

American Psychiatric Association (1994). *Diagnostic and Statistical Manual of Mental Disorders* (4th ed.). Washington, DC: Author.

Baum, C. M. (1991). Addressing the needs of the cognitively impaired elderly from a family policy perspective. *American Journal Occupational Therapy, 45,* 7, 594-606.

Berila, R. A. (1994). Dementia. In B. R. Bonder & M. Wagner (Eds.), *Functional performance in older adults* (pp. 240-255). Philadelphia: F. A. Davis.

Bonder, B. R. (1994). Psychotherapy for individuals with Alzheimer Disease. *Alzheimer Disease and Associated Disorders, 8* (suppl.), 75-81.

Brandt, J., Mellits, E. D., & Rovner, B. (1989). Relation of age at onset and duration of illness to cognitive functioning in Alzheimer's Disease. *Neuropsychiatry, Neuropsychology, and Behavioral Neurology, 2,* 2, 93-101.

Burns, A. (1992). Cause of death in dementia. *International Journal of Geriatric Psychiatry, 7,* 461-464.

Bryant, W. (1991). Creative group work with confused elderly people: A development of sensory integration therapy. *British Journal of Occupational Therapy, 54,* 5, 187-192.

Byrne, E. J., Smith, C. W., & Arie, T. (1991). The diagnosis of dementia —I clinical and pathological criteria: A review of the literature. *International Journal of Geriatric Psychiatry, 6,* 199-208.

Caine, E. D. (1993). Should aging-associated cognitive decline be included in DSM-IV? *Journal of Neuropsychiatry, 5,* 1-5.

Chui, H. C., Teng, E. L., Henderson, V. W., & Moy, A. C. (1985). Clinical subtypes of dementia of the Alzheimer type. *Neurology, 35,* 1544-1550.

Cummings, J. I. (1982). Cortical dementias. In D. F. Benson & D. Blume (Eds.), *Psychiatric aspects of neurologic disease* (Vol. 2, pp. 93-121). New York: Grune and Stratton.

Davis, R. (1989). *My journey into Alzheimer's disease.* Wheaton, IL: Tyndale House Publishers, Inc.

Egan, V. (1992). Neuropsychological aspects of HIV infection. *AIDS Care, 4,* 1, 3-10.

Fenn, H., Luby, V., & Yesavage, J. A. (1993). Subtypes in Alzheimer's Disease and the impact of excess disability: Recent findings. *International Journal of Geriatric Psychiatry, 8,* 67-73.

Fisher, J. E., & Carstensen, L. L. (1990). Behavior management of the dementias. *Clinical Psychology Review, 10,* 611-629.

Hachinski, V. C., Lassen, N. A., & Marshall, J. (1974). Multi-infarct dementia: A cause of mental deterioration in the elderly. *The Lancet.* July 27.

Heston, L. L., Mastri, A. R., Anderson, V. E., & White, J. (1981). Dementia of the Alzheimer type. *Archives of General Psychiatry, 38,* 1085-1090.

Jeste, D. V., Gierz, M., & Harris, M. J. (1990). Pseudodementia: Myths and reality. *Psychiatric Annals, 20,* 2, 71-79.

Josephsson, S., Backman, L., Borell, L., Bernspang, B., Nygard, L., & Ronnberg, L. (1993). Supporting everyday activities in dementia: An intervention study. *International Journal of Geriatric Psychiatry, 8,* 395-400.

LaRue, A. (1982). Memory loss and aging. *Psychiatric Clinics of North America, 5,* 89-103.

Lipowski, Z. J. (1992). Update on delirium. *The Interface of Psychiatry and Neurology, 15,* 335-346.

McGowin, D. F. (1993). *Living in the labyrinth: A personal journey through the maze of Alzheimer's.* San Francisco, CA: Elder Books.

Minthon, L., Gustafson, L., Dalfelt, G., Hagberg, B., Nilsson, K., Risberg, J., Rosen, I., Seiving, B., & Wendt, P. E. (1992). Oral tetrahydroaminoacridine treatment of Alzheimer's disease evaluated clinically and by regional cerebral blood flow and EEG. *Dementia, 4,* 32, 32-42.

Murdoch, B. E., Chenery, H. J., Wilks, V., & Boyle, R. S. (1987). Language in Alzheimer dementia. *Brain and Language, 31,* 122-137.

Navia, B. A., Jordan, B. D., & Price, R. W. (1986). The AIDS dementia complex: I. clinical features. *Annals of Neurology, 19,* 517-524.

Pomeroy, V. M. (1993). The effect of physiotherapy input on mobility skills of elderly people with severe dementing illness. *Clinical Rehabilitation, 7,* 163-170.

Riley, K. P. (1994). Depression. In B. R. Bonder & M. Wagner (Eds.), *Functional performance in older adults* (pp. 256-268) Philadelphia: F. A. Davis.

Rosenberg, R. N. (1993). A causal role for amyloid in Alzheimer's disease: The end of the beginning. *Neurology, 43,* 851-856.

Schneider, L. S., & Sobin, P. B. (1991). Non-neuroleptic medications in the management of agitation in Alzheimer's disease and other dementia: A selective review. *International Journal of Geriatric Psychiatry, 6,* 691-701.

Selkoe, D. J. (1992). Alzheimer's disease: New insights into an emerging epidemic. *Journal of Geriatric Psychiatry, 25,* 2, 211-227.

Seltzer, B. (1988). Organic mental disorders. In A. M. Nicholi (Ed.), *The new Harvard guide to psychiatry* (pp. 358-386). Cambridge, MA: Belknap Press.

Silverman, J. M., Breitner, J. C. S., Mohs, R. C., & Davis, K. L. (1986). Reliability of the family history method in genetic studies of Alzheimer's disease and related dementias. *American Journal of Psychiatry, 143,* 1279-1282.

Steffes, R., & Thralow, J. (1987). Visual field limitation in the patient with dementia of the Alzheimer's type. *Journal of the American Geriatric Society, 35,* 198-204.

Trace, S., & Howell, T. (1991). Occupational therapy in geriatric mental health. *American Journal of Occupational Therapy, 45,* 833-838.

Tucker, G. J., Caine, E. D., Folstein, M. F., et.al. (1992). Introduction to background papers for the suggested changes to DSM-IV: Cognitive disorders. *The Journal of Neuropsychiatry and Clinical Neurosciences, 4,* 360-368.

Van Deusen, J. (1992). Perceptual dysfunction in persons with dementia of the Alzheimer's type: A literature review. *Physical and Occupational Therapy in Geriatrics, 10,* 4, 33-46.

Chapter 5
Substance Related Disorders

In our society, a vast number of substances are abused. Some are illicit, among them cannabis, cocaine, phencyclidine (PCP), hallucinogens, and some opiates. Others are available as prescription medications, useful for specific purposes, but hazardous if misused. This group includes sedatives and other opioids (Figure 5-1). Still other substances are intended for other purposes; glues, paints, and solvents may be inhaled. One of the most commonly abused substances is alcohol, which is legal, widely available, and socially accepted under many circumstances. Similarly, nicotine is a legal and readily available psychoactive substance with potentially devastating health effects. The illegal substances have been recognized as problematic for years, while disapproval of alcohol and nicotine abuse has ebbed and flowed, with Prohibition in the 1920s and 30s, and the current push to reduce smoking.

Figure 5-1. Categories of Abused Substances.

- Alcohol and sedatives
- Cocaine and amphetamines
- Hallucinogens and PCP
- Opioids
- Cannabis
- Inhalants
- Nicotine
- Caffeine

DSM-IV (APA, 1994) has four general categories which apply regardless of the substance being abused, or in cases where several are abused simultaneously. These categories are dependence, intoxication, abuse, and withdrawal. Dependence and abuse are considered "use disorders," intoxication and withdrawal, "substance induced disorders." Each substance is then described separately. It is also possible to diagnose alcohol or drug induced mood, anxiety, and psychotic disorders.

Dependence is diagnosed when at least three of the following signs occur within a 12-month period: 1) the substance is taken in larger amounts or over more time than the individual planned, 2) efforts to cut down are unsuccessful, and 3) much of the person's activity revolves around getting the substance, and other activities are reduced as a result, even though the individual may know that this is a harmful pattern. Obligations are not met, and dangerous behavior may result from intoxication. For example, the individual may miss work, spend paychecks to obtain the substance rather than food, and may drive while intoxicated or begin to steal to have money to pay for the substance. The individual is aware that the problem exists, but develops a tolerance for the substance (i.e., increasing amounts are needed to obtain an effect). In addition, for most of these substances, withdrawal symptoms can occur and the individual may take the substance to avoid these symptoms. Thus, even though the individual knows that he or she has a problem, withdrawal becomes so unpleasant that the individual expends considerable effort to continue the substance.

Some earlier descriptions of substance abuse sought to distinguish between dependence (psychological need for a substance) and addiction (physical need for a substance to avoid physical withdrawal symptoms). DSM-IV handles this by allowing a distinction between dependence with and dependence without physiological characteristics.

Abuse is diagnosed when criteria for dependence are not met, but the individual has noticeable behavioral problems related to substance use. The symptoms are not as global or persistent as those for dependence.

Intoxication describes single episodes of substance use, during which behavior is affected. Behavior during intoxication may include belligerence; emotional lability; cognitive, judgment, social, or vocational impairment, all directly due to recent ingestion of a substance.

Withdrawal describes emotional distress or impairment in functioning directly due to efforts to stop using a substance. This does not include short-term effects (e.g., hangover) which result from single episodes of use and cessation.

Those types of substance abuse which are most likely to come to the attention of the occupational therapist are described in detail, in this chapter, those less common to occupational therapy clinics are discussed briefly. Substances with similar physiological actions are discussed together. Because occupational therapy interventions for substance abuse are similar regardless of substance, these are presented together later in the chapter.

It is important for therapists to remember that individuals with substance abuse disorders may well present in other areas of practice. As one example, an individual in a rehabilitation setting may have been injured in an accident while impaired by substance abuse. Treatment for the other conditions must take the client's substance abuse into consideration.

Alcohol and Sedatives

Both alcohol and sedatives are CNS depressants. While alcohol may cause a brief sense of excitement, both have the effect of slowing responses over time. The "high" which accompanies them is actually a slowing of CNS and autonomic function. In cases of overdose, death may occur as a result of respiratory or cardiac slowing.

Alcohol use and abuse are common in the United States, although different cultural and religious groups vary in their patterns of use, some abstaining totally, others using alcohol in specific ceremonial contexts, others using alcohol liberally (Vega et al., 1993). Among heavy drinkers, three main patterns of abuse appear. One is characterized by daily intake of large amounts of alcohol, the second by regular binges, on weekends, for example. The third pattern is characterized by long periods of abstinence interspersed with heavy binges. Other substance abuse, particularly for nicotine, is frequently present in these individuals.

Sedatives are characterized by two common patterns of abuse. In some individuals, the drug may be prescribed for a specific purpose, but tolerance may develop and symptoms of dependence appear. Cases in which these drugs are prescribed for long periods of time in order to allow an individual to function, as in the case of severe anxiety, do not qualify as substance abuse. In other cases, however, obtaining the drug becomes primary, and function changes in negative ways as a result. The second pattern of abuse is seen in individuals who obtain the drug through illicit means, specifically for purposes of abuse, i.e., for the "high." In both cases, tolerance is marked.

Etiology and Incidence

There are several theories about the emergence of alcoholism. A familial pattern, evident even when children are raised by adoptive parents, suggests some genetic component in at least some cases (Goodwin, 1985). Goodwin (1985) suggests that familial and non-familial alcoholism may be two different diseases. Familial alcoholism seems to have an earlier onset and worse prognosis (Nathan, 1991). During the early part of the century, the pre-Prohibition and Prohibition years, alcoholism was thought to be a moral failure. Since that time, it has come to be viewed as a disease, and that is now the commonly held explanation. One theory holds that a genetic predisposition may be triggered by certain environmental factors (Dantzer & Ollat, 1991). While the origins of alcoholism are not entirely clear, individual and racial differences in alcohol tolerance, separate from dependence and abuse, have been noted. For example, individuals of some races are much more likely to have severe reactions to alcohol than whites, and therefore drink less.

Women who are alcoholic have later onset and drink less, but progress more rapidly through the stages of the disorder (Lex, 1991). Women's alcoholism is of particular concern because of the potential for harm to fetuses during pregnancy. Chronic alcohol abuse is associated with Fetal Alcohol Syndrome, which causes retardation and CNS damage to the infant.

As with other forms of substance abuse, alcoholism is more common in individuals with personality disorders (Grinspoon & Bakalar, 1988). In addition, alcoholics appear more likely to be depressed (Waisberg, 1990) or suicidal (Berglund, 1984).

Alcohol abuse is of particular importance in adolescents, as there is a substantial body of evidence suggesting that it is the first substance abused by almost all adolescents who go on to abuse other drugs (Kandel & Faust, 1975; Yamaguchi & Kandel, 1984). It is worth noting that conduct disorder is predictive of alcohol abuse in adolescents (Boyle et al., 1993). While this does not mean alcohol abuse causes other substance abuse or that all adolescents who use alcohol will escalate to other drugs, it may be an important prognostic sign, and provide a clue that prevention and intervention efforts may be needed.

At the other end of the lifespan, older adults may also abuse alcohol or become alcoholic (Liberto, Oslin, & Ruskin, 1992). Older men become alcoholic more often than women. All older adults who are alcoholic have an increased risk of psychiatric comorbidity, but late onset alcoholism seems to have a better prognosis than early onset.

Dependence on sedatives is less well explained. For individuals who are exposed to the drugs as a result of some other condition, dependence probably results from the effects of the drug itself. Among those who experiment with sedatives as illicit drugs, personality disorders which may predispose to drug experimentation, e.g., antisocial personality, may be precursors of the problem. In addition, sedative abuse may result from efforts to self-treat panic disorder (Cox, Norton, Swinson, & Endler, 1990). Physicians often prescribe sedatives to control anxiety (Miller & Gold, 1990).

Approximately 6% of the adult population of the United States has had problems with alcohol dependence at some point during their lives (Grant, 1992). The incidence of sedative dependence is roughly 1.1% of the population (APA, 1994).

Prognosis

Some individuals simply stop abusing alcohol (Klingemann, 1991) or sedatives. The exact percentage of spontaneous remissions is not known. Others benefit from treatment, while some continue abuse throughout their lives, typically lives shortened by the dependence. It does seem that some alcoholics go on to drink more moderately (Gottheil, Thornton, Skoloda, & Alterman, 1982). This finding is controversial, as the vast majority of treatment programs hold that alcoholics must be totally abstinent to avoid relapse. Without further evidence on the point, the latter view must be taken as accurate.

Follow-up studies suggest that about 50% of alcoholics will continue to have drinking problems while others will be abstinent or controlled drinkers (Polich, Armor, & Braiker, 1980). Gottheil and colleagues (1982) note that individuals may shift between these groups at various times, a finding they could not explain.

Prognosis for sedative abuse is similarly mixed. One study found that approximately half of abusers continued abuse after treatment (Allgulander, Borg, & Vikander, 1984) and another 30% continued to take the drugs. Almost a quarter also abused alcohol.

Alcoholism is a serious problem with major physical consequences. Individuals who continue abuse frequently suffer liver damage and may have signs of organic brain disorders such as Wernicke-Korsakoff's disease, as noted in the previous chapter. There is some evidence of cognitive dysfunction whether or not Wernicke-Korsakoff's disease is diagnosed (Bowden, 1990).

Implications for Function and Treatment

As noted, in order for these diagnoses to be made, functional impairment must be present. Since these substances are all CNS depressants, recent ingestion leads to drowsiness and reduction in perceptual and motor function, with accompanying problems in ability to perform. Vocational and social performance are most commonly affected, although later stages of dependence, particularly if organic signs appear, may result in decrements in all areas of function. Early in the disease, leisure time is most affected, with the individual's primary leisure activity being substance ingestion. Many alcoholics are quite lonely, though cause and effect are hard to determine (Akerlind & Hornquist, 1992). As time goes on, family life suffers as the individual spends more time drinking. Work behavior is impaired as the individual either misses time from work as a result of hangovers or performs poorly because of intoxication on the job.

Of special importance is the likelihood of injury resulting from driving while intoxicated. Industrial accidents may also result from impaired motor and perceptual abilities while under the influence. Withdrawal symptoms may lead the individual to spend a great deal of time obtaining the substance or to become irritable or enraged. ADL and IADL are rarely severely impaired, although some individuals lose interest in eating as the disorder progresses. Nutritional deficiencies may result from poor diet. Similarly, individuals may become forgetful, resulting in chores undone, checkbooks unbalanced, and so on.

Special note should be made of social role performance. Individuals who are dependent on these substances spend much of their leisure time obtaining and using the substance. They prefer the company of others who are dependent. In addition, if their spouses and family members do not desert them, the family members may feel compelled to hide the abuse, thereby supporting it. This pattern has been described as "codependence" and is problematic in efforts to treat dependence.

Performance decrements may well be due to CNS changes. It is clear that intoxication causes such alterations (Cohen, Schandler, & Naliboff, 1983). While the changes diminish to some extent following detoxification, subtle neurological signs may persist and, if abuse continues over time, become more prominent.

A wide variety of treatments have been attempted, including various milieu and behavioral interventions. One of the best known, and apparently most successful treatments is Alcoholics Anonymous (AA). This is a self-help group, which has a philosophy based in a specific set of religious and moral beliefs. AA or other self-help groups may be linked to formal alcoholism treatment programs. Medical interventions include detoxification/withdrawal assistance and relapse prevention (Gorelick, 1993). In addition, various family interventions seem helpful (O'Farrell, 1992). Typically for both sedative and alcohol abuse, recognition of the problem and willingness to do something about it are important first steps.

Cocaine and Amphetamines

Unlike alcohol and sedatives, these substances are stimulants which result in a psychological "high" and psychomotor excitement, both of which are brief, encouraging increasing use. Cocaine is most commonly inhaled, though it may also be smoked (in the case of the "freebase" or "crack" form) or injected.

Etiology and Incidence

Both substances tend to be abused in similar patterns. Two are prominent. The first involves daily use of the substance, the second, binges of varying frequency. Amphetamine abuse can emerge following use of the medications to assist in dieting. Although use of the drug for this purpose has been largely discredited, some physicians still prescribe it. Cocaine is strictly illicit, although it has been considered trendy by middle and upper class individuals. At the same time, the numbers of lower class individuals abusing cocaine increased dramatically as crack has become cheaper and more readily available. Both can be highly addictive, with only a few exposures leading to both withdrawal symptoms and increasing desire for the effects. Cocaine abuse has increased dramatically among adolescents (Washton, Gold, Pottash, & Semlitz, 1984).

Of these two dependencies, cocaine is by far the greater concern at present in this country. Estimates of incidence are probably extremely low. Early in the 1980s it was estimated at .2% of the population, but use increased dramatically until leveling off in the early 1990s (Weddington, 1993).

One additional reason for concern is the teratogenic effect on fetuses (Gingras, Weese-Mayer, Hume, & O'Donnell, 1992). Given the number of pregnant women who abuse cocaine, and the fact that cocaine crosses the placental barrier, increasing numbers of infants are born cocaine-addicted and have lasting neurological damage as a result.

Prognosis

Prognosis for both types of abuse is poor, as they are so highly addictive. In addition, until recently, cocaine enjoyed a somewhat glamorous image. Recent deaths of movie stars and athletes as a result of cocaine ingestion has changed that image somewhat. Although these individuals have received much attention, the problem is probably worst among individuals in lower socioeconomic groups (Smart, 1991). The increased availability of crack and the reductions in cost have increased the probability that individuals will continue to abuse the drug. While the pleasurable effects of these substances diminish over time, the craving does not. In addition, abuse of sedatives or alcohol frequently accompanies abuse of these substances, to reduce some of the undesirable effects of the drugs such as anxiety and insomnia. Thus the picture is complicated by addiction to several substances at once.

Implications for Function and Treatment

As with alcohol and sedative dependence, abuse of these substances is most likely to affect vocational and social performance. Irritability is pronounced and social withdrawal may develop and become severe. Use of the drug becomes the primary avocational interest, thus affecting function in this sphere as well. ADL and IADL are affected as organic (CNS) signs begin to appear, or as need for the drug begins to supersede the wish to attend to these activities.

Some individuals who abuse these drugs turn to criminal activity to support the habit. They may steal or become prostitutes to pay for the drug, as their ability to hold jobs decreases and their need for the drug increases. Others become drug pushers themselves.

Treatment is problematic and still poorly developed. AA type interventions may be valuable. Some medical attention may be necessary to prevent complications during withdrawal. The array of treatments includes medications to avoid withdrawal symptoms and reduce anxiety (Tutton & Crayton, 1993), 28-day inpatient stays, 12-step programs modeled after Alcoholics Anonymous, and outpatient group and individual therapy (Rawson et al., 1993). The last of these is the only one with any systematic evaluation demonstrating positive results.

In general, however, current efforts to treat these types of abuse are not particularly effective. Several problems have been noted in treatment efforts. First, there is no medication to ameliorate withdrawal effects. Second, unlike some other substances, the pleasurable effect, though diminished over time, continues to occur. Third, there is an increasingly well-developed culture around these drugs, particularly in ghetto environments. Thus, there may be little motivation to withdraw, and little medical help for those who do wish to do so.

Hallucinogens and PCP

Etiology and Incidence

Abuse of these substances appears to be somewhat less than it was two decades ago. Initial contact usually occurs as a result of experimentation with drugs. Thus, personality disorders or adjustment problems must be considered as predisposing factors because they might encourage such experimentation. Hallucinogens and PCP are often contaminated with or taken with other substances, particularly cannabis and alcohol.

Users generally find the effects unpredictable. For some individuals, one exposure to the negative effects, particularly during an early experience with the drug, is sufficient to end its use. Occasionally, a pattern of long-term abuse may emerge. Heavier use has been correlated with flashbacks, although the exact nature/cause of this phenomenon is not clear (Naditch & Fenwick, 1977). It may be the result of neurological changes caused by the drug or a hysterical phenomenon.

Prognosis

Most individuals abuse these drugs for relatively short periods of time before resuming previous activities. For most people these are drugs that prompt experimentation, but not usually long-term addition. PCP is the more dangerous, as it is easily produced in a laboratory, thus it is readily available. It has particularly damaging consequences, including the potential for brain damage, sometimes after very few uses (Lewis & Hordan, 1986), and psychotic reactions, and violent rage (Young, Lawson, & Gacono, 1987).

Implications for Function and Treatment

While the drugs are being abused, performance is severely impaired in all spheres. This is a direct result of the effects of the drugs, which cause hallucinations and cognitive and perceptual dysfunction. It is rare, however, to see such individuals in treatment as a result of dependence or abuse of these two classes of drugs. The exception is when an organic mental disorder appears, as is more likely to be the case with PCP.

Treatment seems most likely to be successful when medical management of acute intoxication is followed by psychotherapy (Young et al., 1987).

Opioids

Among this group of drugs are some that are clearly illicit, such as heroin and morphine, and others which may be prescribed as analgesics, anesthetics, or cough-suppressants. The latter group includes codeine, hydromorphone, and methadone. Used in properly supervised medical settings, none of the latter group should lead to dependence, but many of them are used without supervision or obtained through illicit sources. Methadone is a special problem. Used as a treatment for opioid addiction, it is itself addicting, though it does not cause a "high." It is, however, abused in some situations and does have a street value.

Etiology and Incidence

In almost all cases, dependence on these substances is a reflection of other problems in an individual's life. These may be related to a preexisting or coexisting character disorder, situational problems, or adjustment difficulties. For example, Vietnam veterans who were substance abusers were found to have been subjected to higher levels of stress than those who were not (Penk et al., 1981). Since abuse of these substances requires contact with illicit sources, establishment of a dependence requires action on the part of the individual. It is common, for example, to find this sort of addiction in individuals with prior histories of delinquency, or from unstable home situations. Almost all have a history of other prior substance abuse (Dinwiddie, Reich, & Cloninger, 1992). It should be noted, however, that these addictions can be found in individuals from all sorts of life circumstances (Penk et al., 1981).

Incidence appears to be roughly .7% of the population, i.e., this number of adults in the United States have abused opioids at some point in their lives (APA, 1994).

Prognosis

Dependence on these drugs is intractable, although apparently less so than cocaine. The drugs cause significant tolerance effects fairly rapidly, and withdrawal symptoms are severe and unpleasant. Thus, after initial experiences with the drugs for the "high" they cause, later experiences are often attempts to avoid withdrawal symptoms. In addition, since these drugs are related to lifestyle and personality characteristics, the environment tends to support the addiction. In order to successfully withdraw, individuals may have to cope not only with withdrawal, but also with making necessary changes in lifestyle to avoid encouragement to continue abusing the substance. Tolerance of the drugs is a particular problem. As it develops, increasing amounts are required to experience the euphoria it causes. However, these drugs are also CNS depressants. Many individuals die of an overdose, particularly of heroin.

While prognosis is generally thought to be poor, there is not absolute agreement on this. Cottrell, Childs-Clarke, and Ghodse (1985) found that less than half of a group of 83 drug abusers were still using heroin/methadone 11 years later. Among those individuals, deviant behavior had diminished. Klingemann (1991) also reports instances of "auto-remission" although the reasons for this occurrence are not clear. As with other abuse, coexisting psychosis is a predictor of poor prognosis (Perkins, Simpson, & Tsuang, 1986).

Implications for Function and Treatment

These addictions have a particularly severe impact on function. The drugs are illicit and expensive, and tolerance develops quickly. Thus individuals who become dependent on these substances are likely to spend much of their time in pursuit of their next "fix." Once ingested, the drugs cause lethargy and withdrawal, making it difficult to maintain stable employment. The need for money to purchase the drug, accompanied by its effects, means that these individuals often turn to crime as a means to support a habit. Stealing and prostitution are common among addicts.

In addition to impact on ability to maintain vocational function, dependence has a severe impact on social function. Social life also focuses on the drug, friends tend to be involved with it, and relationships are tenuous, as the drug assumes primary importance in the individual's life. Similarly, leisure activities are replaced by the drug, which becomes the individual's vocation, avocation, and social life.

ADL and IADL function become impaired as dependence increases. The lethargy while under the influence of the drug leads to lessened interest in self-maintenance and maintenance of the surroundings. Individuals may have little interest in appearance and hygiene or in the environment. In addition, financial woes tend to be severe, leaving little money for food, shelter, or clothing.

Treatment often begins in inpatient settings. "Cold turkey" withdrawal is held by some to be most effective, i.e., the individual must simply stop taking the substance, rather than withdrawing from it gradually. For most individuals, withdrawal is aided by use of medications such as methadone or buprenorphine (Kosten, Schottenfeld, Ziedonis, & Falcioni, 1993), which is discussed below. Medical management may be necessary to deal with complications of withdrawal. At the same time, other interventions must be made. Approaches similar to AA have been reported to be successful with some individuals.

A dilemma with inpatient withdrawal is that some individuals use it as a way to lower their tolerance for the drug, so that when they leave the inpatient setting, their dose requirement of the drug will be less.

In some cases, outpatient treatment may be an option. Methadone, which can cause dependence if taken in an unsupervised setting, is often used as a mechanism for withdrawing individuals from opioids. It prevents the withdrawal symptoms, without providing a "high." However, once started, it must be continued for some time, or withdrawal symptoms will occur. Methadone is generally administered in highly structured settings which require the individual to come in regularly to obtain the drug and psychotherapeutic interventions. Eventually, gradual tapering may be attempted (Sorenson, Trier, Brummett, Gold, & Dumontet, 1992). Those who finish treatment tend to remain abstinent (Stimmel, Goldberg, Rotkopf, & Cohen, 1977).

Social circumstances also affect outcomes. Those individuals who have supportive and involved families do better than others (Kosten, Jalali, Hogan, & Kleber, 1983). This is problematic, however, as opioid addiction often involves a whole lifestyle supported and is encouraged by the social system.

Cannabis

This is probably the most commonly used illicit substance (Hollister, 1988). It is popularly conceived as one of the less dangerous drugs. Many individuals begin using marijuana and hashish in social settings, believing them to be relatively harmless. Psychoactive symptoms appear to be less than those of other substances, making it unlikely that individuals with dependence will be seen in treatment. Chronic cannabis use seems to interfere with motivation, and therefore with function. In addition, a fairly high proportion of individuals with other psychiatric disturbances and alcoholics are also problematic cannabis abusers and these individuals have a much worse course. The best documented negative effects of cannabis are delirium, panic, and acute paranoia or mania. No catastrophic health effects have been found (Hollister, 1988), except that smoking pot contributes to lung cancer.

Dependence and abuse generally develop over a relatively long period of time. They are characterized by increasing frequency of use, rather than increased amounts at a given time. Prolonged use may lead to lethargy, anhedonia, and memory and attention deficits. Some changes in perceptual skills have also been noted. However, function is not as severely impaired as in other forms of substance abuse.

Data about marijuana use are conflicting. While some researchers have found most mental processes to be impaired in experienced cannabis users (Klonoff, Low, & Marcus, 1973), others have noted such changes only in those who are not experienced users (Weil, Zinberg, & Nelson, 1968). Weil and colleagues (1968) found impairment on digit symbol and pursuit rotor performance in their naive subjects; experienced subjects had no performance decrements.

Kandel (1984) found that marijuana users were more likely to abuse other substances and to have poorer adjustment to normal adult roles. They were more likely to participate in deviant activities and to have psychiatric hospitalizations. It is unclear, however, whether the marijuana led to deviant behavior or the reverse.

There is one situation in which cannabis poses clear risk, and that is in schizophrenics (Treffert, 1978). Schizophrenic cannabis users were very likely to have psychotic episodes requiring hospitalization as a result of this use.

Inhalants

A wide variety of substances may be inhaled, including gasoline, paint thinners, glue, and various cleaners. The active ingredients are aliphatic and aromatic hydrocarbons which cause intoxication, resulting in a "high."

This type of substance abuse most often appears in children and adolescents, particularly those from disadvantaged backgrounds. These children are typically from dysfunctional families, and show significant adjustment problems, including truancy, poor grades, delinquency, and so forth. It appears that these adjustment problems predate the substance abuse. It also appears that abuse of inhalants leads to abuse of other substances. Inhalants are extremely dangerous, leading to physical and mental problems, including kidney and liver disease, even when used for only short periods of time.

Tolerance and withdrawal symptoms have been reported, but it is not clear why either phenomenon occurs. It is clear, however, that this type of abuse is intractable, recurring even after treatment. Furthermore, the effects of the drugs exacerbate existing functional difficulties. Performance of vocational, leisure, and self-care are all affected, probably with some coexisting decrements in cognitive and psychological skills due to CNS damage.

Nicotine

Nicotine is the drug that makes cigarette smoking appealing. It is a highly addicting substance. It is a mild stimulant that is difficult to stop once an addiction has developed, usually over the course of time. Smoking is a leading cause of preventable disease (Sees & Clark, 1993).

While some individuals are able to withdraw from smoking, the majority have considerable difficulty doing so. Behavioral techniques are effective in highly motivated individuals, but for many, the effects of nicotine are too reinforcing to be given up.

For most, however, symptoms and interference with function are minimal, at least from a psychological perspective. Some individuals may have increasing problems in work situations as smoking is increasingly prohibited. Most, however, continue to perform well. Major problems with this type of addiction are physical and appear over long periods of time. Development of lung, larynx, and oral cancer, as well as cardiovascular problems, is common, but usually occurs after decades of smoking. Such long-term hazards tend to be disregarded by smokers or provide insufficient motivation to stop a severe addiction. Other hazards, e.g., fire from careless smoking, are less publicized. It does appear that some CNS function is compromised, possibly leading to such problems as auto accidents.

Caffeine

Caffeine is newly included in DSM-IV (APA, 1994) as an abused substance. It is the most widely used psychoactive substance in the United States and elsewhere (Heishman & Henningfield, 1992). It is a mild stimulant, but has the potential for excessive doses, resulting in jitteriness, anxiety, insomnia, and tachycardia. It also has withdrawal symptoms, most notably fatigue and headache.

However, caffeine is rarely addressed as a drug in treatment settings. As compared with other drugs, its negative consequences are minimal, thus treatment is rare. Pregnant women are encouraged to limit consumption, although even the evidence about potential harm to a fetus is equivocal.

General Treatment Considerations

Many reports of addiction note the clustering of substance use (Strain, Brooner, & Bigelow, 1991). For this reason, treatment may be described for substance abuse overall, rather than by substance. For example, Flores and Mahon (1993) describe the effectiveness of group psychotherapy as a means to enhance self-concept and improve social supports. Similarly, Pettinati, Meyers, Jensen, and their colleagues (1993) note that regardless of the type of substance, outpatient treatment leads to four times more treatment failures than inpatient.

This latter finding has resulted in development of specific relapse prevention strategies in outpatient care (Rawson et al., 1993). These include education, identification of strategies for dealing with high risk situations, development of coping skills, and developing new lifestyle behaviors. Clearly, these strategies are of importance in occupational therapy, where pursuit of these goals is likely to be a central focus of treatment.

Similarly, prevention of substance abuse is a central focus of many programs (Dusenbury & Botvin, 1992). As in relapse prevention, emphasis on lifestyle is crucial in efforts to prevent substance abuse.

Dual Diagnosis

Substance abuse can coexist with conduct disorder, depression (Neighbors, Kempton, & Forehand, 1992), developmental disabilities (Moore & Polsgrove, 1991), schizophrenia (Arndt, Tyrrell, Flaum, & Andreasen, 1992), manic depressive disorder, and personality disorders (Cohen & Henkin, 1993).

This so-called "dual diagnosis" is extremely problematic (Robertson, 1992) in that treatment efforts are confounded by the combination of problems. In general, such patients have very poor problem-solving ability which complicates intervention. It is also difficult to know which condition led to the other, or whether they emerged separately from each other. Popkin and Tucker (1992) note that substance abuse can lead to mood, anxiety, and psychotic disorders. It is also possible that individuals abuse substances secondary to, or as a result of, another disorder. Alcohol abuse may emerge as a means to self-treat anxiety, for example. Understanding the etiology of the coexisting disorders is essential to satisfactory intervention.

Treatment recommendations vary. Shilony, Lacey, O'Hagen, & Curto (1993) recommend a continuum from 6 months to 1 year of residential treatment to sheltered housing to outpatient aftercare. They note that lack of housing and aftercare presents significant problems. Care must include stabilization, engagement in treatment, persuasion to continue care, active treatment, and relapse prevention (Robertson, 1992). However, data regarding effectiveness of various forms of treatment are sparse, with preliminary studies showing no increased positive effect when programs are specially planned for individuals with dual diagnosis (Lehman, Herron, Schwartz, & Myers, 1993). It is also important to recognize that changes in health care insurance have resulted in reduced coverage for inpatient treatment of substance abuse. Long-term consequences of this change are unknown.

Implications for Occupational Therapy

All substance abuse can interfere with accomplishment of ADL/IADL, vocational, and leisure activities. In addition, there is reason to believe that CNS processing is impaired by some of the substances discussed in this chapter. Thus, intervention must occur at the level of both skill and performance.

Van Deusen (1989) discusses the impact of alcohol abuse on fine motor skills, tactile and figure-ground perception, and visual spatial function. She notes that there seems to be some spontaneous recovery of these skills in individuals who abstain from drinking, but that practice may enhance this recovery. Her recommendation is that occupational therapists focus on remediating motor and sensory-motor deficits by way of sports activities, computer games, and so on. It is reasonable to assume that other substance abusers might respond to similar intervention.

A second area of focus for intervention is expression of emotion. Many substance abusers have difficulty verbalizing their feelings, and the expressive arts (e.g., drawing, painting) have been suggested as modalities (Smith & Glickstein, 1980). Individuals who use drugs to block emotion may benefit.

A third area of concern is use of time, particularly leisure time (Mann & Talty, 1990; Van Deusen, 1989). Substance abuse often becomes the primary focus of activity, and individuals with abuse disorders need to learn through education and experimentation about alternative uses of time. Identification of new and satisfying leisure activities (Cassidy, 1988) can have a significant impact on outcomes of treatment. The individual must learn to fill new free time with activities that will divert attention from the desire for the abused substance, and provide enjoyment. In addition, social skills training may help the individual to acquire new friends to replace those who were fellow alcoholics. Because loneliness is such a problem (Akerlind & Hornquist, 1992) this may be essential. Family treatment can also be helpful in resolving feelings of loneliness, and enhancing relationships which are almost certainly damaged by substance abuse (Moyer, 1992).

The issue of time use is closely related to sociocultural considerations about work and work skills. Many substance abusers lose their jobs because of their addiction and must relearn job skills, as well as work-related skills such as following directions and relating to supervisors. Time management is a particular problem related to work as well as other activities (Scaffa, 1991).

More problematic is the issue of individuals who turn to substance abuse specifically because they feel hopeless about future prospects. In inner city areas, substance abusers often have no job experience or skills and no hope of acquiring them. Training in work and work-related skills may mean starting at square one with reading and writing. Although this approach can be very valuable, it is time- and cost-intensive. Linkage with community services and constant follow-up is vital. All these difficulties contribute to, or are caused by, poor self-esteem. Experiences that can provide both motivation and hope are essential.

Finally, learning new methods for managing stress and experiencing successes which build self-esteem can assist individuals to remain substance free. Beck (1993) notes that all these approaches can be used successfully in group treatment, and that the group itself may have positive benefit in terms of providing realistic feedback, as well as an opportunity to practice interpersonal skills.

References

Akerlind, I., & Hornquist, J. O. (1992). Loneliness and alcohol abuse: A review of evidences of an interplay. *Social Science and Medicine, 34,* 405-414.

Allgulander, C., Borg, S., & Vikander, B. (1984). A 4-6 year follow-up of 50 patients with primary dependence on sedative and hypnotic drugs. *American Journal of Psychiatry, 141,* 1580-1582.

American Psychiatric Association (1994). *Diagnostic and Statistical Manual of Mental Disorders* (4th ed.). Washington, DC: Author.

Arndt, S., Tyrrell, G., Flaum, M., & Andreasen, N. C. (1992). Comorbidity of substance abuse and schizophrenia: The role of pre-morbid adjustment. *Psychological Medicine, 22,* 379-388.

Beck, N. L. (1993). Substance abuse: Drug addiction and alcoholism. In H. L. Hopkins & H. D. Smith (Eds.), *Occupational therapy* (8th ed.). Philadelphia: J. B. Lippincott.

Berglund, M. (1984). Suicide in alcoholism. *Archives of General Psychiatry, 41,* 888-891.

Bowden S. C. (1990). Separating cognitive impairment in neurologically asymptomatic alcoholism from Wernicke-Korsakoff syndrome: Is the neuropsychological distinction justified? *Psychological Bulletin, 107,* 355-366.

Boyle, M. H., Offord, D. R., Racine, Y. A., et al. (1993). Predicting substance use in early adolescence based on parent and teacher assessments of childhood psychiatric disorder: Results from the Ontario Child Health Study follow-up. *J. Child Psychol. Psychiat. 34,* 535-544.

Cassidy, C. L. (1988). Occupational therapy intervention in the treatment of alcoholics. *Occupational Therapy in Mental Health, 8,* 17-26.

Cohen, E., & Henkin, I. (1993). Prevalence of substance abuse by seriously mentally ill patients in a partial hospital program. *Hospital and Community Psychiatry, 44,* 178-180.

Cohen, M. J., Schandler, S. L., & Naliboff, B. D. (1983). Psychophysiological measures from intoxicated and detoxified alcoholics. *Journal of Studies on Alcohol, 44,* 271-282.

Cottrell, D., Childs-Clarke, A., & Ghodse, A. H. (1985). British opiate addicts: An 11-year follow-up. *British Journal of Psychiatry, 146,* 448-450.

Cox, M. J., Norton, G. R., Swinson, R. P., & Endler, N. S. (1990). Substance abuse and panic-related anxiety: A critical review. *Behavioral Research Therapy, 28,* 385-393.

Dantzer, R., & Ollat, H. (1991). Alcoholism: A psychobiological perspective. *European Psychiatry, 6,* 209-215.

Dinwiddie, S. H., Reich, T., & Cloninger, C. R. (1992). Patterns of lifetime drug use among intravenous drug users. *Journal of Substance Abuse, 4,* 1-11.

Dusenbury, L., & Botvin, G. J. (1992). Substance abuse prevention: Competence enhancement and the development of positive life options. *Journal of Addictive Diseases, 11,* 29-45.

Flores, P. J., & Mahon, L. (1993). The treatment of addiction in group psychotherapy. *International Journal of Group Psychotherapy, 43,* 143-156.

Gingras, J. L., Weese-Mayer, D. E., Hume, R. F., & O'Donnell, K. J. (1992). Cocaine and development: Mechanisms of fetal toxicity and neonatal consequences of prenatal cocaine exposure. *Early Human Development, 31,* 1-24.

Goodwin, D. W. (1985). Alcoholism and genetics: The sins of the fathers. *Archives of General Psychiatry, 42,* 171-174.

Gorelick, D. A. (1993). Overview of pharmacologic treatment approaches for alcohol and other drug addiction. *Psychiactric Clinics of North America, 16,* 141-156.

Gottheil, E., Thornton, C. C., Skoloda, T. E., & Alterman, A. I. (1982). Follow-up of abstinent and nonabstinent alcoholics. *American Journal of Psychiatry, 139,* 560-565.

Grant, B. F. (1992). Prevalence of the proposed DSM-IV alcohol use disorders: United States, 1988. *British Journal of Addiction, 87,* 309-316.

Grinspoon, L., & Bakalar, J. (1988). Substance use disorders. In A. M. Napoli (Ed.), *The new Harvard guide to psychiatry* (pp. 418-433). Cambridge, MA: Belknap Press.

Heishman, S. J., & Henningfield, J. E. (1992). Stimulus functions of caffeine in humans: Relation to dependence potential. *Neuroscience and Biobehavioral Reviews, 16,* 273-287.

Hollister, L. E. (1988). Cannabis-1988. *Acta Psychiatrica Scandinavia, 345,* 108-118 (Suppl.).

Kandel, D. B. (1984). Marijuana users in young adulthood. *Archives of General Psychiatry, 41,* 200-209.

Kandel, D., & Faust, R. (1975). Sequence and stages in patterns of adolescent drug use. *Archives of General Psychiatry, 32,* 923-932.

Klingemann, H. K. H. (1991). The motivation for change from problem alcohol and heroin use. *British Journal of Addiction, 86,* 727-744.

Klonoff, H., Low, M., & Marcus, A. (1973). Neuropsychological effects of marijuana. *Canadian Medical Association Journal, 108,* 150-156, 165.

Kosten, T. R., Jalali, B., Hogan, I., & Kleber, H. D. (1983). Family denial as a prognostic factor in opiate addict treatment outcome. *Journal of Nervous and Mental Disease, 171,* 611-616.

Kosten, T. R., Schottenfeld, R., Ziedonis, D., & Falcioni, J. (1993). Buprenorphine versus methadone maintenance for opioid dependence. *The Journal of Nervous and Mental Disease, 181,* 358-364.

Lehman, A. F., Herron, J. D., Schwartz, R. P., & Myers, C. P. (1993). Rehabilitation for adults with severe mental illness and substance use disorders. *Journal of Nervous and Mental Disease, 181,* 86-90.

Lewis, J. E., & Hordan, R. B. (1986). Neuropsychological assessment of phencyclidine abusers. *National Institute on Drug Abuse, 64,* 190-208.

Lex, B. W. (1991). Some gender differences in alcohol and polysubstance users. *Health Psychology, 10,* 121-132.

Liberto, J. G., Oslin, D. W., & Ruskin, P. E. (1992). Alcoholism in older persons: A review of the literature. *Hospital and Community Psychiatry, 43,* 975-984.

Mann, W. C., & Talty, P. (1990). Leisure activity profile measuring use of leisure time by persons with alcoholism. *Occupational Therapy in Mental Health, 10,* 31-42.

Miller, N. S., & Gold, M. S. (1990). Benzodiazepines: Reconsidered. *Advances in Alcohol & Substance Abuse, 8,* 67-84.

Moore, D., & Polsgrove, L. (1991). Disabilities, developmental handicaps, and substance misuse: A review. *The International Journal of the Addictions, 26,* 65-90.

Moyer, P. A. (1992). Occupational therapy intervention with the alcoholic's family. *American Journal of Occupational Therapy, 46,* 105-111.

Naditch, M. P., & Fenwick, S. (1977). LSD flashbacks and ego functioning. *Journal of Abnormal Psychology, 86,* 352-359.

Nathan, P. E. (1991). Substance use disorders in the DSM-IV. *Journal of Abnormal Psychology, 100,* 356-361.

Neighbors, B., Kempton, T., & Forehand, R. (1992). Co-occurrence of substance abuse with conduct, anxiety, and depression disorders in juvenile delinquents. *Addictive Behaviors, 17,* 379-386.

O'Farrell, T. J. (1992). Families and alcohol problems: An overview of treatment research. *Journal of Family Psychology, 5,* 339-359.

Penk, W. E., Robinowitz, R., Roberts, W. R., Patterson, E. T., Dolan, M. P., & Atkins, H. S. (1981). Adjustment differences among male substance abusers varying in degree of combat experience in Vietnam. *Journal of Consulting and Clinical Psychology, 49,* 426-437.

Perkins, K. A., Simpson, J. C., & Tsuang, M. T. (1986). Ten-year follow-up of drug abusers with acute or chronic psychosis. *Hospital and Community Psychiatry, 37,* 581-484.

Pettinati, H. M., Meyers, K., Jensen, J. M., et al. (1993). Inpatient vs. outpatient treatment for substance dependence revisited. *Psychiatric Quarterly, 64,* 173-182.

Polich, J. M., Armor, D. J., & Braiker, H. B. (1980). *The course of alcoholism: Four years after treatment.* Santa Monica, CA: Rand Corporation.

Popkin, M. K., & Tucker, G. J. (1992). "Secondary" and drug-induced mood, anxiety, psychotic, catatonic, and personality disorders: A review of the literature. *Journal of Neuropsychiatry, 4,* 369-385.

Rawson, R. A., Obert, J. L., McCann, M. J., et al. (1993). Cocaine abuse treatment: A review of current strategies. *Journal of Substance Abuse, 3,* 457-491.

Robertson, E. C. (1992). The challenge of dual diagnosis. *Journal of Health Care for the Poor and Underserved, 3,* 198-207.

Scaffa, M. E. (1991). Alcoholism: An occupational behavior perspective. *Occupational Therapy in Mental Health, 11,* 99-112.

Sees, K. L., & Clark, H. W. (1993). When to begin smoking cessation in substance abusers. *Journal of Substance Abuse Treatment, 10,* 189-195.

Shilony, E., Lacey, D., O'Hagen, P., & Curto, M. (1993). All in one neighborhood: A community-based rehabilitation treatment program for homeless adults with mental illness and alcohol/substance abuse disorders. *Psychosocial Rehabilitation Journal, 16,* 103-116.

Smart, R. G. (1991). Crack cocaine use: A review of prevalence and adverse effects. *Am. J. Drug Alcohol Abuse, 17,* 13-26.

Smith, T. M., & Glickstein, C. S. (1980). Art as a therapeutic modality for individuals with alcohol related problems in a milieu setting. *Occupational Therapy in Mental Health, 1,* 33-44.

Sorenson, J. L., Trier, M., Brummett, S., Gold, M. L., & Dumontet, R. (1992). Withdrawal from methadone maintenance: Impact of a tapering network support program. *Journal of Substance Abuse Treatment, 9,* 21-26.

Stimmel, B., Goldberg, J., Rotkopf, E., & Cohen, M. (1977). Ability to remain abstinent after methadone detoxification. *Journal of American Medical Association, 237,* 1216-1220.

Strain, E. C., Brooner, R. K., & Bigelow, G. E. (1991). Clustering of multiple substance use and psychiatric diagnoses in opiate addicts. *Drug and Alcohol Dependence, 27,* 127-134.

Treffert, D. A. (1978). Marijuana use in schizophrenia: A clear hazard. *American Journal of Psychiatry, 135,* 1213-1215.

Tutton, C. S., & Crayton, J. W. (1993). Current pharmacotherapies for cocaine abuse: A review. *Journal of Addictive Diseases, 12,* 109-126.

Van Deusen, J. (1989). Alcohol abuse and perceptual-motor dysfunction: The occupational therapist's role. *American Journal of Occupational Therapy, 43,* 384-390.

Vega, W. A., Zimmerman, R. S., Warheit, G. J., et al. (1993). Risk factors for early adolescent drug use in four ethnic and racial groups. *American Journal of Public Health, 83,* 185-189.

Waisberg, J. L. (1990). Patient characteristics and outcome of inpatient treatment for alcoholism. *Advances in Alcohol & Substance Abuse, 8,* 9-32.

Washton, A. M., Gold, M. S., Pottash, A. C., & Semlitz, L. (1984). Adolescent cocaine abusers. *The Lancet,* September 29, 746.

Weil, A. T., Zinberg, N. E., & Nelson, J. M. (1968). Clinical and psychological effects of marijuana in man. *Science, 162,* 1234-1242.

Yamaguchi, K., & Kandel, D. B. (1984). Patterns of drug use from adolescence to young adulthood: III. Predictors of progression. *American Journal of Public Health, 74,* 673-680.

Young, T., Lawson, G. W., & Gacono, C. B. (1987). Clinical aspects of Phencyclidine (PCP). *The International Journal of the Addictions, 22,* 1-15.

Chapter 6
Schizophrenia and Other Psychotic Disorders

The psychotic disorders, including schizophrenia, are among the most disabling, and perhaps for that reason have received a great deal of attention. The clinical definition of schizophrenia has been narrowed considerably in the most recent diagnostic manuals, resulting in, among other things, a poorer prognosis (Harrow, Carone, & Westermeyer, 1985). DSM-IV (APA, 1994) identifies characteristics that must be present for the diagnosis to be made, including a minimum duration, and a specific constellation of symptoms (Figure 6-1).

Figure 6-1. Common Types of Schizophrenia.

- Paranoid type
- Disorganized type
- Catatonic type
- Undifferentiated type
- Residual type

Schizophrenia

This is one of the mental disorders that is defined relative to function. In order for the diagnosis to be made, functional level must be below the highest level previously achieved in one or more areas. In addition, thought, including both content and form, is disturbed. Delusions, beliefs that are firmly held but not true, are frequently found in these individuals. The most common types of delusions are delusions of persecution (fear that one is being followed or will be harmed by others), delusions of reference (the belief that one is being talked about by others), or delusions of grandeur (the belief that one possesses special powers, abilities, or gifts). Loosening of associations, incoherence, or excessively concrete or abstract thought are also characteristic. Someone with loose associations might answer a question about the weather by launching into a discussion of weather patterns in outer space. An excessively concrete response might be that there are two rain drops on the window of a red car outside, and an excessively abstract answer might be that weather is in the eye of the beholder and relates to the meaning of life.

Perception and affect are also disturbed. Hallucinations, experiences such as hearing voices or feeling ants crawling under the skin, are typical. Auditory hallucinations, hearing voices, are most common, although any sense may be involved. The individual may smell peculiar smells and think that poison gas is in the room, or see strange figures in the mirror. Affect is either flat or inappropriate. Some of these individuals are totally expressionless, while others may have bizarre smiles, laugh inappropriately, and so on.

Peculiar psychomotor behavior may be present. Odd mannerisms, grimacing, hyperactivity or, conversely, waxy rigidity may be observed. Sense of self is also impaired. The individual may have difficulty discriminating between self and others or between self and the environment.

Most often, the disorder appears during adolescence or early adulthood. Less often, the schizophrenia develops in childhood (McClellan & Werry, 1992) or in late life (Lacro, Harris, & Jeste, 1993). In order for the diagnosis to be made, symptoms must continue for at least 6 months. Within the most recent month, the individual must experience at least two of the following: delusions, hallucinations, disorganized speech or behavior, catatonic symptoms, or negative symptoms such as flat affect or avolition.

Schizophrenia is usually characterized by a prodromal phase, in which function begins to deteriorate. The individual withdraws from friends and family, and work, self-care, and avocational activities suffer. The individual may begin to have trouble relating to people at work or school, stop bathing, and spend most free time staring in a mirror or just sitting. The active phase is characterized by delusions and hallucinations, thought disorder, and other psychotic symptoms. This phase may occur spontaneously, or as a result of stress. The residual phase is the third phase. It is often similar to the prodromal phase in terms of symptomatology. During this phase functional level continues to be below the highest level ever achieved by the individual. Most individuals continue to have flat affect, peculiar behavior, and functional difficulties between active phases. They usually have few friends or interests, ignore self-care, and may have problems concentrating well enough to work.

The diagnosis may include indication of an episodic pattern, continuous symptoms, or single episodes.

Several types of schizophrenia are identified in DSM-IV (APA, 1994), with differing constellations of symptoms (Figure 6-2). Catatonic schizophrenia is characterized by immobility or catatonic excitement (motor excitation that is purposeless and not affected by external stimuli), echolalia or echopraxia, negativism to external stimuli which should encourage movement, peculiar movements, or mutism. Individuals with catatonic schizophrenia may sit rigid for hours without moving, often in positions that appear very uncomfortable. They may not eat, speak, or in any way acknowledge the environment during these periods. This is an uncommon type of schizophrenia, occurring in approximately 10% of all cases (Fink & Taylor, 1991).

Figure 6-2. Schizophrenia: Symptoms and Deficits.

Disorder	Symptoms	Functional Deficits
Duration at least 6 months with 2 or more symptoms for at least 1 month		
Schizophrenia	1. Delusions 2. Hallucinations 3. Disorganized speech 4. Disorganized behavior 5. Negative symptoms 6. Flat or inappropriate affect 7. Episodic deterioration of function	Global, with exacerbations and remissions
A. Catatonic Type	1. Catatonia is most marked symptom	Global with exacerbations and remissions
B. Disorganized	1. Above symptoms plus disorganized speech 2. Incoherence or severely disorganized behavior 3. Flat affect	Global with exacerbations and remissions
C. Paranoid	1. Preoccupation with delusional system and/or auditory hallucinations 2. Absence of loose associations, flat or inappropriate affect, catatonic or disorganized behavior	Usually less impaired ADL/IADL Usually little motor impairment

Disorganized type is characterized by flat or inappropriate affect and disorganization of behavior or speech. Individuals who are diagnosed with this type of schizophrenia are usually unkempt and disheveled, walk with a shuffling gait and stooped posture, and may mutter unintelligibly. Conversations with such individuals may be incomprehensible, or they may exclaim with great fear about voices telling them terrible things, or figures appearing to them. They tend to be lethargic and difficult to engage in activity, or occasionally, to be excessively active, but not engaged in any purposeful activity.

Paranoid type is noticeably different from the other schizophrenias, as catatonic behavior, inappropriate affect, disorganized behavior, and loose associations are not present. The presenting features are auditory hallucinations with disorganized, catatonic, or flat or inappropriate affect. Hallucinations tend to feed into a sense of persecution. These are the individuals who, if willing to discuss their fears at all, may complain of being followed by the FBI, for example. This type appears less likely to have a genetic component (McGlashan & Fenton, 1991) and to have onset later in life than other types of schizophrenia. Typically these individuals have better premorbid social, marital, and instrumental functioning, and the diagnosis is more stable than other types (McGlashan & Fenton, 1991).

Residual type is diagnosed when the individual has psychotic symptoms but does not fit the criteria for other forms of schizophrenia. Catatonic and undifferentiated schizophrenia may develop over time into the residual type (McGlashan & Fenton, 1991), while paranoid type does not.

Etiology and Incidence

There are a variety of theories about the emergence of schizophrenia. There is a family pattern which can be demonstrated even when the individual is not raised by the biological family (Onstad, Skre, Torgersen, & Kringlen, 1991). Thus a genetic component is evident (Guze, Cloninger, Martin, & Clayton, 1983). Individuals with close relatives with schizophrenia have a 3.2% risk (Tsuang, Winokur, & Crowe, 1980) as compared with a risk of less than .6% for the general population. Monozygotic (identical) twins have up to six times the normal risk (Gottesman & Shields, 1972), if their twin has the disorder.

However, the genetic component does not seem sufficient to cause the emergence of the disease, since not all individuals who are genetically predisposed develop schizophrenia, even if they are identical twins. Some theorists suggest that environmental factors including a variety of psychosocial stressors such as maladjusted family relationships contribute as well. Stress has been examined as an etiologic factor, and while it seems unlikely that it causes schizophrenia, it appears to be a factor in exacerbations (Tsuang, Faraone, & Day, 1988). Dohrenwend and Ergi (1981) feel stress is a significant contributing factor in the emergence of the disease. There is evidence that the diagnosis is more common in lower socioeconomic groups, but this may be an outcome of the disease, rather than a predisposing factor.

Since the disease is marked by functional decline, the individual may move downward in terms of socioeconomic factors. Premorbid social anhedonia (Mishlove & Chapman, 1985) and poor interpersonal competence (Beckfield, 1985) are associated with schizophrenia.

Recent explanations have focused on biological factors in schizophrenia. A variety of studies have examined the role of biochemical changes, neurological factors, and other physical agents in the emergence of the disorder (Szymanski, Kane, & Lieberman, 1991). Conflicting findings in this sphere have led some to theorize that schizophrenia may be more than one disease (Kety & Matthysse, 1988). Biological factors discussed include brain abnormalities, genetic disorders, and neurotransmitter disorders (Lieberman & Koreen, 1993) as well as the possibility of an autoimmune disorder (Knight, 1985). Physical markers include abnormal eye movements, electrodermal activities, event related brain potentials, and brain imaging, but none of these is sufficient to clearly determine risk (Szymanski et al., 1991).

Another biological factor examined in some detail is the role of neurotransmitters. The phenothiazines, drugs commonly used to treat psychotic disorders, block dopamine receptors, suggesting elevated dopamine transmission as a causative factor. In addition, structural abnormalities have been found in the brains of some schizophrenic individuals. Ventricular enlargement has been noted (Andreasen, Smith, Jacoby, Dennert, & Olsen, 1982), although the frequency and impact of this finding have been debated. In addition, as a group, individuals with schizophrenia have smaller frontal lobes, cerebrums, and crania, suggesting early developmental abnormalities (Andreasen et al., 1986). Various forms of neuropsychological deficit are well documented (Bornstein et al., 1990), although it is not clear whether these are cause or effect.

Prevalence of schizophrenia is approximately .5% to 1% of the adult population (APA, 1994). Full-blown catatonic schizophrenia is the least common, but these symptoms may be seen in other forms of schizophrenia (McGlashan & Fenton, 1991).

Prognosis

Reviews of literature related to prognosis suggest variable outcomes (Ram, Bromet, Eaton, Pato, & Schwartz, 1992). For many individuals, the prognosis for schizophrenia must be considered poor. Tsuang, Woolson, Winokur, & Crowe, (1981) found schizophrenia to be a stable diagnosis over 30 to 40 years, although they noted that some of the symptoms are ameliorated over time. Diminution of function continues, but this may become less prominent. The individual may have fewer active episodes, and remain in the residual phase for long periods.

A variety of factors have been examined to determine their value as predictors of outcome. Tsoi and Kua (1992) found marital status and duration of illness to be good predictors; age, sex, and education somewhat useful; and race, family history, and symptoms to be poor predictors. It appears that prognosis is reasonably good on a first hospital admission, and worsens with subsequent admissions (Ram et al., 1992). Subtype may affect outcome, although the research is conflicting, with some researchers finding that paranoid schizophrenia is predictive of better outcome (Opjordsmoen, 1991), while others find no difference (Marengo, Harrow, & Westermeyer, 1991). Overall, it appears that about one third of schizophrenics have good outcomes, one third continue to experience some difficulties, and one third continue to have severe symptoms or frequent relapses (Ram et al., 1992). Combined drug treatment and psychotherapeutic intervention is related to better outcomes (Ram et al., 1992).

A special problem is the coexistence of secondary depression (Sirls, 1991). There is evidence that this is a fairly common occurrence, and outcomes can be particularly problematic in these cases. Suicide occurs in approximately 10% to 13% of individuals with schizophrenia (Caldwell & Gotesmann, 1992). In particular, risk is high when the individual is showing some improvement. Suicide is discussed in greater detail in the next chapter, but should be remembered as a significant risk in working with individuals with schizophrenia.

Implications for Function and Treatment

As noted, functional impairment is a defining characteristic of schizophrenia. Social, vocational, avocational, and self-care abilities are markedly affected, leading to a global picture of disability. It is important to note, however, that the degree of impairment is variable, dependent on severity of the illness, phase, and type of illness.

During the prodromal and residual phases, function may be minimally impaired. This is particularly true when supportive treatment such as outpatient counseling is available. Individuals who can identify environments in which demand and stress are reduced may do well. They may regain reasonable measures of social and self-care function. In addition, if a supportive work environment can be found, with low levels of stress and an understanding supervisor, individuals with schizophrenia may be able to hold jobs.

For others, however, the prodromal and residual phases are characterized more by functional impairment than by psychological symptoms. Thus even though their delusions and hallucinations may disappear and their thought processes clear, they may continue to demonstrate severe social and vocational impairment. This is particularly true for individuals whose premorbid functioning was poor. As was noted in an earlier section, individuals who develop schizophrenia often were isolated, anhedonic (lacking the ability to enjoy events), and lacking in motivation prior to the onset of the disorder. An additional factor in probable level of function during the residual phase is the time of onset of the disorder. If the individual develops schizophrenia during adolescence, he or she may miss important milestones in normal development. This makes it more difficult to function well later, even when acute symptoms abate.

As an example, a young adult who was isolated and lethargic as a teenager, had few friends, and did poorly in school might develop schizophrenia and, even during the residual phase, continue to have few friends and find work difficult. By contrast, someone who held a job, had a social circle, and developed schizophrenia in his or her late 20s would be likely to do much better during residual phases.

For both children and adolescents with schizophrenia, treatment should include medication and psychosocial interventions (McClellan & Werry, 1992). In addition, educational and vocational habilitation or rehabilitation will be required to improve outcomes.

During active phases of the disease, functional impairment is much more severe. It is rare that these individuals can work, they demonstrate very little motivation to engage in other activities, and they tend to be severely withdrawn socially. Personal hygiene suffers, as do other self-care activities.

Impairments occur at the skill level, as well as the performance level, probably contributing to overall poor function. A whole variety of cognitive decrements have been found. IQ is thought to be lower among schizophrenics (Aylward, Walker, & Bettes, 1984) and to become worse as the disease progresses. This is most prominent in hospitalized individuals, but is true of others as well.

Among the other cognitive impairments noted are disturbances of will and volition (Frith, 1987), poor spatial and nonspatial associative learning (Kemali, Maj, Galderisi, Monteleone, & Mucci, 1987), difficulty with color perception (David, 1987), and poverty of written response (Manschreck, Ames, Maher, & Schneyer, 1987).

Taylor and Abrams (1987) found moderate to severe global cognitive impairment, which they later divided into two subtypes (Taylor & Abrams, 1987). One pattern is a bifrontal and nondominant hemisphere dysfunction, impacting personality and affect among other factors; the other, dominant temporo-parietal-occipital, impacts on the senses and ability to process sensory information. This second pattern is consistent with symptoms of thought disorder.

Other dysfunctions identified include poor visuomotor tracking (Gaebel & Ulrich, 1987) even during periods of remission, and disturbed voluntary motor performance (Manschreck, Maher, Rucklos, & Vereen, 1982).

Unfortunately, all these problems are compounded when tardive dyskinesia appears as a side effect of psychopharmacologic treatment (DeWolfe, Ryan, & Wolf, 1988). TD is a motor impairment which includes facial grimacing, tongue thrusting, tremors, and shuffling gait. It is a side effect of several antipsychotic medications. Motor performance, sensory processing, learning, and reasoning are all even worse in these individuals. In addition, long-term hospitalization may also have a negative impact on these skills.

An additional skill area of particular importance is the social sphere. As noted earlier, poor social skills may be among the predictors of schizophrenia. They are a good prognostic indicator as well (Morrison & Bellack, 1987). During periods of florid illness, social skills may be almost totally absent, and even during remission, social interactions may be awkward, unskilled, or contentious.

An exception to this picture is noted among individuals with paranoid schizophrenia. These individuals tend to be much better organized, and to demonstrate less cognitive impairment even during active phases of the disease. They may be able to work, are usually reasonably competent in self-care activities, and may even have avocational interests (although those activities might relate to escaping persecution, building "security systems" for the home, for example). Social functioning is impaired as a result of persecutory fears, but superficial social skills are often maintained. Work and social activities are interfered with as a result of suspicions, which often lead to angry exchanges with supervisors and neighbors who are believed to harbor wishes to harm the individual. These fears may be well masked, however. In some cases, the masking is symptomatic of the disorder, as the individual does not trust anyone enough to confide about his or her concerns. Some research suggests that almost half of individuals with paranoid schizophrenia may recover well (Opjordsmoen, 1991), as compared with one third of schizophrenics overall.

Schizophrenia is generally treated through a combination of modalities. It is a disorder in which psychotropic drugs are clearly effective (Kane & Marder, 1993). Drugs minimize thought disorder and sensory impairment during the active phase of the illness. In addition, medication may reduce the number of exacerbations and lengthen the intervals between active periods of the disease. Use of medication for schizophrenia is discussed further in Chapter 11.

Another biological treatment which seems helpful for some individuals with schizophrenia is electroconvulsive treatment (ECT). Reasons for its effectiveness are not clear, but particularly with older individuals with schizophrenia, it can have substantial impact in reducing symptoms (Lacro et al., 1993).

Other treatments include behavior, environmental, and social interventions (Birchwood, 1992; McClellan & Werry, 1992). During the active period of the disorder, individuals with schizophrenia often require hospitalization. While drug treatment is instituted, the individual may also be placed in a therapeutic milieu, or in some sort of behavioral program. Brief hospital stays may be beneficial, particularly if community follow-up is available.

In addition, skill training is often introduced. Many of these individuals never had the opportunity to acquire skills because symptoms of the disorder intervened in the normal developmental process (McClellan & Werry, 1992). Others, typically those who have been hospitalized frequently or for long periods, lose skills as a result of environmental deprivation. Social skills training is a patterned set of interventions designed to assist individuals in enhancing relationships. It has been developed as a way to deal with the frequent social impairment noted in individuals with schizophrenia. Research on the subject suggests that social skills training can improve specific behaviors, but has less impact on overall quality of life (Wallace et al., 1980).

ADL and IADL training may also be employed. Vocational assessment and work skills training are also part of intervention, particularly as individuals prepare for discharge. Work as an activity is clearly important as an intervention (Bebbington & Kuipers, 1982; McClellan & Werry, 1992).

A variety of types of psychotherapy, individual and group, have been attempted with schizophrenics, with reports of varying degrees of success. While Freud felt that psychoanalysis was not useful with schizophrenics, it has nonetheless been attempted. Other forms of verbal therapy have also been employed, largely as adjuncts to more structured treatments and medication.

In addition, family therapy is often employed, both to assist the family in dealing with the problem, and to remediate psychosocial stressors related to family interaction. Some theorists have suggested that schizophrenia is a rational adaptation to an irrational environment (c.f. Henry, 1971; Laing, 1969). The correlate to this belief is the need to treat the environment as well as the individual. It seems clear that family interactions are important in development of the disorder (Doane, Falloon, Goldstein & Mintz, 1985). Thus family therapy is a logical choice for intervention. Studies have found it to be helpful, particularly in combination with other approaches (Falloon et al., 1985; Hogarty et al., 1986).

In general, a combination of medication and a variety of psychotherapeutic interventions seems to yield the best outcomes (Birchwood, 1992).

During the prodromal and residual phases of the disease, a variety of approaches are employed to minimize risk of exacerbation. Medications may be continued, though it is not uncommon for the individual to stop taking them. In some instances, this appears to be sufficient to cause the disease to enter its active phase. A variety of environmental supports have been developed. Among them are community mental health centers which provide ongoing therapy, medication, and social support. Some schizophrenics do well in sheltered environments such as group homes and sheltered workshops. Halfway houses may ease the transition to the community.

Issues relative to management of individuals with schizophrenia in the community have received increasing notice in recent years. In the early 60s, a move began toward deinstitutionalization of individuals with schizophrenia and other chronic mental illnesses. The original intent of this move was quite humane and logical. Prior to that time, long-term institutionalization, often lasting throughout the individual's life, was common. The idea for the change related to a desire to maximize function and quality of life for these patients. The development of community mental health centers, which occurred at the same time, was intended as a means for providing support for these individuals as they returned to their communities.

The realities of deinstitutionalization have proved less satisfactory, however. Funding for community programs has been cut, and other bridges to the community have been slow to develop. Communities have been less than welcoming of these initiatives, as the patients may continue to demonstrate peculiar behaviors. In addition, fears that individuals with schizophrenia may be dangerous are common among the general population. While these fears do not appear to be borne out by reality, they have led to resistance to establishment of group homes and halfway houses.

Thus, after being discharged from inpatient care, individuals with schizophrenia or other chronic mental illnesses often end up in boarding houses, nursing homes, or in the streets. The growing problem of the homeless is, at least in part, a problem caused by deinstitutionalization (Scott, 1993), as a disproportionate number of homeless individuals have mental disorders of various types. Not only have community supports remained scarce, funds for inpatient treatment have been cut. Length of stay in inpatient settings has been drastically reduced, meaning that some of these individuals may be discharged prematurely. For many, a "revolving door" pattern of admissions is apparent. They are admitted, treated, and discharged, are unable to cope in the community, and must be readmitted.

The problems of deinstitutionalization relate to any of the chronic mental disorders, not just to schizophrenia. Individuals with chronic depression, manic depressive disorders, and substance abuse disorders, among others, may have chronic courses which present intervention difficulties similar to those described above.

Clearly, schizophrenia presents significant treatment dilemmas which have yet to be well addressed through public policy. Efforts to improve treatment outcomes continue, and certainly the development of more effective psychotropic medications has improved the picture. However, for these individuals, the outlook continues to be bleak.

Implications for Occupational Therapy

Like many of the organic mental disorders, schizophrenia affects all performance areas, and many underlying skills. Because of this, occupational therapy intervention must be comprehensive. Motor, sensory, sensorimotor, and psychosocial skills must be assessed, and history and current status of performance in self-care, leisure, and work must be considered.

Strengths as well as weaknesses should be assessed. There is a tendency to ignore strengths when dealing with someone who has a disorder with a poor prognosis, but often important assets do exist that can be built upon. For example, one patient was quite artistic and creative. As he improved, he was able to find work as a greeting card artist for a company noted for its somewhat "off the wall" cards.

Another young woman with a long history of psychosis simply decided one day that the other patients on her ward at the state hospital were depressing, and that she did not want to be like them. Her recovery was long and arduous, but she eventually went back to school and became an effective psychotherapist. Her case illustrates, among other things, the importance of motivation as a crucial asset.

Motivating clients with schizophrenia is no easy matter, as many are quite discouraged. Frequently, careful probing is necessary to uncover activities that have meaning for the person, and the ways in which they can be therapeutic. For the woman described above, school was that activity. She wanted to understand as much as possible about her own condition.

Remediating skill deficits through education, behavioral, or sensorimotor approaches is vital. The woman described above had few social skills. She had to learn to make eye contact and engage in social interaction before she could consider going to school. While social skills training has demonstrated effectiveness in the short-term, the ability of clients to generalize to new situations has not been demonstrated (Hayes, Halford, & Varghese, 1991). Therapists should make sure that the individual can function in a variety of settings to address this concern.

Not only must skills and performance be remediated, but self-esteem must be addressed, since these individuals often feel a profound sense of despair. Activities that provide success and social reinforcement (making cookies for others in the treatment program, for example) can be helpful.

Another dominant emotion is fear. Many hallucinations and delusions are quite frightening, as are the reactions of people in the community to these individuals, whose appearance and behavior may seem quite odd. Opportunities to express these fears are important.

Function in the community may require considerable skill training and support for the individual. Sheltered living may be of value for some. For others, relatively simple strategies are effective. A dentist diagnosed as paranoid schizophrenic was able to return to independent living once he learned by way of a behavioral program to discuss his delusions only with his therapist and family.

The occupational therapist should also place particular emphasis on leisure, as unstructured time may be hardest for these individuals to manage. In the hospital, individuals demonstrate a strong focus on the present, with little ability to plan ahead (Suto & Frank, 1994). This may reduce their ability to plan for satisfying activities. One woman whose only leisure activity was watching television had frequent remissions as she came to believe that the TV was talking directly to her and telling her she was an evil person. She needed to find other ways to fill her time.

A number of occupational therapy theories relate directly to schizophrenia and its treatment. Therapists who subscribe to the cognitive model (Allen, 1985) will make different assessment and treatment choices than those who subscribe to the Model of Human Occupation (Kielhofner, 1985). Differences among theories are considered briefly in Chapter 2 of this text. It is beyond the scope of this text to deal with the subject in detail; however, therapists should inform themselves about differing theories, and evidence which supports and refutes each of them. While much research remains to be done to validate specific theories, there is evidence that overall, occupational therapy is helpful in addressing the problems of individuals with schizophrenia (Brown, Harwood, Hays, Heckman, & Short, 1993; Reisman & Blakeney, 1991).

Delusional Disorder

As with paranoid schizophrenia, the primary feature of this disorder is the existence of a persistent, non-bizarre delusion (APA, 1994). The diagnosis is made only in the absence of any identifiable organic problem that caused the disorder. The delusion may have any content, most prominent being:

- erotomanic, in which the individual believes that he or she is loved by someone else, usually a prominent figure whom the individual does not actually know
- grandiose, a belief that the individual has some special, great characteristic
- jealous, in which the individual is convinced that a spouse or lover is unfaithful
- persecutory, a belief that the individual is being conspired against
- somatic, a belief that the individual has some gross physical problem.

Persecutory delusions are most common.

The disorder most often occurs in middle or later life, and is more common among deaf or immigrant individuals. Cause is not established.

The course of the disease is variable, although most commonly chronic, with exacerbations and remissions. Impairment of vocational, avocational, and self-care are rare, while social impairment is frequent and often severe. Outcome appears worst in cases where erotomanic or paranoid content is prevalent (Kaschka, Negele-Anetsberger, & Joraschky, 1991).

Other Psychotic Disorders

There are several categories of diagnosis which are made when the disorder does not fit the criteria for schizophrenia, paranoid disorder, or mood disorders that have psychotic features (APA, 1994). In particular, these diagnoses may be made when criteria of duration, symptom constellation, or functional impairment are not met. They include brief reactive psychosis, a label applied when the psychosis clearly relates to a psychosocial stressor and is of brief (1 month maximum) duration. Schizophreniform disorder is identical to schizophrenia, without meeting the criterion of duration. Thus psychoses which manifest with schizophrenia-like symptoms, but last from 1 to 6 months, will be called schizophreniform. If it persists for 6 months, the diagnosis will be changed to schizophrenia.

Schizoaffective disorder does not meet the criteria for either schizophrenia or a psychotic mood disorder, but has characteristics of both. In many ways it represents a hybrid of the two kinds of disorder. For example, the course of the disease is typically chronic, but prognosis is better than for schizophrenia, worse than for a mood disorder (Lapensee, 1992a; 1992b).

Finally, shared psychotic disorder (folie a deux) is a psychosis that occurs as a result of association with someone else who is psychotic. Most typically an individual will be drawn into the delusional system of a significant other. In these cases, impairment is not as severe as for the first individual, but the disorder is amenable to treatment only if the relationship can be altered.

None of these disorders is well understood. Etiological factors are not clear. While all have better prognoses than schizophrenia, the course of each is variable. Treatment is employed on the basis of symptoms exhibited, with drugs, hospitalization, psychotherapy, behavioral therapy, and so on being attempted with varying degrees of success.

References

Allen, C. (1985). *Occupational therapy for psychiatric diseases: Measurement and management of cognitive disorders.* Boston: Little, Brown & Co.

American Psychiatric Association (1994). *Diagnostic and Statistical Manual of Mental Disorders (4th ed.).* Washington, DC: Author.

Andreasen, N. C., Smith, M. R., Jacoby, C. G., Dennert, J. W., & Olsen, S. A. (1982). Ventricular enlargement in schizophrenia: Definition and prevalence. *American Journal of Psychiatry, 193,* 292-296.

Andreasen, N. C., Nasrallah, H. A., Dunn, V., Olson, S. C., Brove, W. M., Ehrhardt, J. C., Coffman, J. A., & Crossett, J. H. W. (1986). Structural abnormalities in the frontal system in schizophrenia. *Archives of General Psychiatry, 43,* 136-144.

Aylward, E., Walker, E., & Bettes, B. (1984). Intelligence in schizophrenia: Meta-analysis of the research. *Schizophrenia Bulletin, 10,* 430-459.

Bebbington, P., & Kuipers, L. (1982). Social management of schizophrenia. *British Journal of Hospital Medicine, 28,* 399-402.

Beckfield, D. F. (1985). Interpersonal competence among college men hypothesized to be at risk for schizophrenia. *Journal of Abnormal Psychology, 94,* 397-404.

Birchwood, M. (1992). Early intervention in schizophrenia: Theoretical background and clinical strategies. *British Journal of Clinical Psychology, 31,* 257-278.

Bornstein, R. A., Nasrallah, H. A., Olson, S. C., Coffman, J. A., Torello, M., & Schwarzkopf, S. B. (1990). Neuropsychological deficit in schizophrenic subtypes: Paranoid, nonparanoid, and schizoaffective subgroups. *Psychiatry Research, 31,* 15-24.

Brown, C., Harwood, K., Hays, C., Heckman, J., & Short, J. E. (1993). Effectiveness of cognitive rehabilitation for improving attention in patients with schizophrenia. *Occupational Therapy Journal of Research, 13,* 71-86.

Caldwell, C. B., & Gotesmann, I. I. (1992). Schizophrenia-A high-risk factor for suicide: Clues to risk reduction. *Suicide and Life-Threatening Behavior, 22,* 479-493.

David, A. S. (1987). Tachistoscopic tests of colour naming and matching in schizophrenia: Evidence for posterior callosum dysfunction? *Psychological Medicine, 17,* 621-630.

DeWolfe, A. S., Ryan, J. J., & Wolf, M. W. (1988). Cognitive sequelae of tardive dyskinesia. *Journal of Nervous and Mental Disease, 176,* 270-274.

Doane, J. A., Falloon, I. R. H., Goldstein, M. J., & Mintz, J. (1985). Parental affective style and the treatment of schizophrenia. *Archives of General Psychiatry, 42,* 34-42.

Dohrenwend, B. P., & Egri, G. (1981). Recent stressful life events and episodes of schizophrenia. *Schizophrenia Bulletin, 7,* 12-23.

Falloon, I. R. H., Boyd, J. L., McGill, C. et al. (1985). Family management in the prevention of morbidity of schizophrenia. *Archives of General Psychiatry, 42,* 887-896.

Fink, M., & Taylor, M. A. (1991). Catatonia: A separate category in DSM-IV. *Integrative Psychiatry, 7,* 2-10.

Frith, C. D. (1987). The positive and negative symptoms of schizophrenia reflect impairments in the perception and initiation of action. *Psychological Medicine, 17,* 631-648.

Gaebel, W., & Ulrich, G. (1987). Visuomotor tracking performance in schizophrenia: Relationship with psychopathological subtyping. *Neuropsychobiology, 17,* 66-71.

Gottesman, T. T., & Shields, J. (1972). *Schizophrenia and genetics: A twin study vantage point.* New York: Academic Press.

Guze, S. B., Cloninger, R., Martin, R. L., & Clayton, P. J. (1983). A follow-up and family study of schizophrenia. *Archives of General Psychiatry, 40,* 1273-1276.

Harrow, M., Carone, B. J., & Westermeyer, J. F. (1985). The course of psychosis schizophrenia: Relationship with psychopathological subtyping. *Neuropsychobiology, 17,* 66-71.

Hayes, R. L., Halford, W. K., & Varghese, F. N. (1991). Generalization of the effects of activity therapy and social skills training on the social behavior of low functioning schizophrenic patients. *Occupational Therapy in Mental Health, 11,* 3-20.

Henry, J. (1971). *Pathways to madness.* New York: Vintage Press.

Hogarty, G. E., Anderson, C. M., Reiss, D. J., Kornblith, S. J., Greenwald, D. P., Javna, C. D., & Madonia, M. J., (1986). Family psychoeducation, social skills training, and maintenance chemotherapy in the aftercare treatment of schizophrenia. *Archives of General Psychiatry, 43,* 633-642.

Kane, J. M., & Marder, S. R. (1993). Psychopharmacologic treatment of schizophrenia. *Schizophrenia Bulletin, 19,* 287-302.

Kaschka, W. P., Negele-Anetsberger, J., & Joraschky, P. (1991). Treatment outcome in patients with delusional (paranoid) disorder. *European Journal of Psychiatry, 5,* 30-34.

Kemali, D., Maj, M., Galderisi, S., Monteleone, P., & Mucci, A. (1987). Conditional associative learning in drug-free schizophrenic patients. *Neuropsychobiology, 17,* 30-34.

Kety, S. S., & Matthysse, S. (1988). Genetic and biochemical aspects of schizophrenia. In A. M. Nicholi (Ed.), *The new Harvard guide to psychiatry* (pp. 139-151). Cambridge, MA: Belknap Press.

Kielhofner, G. (Ed.) (1985). *A model of human occupation: Theory and application.* Baltimore: Williams and Wilkins.

Knight, J. G. (1985). Possible autoimmune mechanisms in schizophrenia. *Integrated Psychiatry, 3,* 134-143.

Laing, R. D. (1969). *The politics of the family.* New York: Vantage Press.

Lapensee, M. A. (1992a). A review of schizoaffective disorder: I. Current concepts. *Canadian Journal of Psychiatry, 37,* 335-346.

Lapensee, M. A. (1992b) A review of schizoaffective disorder: II. Somatic treatment. *Canadian Journal of Psychiatry, 37,* 347-349.

Lacro, J. P., Harris, M. J., & Jeste, D. V. (1993). Late life psychosis. *International Journal of Geriatric Psychiatry, 8,* 49-57.

Lieberman, J. A., & Koreen, A. R. (1993). Neurochemistry and neuroendocrinology of schizophrenia: A selective review. *Schizophrenia Bulletin, 19,* 371-429.

Manschreck, T. C., Ames, D., Maher, B. A., & Schneyer, M. L. (1987). Impoverished written responses and negative features of schizophrenia. *Perceptual and Motor Skills, 64,* 1163-1169.

Manschreck, T. C., Maher, B. A., Rucklos, M. E., & Vereen, D. R. (1982). Disturbed voluntary motor activity in schizophrenic disorder. *Psychological Medicine, 12,* 73-84.

Marengo, J. T., Harrow, M., & Westermeyer, J. F. (1991). Early longitudinal course of acute-chronic and paranoid-undifferentiated schizophrenia subtypes and schizophreniform disorder. *Journal of Abnormal Psychology, 100,* 600-603.

McClellan, J. M., & Werry, J. S. (1992). Schizophrenia. *Pediatric Psychopharmacology, 15,* 131-148.

McGlashan, T. H., & Fenton, W. S. (1991). Classical subtypes for schizophrenia: Literature review for DSM-IV. *Schizophrenia Bulletin, 17,* 609-632.

Mishlove, M., & Chapman, L. J. (1985). Social anhedonia in the prediction of psychosis proneness. *Journal of Abnormal Psychology, 94,* 384-396.

Morrison, R. L., & Bellack, A. S. (1987). Social functioning of schizophrenic patients: Clinical and research issues. *Schizophrenia Bulletin, 13,* 715-725.

Onstad, S., Skre, I., Torgersen, S., & Kringlen, E. (1991). Subtypes of schizophrenia: Evidence from a twin-family study. *Acta Psychiatrica Scandinavia, 84,* 203-206.

Opjordsmoen, S. (1991). Paranoid (delusional) disorders in the light of a long-term follow-up study. *Psychopathology, 24,* 287-292.

Ram, R., Bromet, E. J., Eaton, W. W., Pato, C., & Schwartz, J. E. (1992). The natural course of schizophrenia: A review of first-admission studies. *Schizophrenia Bulletin, 18,* 185-207.

Reisman, J. E., & Blakeney, A. B. (1991). Exploring sensory integrative treatment in chronic schizophrenia. *Occupational Therapy in Mental Health, 11,* 25-44.

Scott, J. (1993). Homelessness and mental illness. *British Journal of Psychiatry, 162,* 314-324.

Sirls, S. G. (1991). Diagnosis of secondary depression in schizophrenia: Implications for DSM-IV. *Schizophrenia Bulletin, 17,* 75-98.

Suto, M., & Frank, G. (1994). Future time perspective and daily occupations of persons with chronic schizophrenia in a board and care home. *American Journal of Occupational Therapy, 48,* 7-18.

Szymanski, S., Kane, J. M., & Liberman, J. A. (1991). A selective review of biological markers in schizophrenia. *Schizophrenia Bulletin, 17,* 99-111.

Taylor, M. A., & Abrams, R. (1987). Cognitive impairment patterns in schizophrenia and affective disorder. *Journal of Neurology, Neurosurgery, and Psychiatry, 50,* 895-899.

Tsoi, W. F., & Kua, E. H. (1992). Predicting the outcome of schizophrenia ten years later. *Australian and New Zealand Journal of Psychiatry, 26,* 257-261.

Tsuang, M. T., Faraone, S. V., & Day, M. (1988). Schizophrenic disorders. In A. M. Nicholi (Ed.),*The new Harvard guide to psychiatry* (pp. 761-779). Cambridge, MA: Belknap Press.

Tsuang, M. T., Winokur, G., & Crowe, R. R. (1980). Morbidity risks of schizophrenia and affective disorder among first degree relatives of patients with schizophrenia. In R. R. Fieve, D. Rosenthal, & H. Brill (Eds.), *Genetic research in psychiatry.* Baltimore: Johns Hopkins University Press.

Tsuang, M. T., Woolson, R. F., Winokur, G., & Crowe, R. R. (1981). Stability of psychiatric diagnosis: Schizophrenia and affective disorders followed up over a 30- to 40-year period. *Archives of General Psychiatry, 38,* 535-539.

Wallace, C. J., Nelson, C. J., Liberman et al., (1980). A review and critique of social skills training with schizophrenic patients. *Schizophrenia Bulletin, 6,* 64-69.

Chapter 7
Mood Disorders

Each of the disorders in this group is characterized by a disturbance of mood: excessive elation, depression, or some combination of these. The disorder may be a single episode, periodic changes, either in one direction or fluctuating between the two extremes, or a chronic pattern of affect disturbance. Because mood impacts on one's world view, these disorders tend to affect functional ability in global fashion.

Mood disorders are usually categorized either as depressive or bipolar. The bipolar disorders are those which fluctuate between mania and depression. It is rare to find an individual whose mood disorder is characterized only by manic episodes, i.e., episodes of extreme elation, although such a pattern is occasionally seen and will be diagnosed as manic episode. The depressive disorders, however, are the most common of psychiatric disorders. These may be either chronic, or periodic depressions caused by seasonal changes, stressful events, etc.

DSM-IV (APA, 1994) groups the various mood disorders in three categories: mood episodes, depressive disorders, and bipolar disorders. This chapter will discuss the more severe mood disorders: manic episode, major depressive episode, and bipolar disorder, as well as the less severe but similar disorders: hypomanic disorder, dysthymic disorder, and cyclothymic disorder. The first group will be discussed in detail, the second, more briefly (Figure 7-1).

Figure 7-1. Mood Disorders (More Severe and Less Severe Forms).

Manic episode	Bipolar disorder	Major depressive episode
⬦	⬦	⬦
Hypomanic disorder	Cyclothymic disorder	Dysthymic disorder

Major Depressive Episode

This disorder represents an episode of extreme depressed mood (Figure 7-2). In order to be given this diagnosis, an individual must exhibit at least five symptoms of depressed mood. Possible symptoms include irritability, anhedonia, unintentional weight loss or gain, insomnia or hypersomnia

Figure 7-2. Mood Disorders: Symptoms and Deficits.

Disorder	Symptoms	Functional Deficits
Major depressive episode	1. Depressed mood 2. Anhedonia 3. Appetite/weight change 4. Insomnia/hypersomnia 5. Lack of energy 6. Feelings of worthlessness/ guilt 7. Possible suicidal ideation 8. Impaired function	Social; work, leisure Cognitive; psychological Improves between episodes
Manic episode	1. Abnormally elevated or irritable mood 2. Grandiosity 3. Decreased sleep 4. Distractibility, flight of ideas 5. Poor judgement 6. Impaired function 7. May be delusions or hallucinations	Work; social, leisure Cognitive; psychological May be mild-severe Improves following/between episodes
Bipolar disorder	1. Recent alternating symptoms of both manic and major depressive episodes	As above
Dysthymia	1. Same as major depressive, but less severe 2. Duration at least 2 years (1 for children)	Same as major depressive, but less severe More chronic
Hypomanic episode	1. Same as manic, but less severe	Same as manic but less severe
Cyclothymia	1. Fluctuating hypomanic episodes and periods of depressed mood 2. Duration at least 2 years (1 for children). No more than 2 months symptom free.	Same as bipolar disorder, less severe

(excessive sleeping), psychomotor agitation or retardation, fatigue, feelings of guilt or worthlessness, poor concentration, and frequent thoughts of death or suicidal ideation may occur. As with a manic episode, hallucinations or delusions may be present, but the diagnosis is made only in the presence of depressed mood. In cases where psychotic symptoms appear without depressed mood, a diagnosis of schizophrenia or some other psychotic disorder would be considered. It is believed by some that "delusional depression" is more common in individuals with bipolar disorder (Weissman, Prusoff, & Merikangas, 1984).

This diagnosis will be made only in the absence of organic causes, and, more significantly, major depressive episode is distinguished from bereavement. In cases where an individual has recently lost a loved one, it would be considered normal to demonstrate the symptoms listed above. However, the therapist may need to identify a time period beyond which major depressive episode as a diagnosis would be considered. This is somewhat problematic, as a wide range of opinion exists about the "normal" duration of bereavement.

With regard to diagnoses of depression, DSM-III-R and DSM-IV mark significant departures from previous diagnostic listings. Most notably, they delete the prior distinction between endogenous and reactive depressions. In earlier editions, reactive depressions were described as those which had a clear cause, e.g., a significant loss or psychosocial stressor such as divorce or loss of a job. Endogenous depressions were thought to be those in which no clear and immediate cause for the depression was evident. It is now thought that this distinction is inaccurate, as many depressions appear to have some identifiable major precipitating stressor (Alnaes & Torgersen, 1993). Further, most have some identifiable biological component (Beats, 1991; Bolwig, 1993; Grahame-Smith, 1992). Thus the diagnostic distinctions among various kinds of depression are now made on the basis of specific symptoms and the pattern of appearance of depression in the individual's life.

Some major depression has a seasonal pattern (sometimes referred to as seasonal affective disorder, or SAD) (Faedda et al., 1993). In these cases, there is a specific pattern to depressive, and sometimes manic, episodes. Typically, these individuals become depressed in the fall and improve in the spring. This pattern must occur for several years before the SAD diagnosis will be made. If regular seasonal changes in life circumstances such as regular winter unemployment or return to school in the fall accompany the mood change, SAD will not usually be diagnosed. One treatment for this type of depression is phototherapy (Hill, 1992), in which the individual is exposed to light for specified periods of time during the winter when there is less natural daylight.

Major depressive episodes may be accompanied by tearfulness, phobias, panic attacks, or excessive brooding. In addition, there may be somatic complaints. Major depressive episodes may occur in individuals of any age, and have somewhat different characteristics among different age groups. Children often have accompanying somatic complaints and psychomotor agitation, while adolescents often engage in substance abuse or antisocial behavior. In elderly individuals depression may present with symptoms of dementia, an important issue for differential diagnosis.

One or more major depressive episodes, in the absence of any manic or hypomanic episode, will be called a major depression, either single episode or recurrent. Some individuals will have only one episode, while others have periodic episodes, sometimes developing into bipolar disorder. While most individuals with depressive disorders return to their prior level of function between episodes, some have chronic form which is reflected by continuing low level depression and mild functional impairment between episodes.

Etiology and Incidence

The precise etiology of depression is poorly understood, but as noted above, it does appear that there is a biological component to depression (Karasu et al., 1993). There is some argument whether biological patterns noted are a cause or a result of the depressive episode. As with mania, there is a familial pattern to depression, arguing for a genetic component (Faraone, Kremen, & Tsuang, 1990; Klerman, 1988). Other biological explanations focus on sensory changes (Amsterdam, Settle, Doty, Abelman, & Winokur, 1987), and on other CNS factors (Klerman, 1988). It appears, for instance, that depression is a common consequence of stroke, and that this type of depression is identical to other major depressive episodes (Lipsey, Spencer, Rabins, & Robinson, 1986).

It is also apparent, however, that depressive episodes correlate with psychosocial stressors. Chronic physical illness, substance abuse, and stressors such as divorce and childbirth have all been associated with depression. Early stressors such as loss of a parent are also predictive of later depression (Alnaes & Torgersen, 1993).

There is a reasonable amount of support for the notion of stress as a risk/precipitant of depression in general (Hirschfeld & Cross, 1982), particularly for "undesirable" life events. However, life events alone do not cause depression. There seems to be an interaction between undesirable life events and inadequate coping responses in people who are biologically prone to depression (Hirshfeld & Cross, 1982). This means individuals with biological predisposition to depression with high stress levels and poor personal resources (e.g., few social contacts) may be most likely to develop depression.

Psychosocial risk factors include early separation from parents (Roy, 1985; Alnaes & Torgersen, 1993). Marital status is also a factor (Hirschfeld & Cross, 1982), with separated and divorced individuals having greater risk for depression. Mothers at home with small children are also particularly subject to depression (Brown & Harris, 1978).

Other explanations of depression are behavioral and cognitive (Karasu et al., 1993). It is possible that peculiar perceptions of the world, faulty interpretations of those perceptions, or an inadequate repertoire of responses may figure in the disorder.

Major depressive episodes occur in roughly 6% of adults (Karasu et al., 1993). It is much more likely that an individual will have only major depressive episodes than only manic episodes. The disorder is much more common in women, as are all types of depression. It is also more common among older adults (Addonizio & Alexopoulos, 1993). The reasons for these differences are not known.

Prognosis

Prognosis for a specific depressive episode is generally good. Since Eysenck (1952) published his landmark work on the effectiveness of psychotherapy, it has been understood that some depressions will resolve within several months, with or without treatment. Some episodes, however, are chronic, persisting for years. Onset of an episode may be gradual over several days or weeks, or may be sudden. Some individuals may have one episode without recurrence, but about 50% of individuals will have recurring episodes (Karasu et al., 1993), each of which resolves with return to premorbid function. The episodes may vary in frequency, or in the case of SAD, may be quite predictable in frequency, severity, and duration. It appears that untreated depressions are likely to improve within 6 months (Karasu et al., 1993). More chronic patients had longer illness prior to treatment, other inpatient hospitalizations, intact marriages (a finding in conflict with the research reported above), low income, and other psychiatric disorders. Gonzalez, Lewinsohn, and Clark (1985) found family history to be a predictor of prognosis, that is, if relatives had the disorder, their course suggests what will happen to the individual.

Implications for Function and Treatment

Function in depressed individuals is greatly dependent on the severity of the episode. Some individuals may be able to manage nearly normal activity, while others may be totally unable to function. Occupational and social dysfunction are defining characteristics of the diagnosis.

At the level of specific skills, it is clear that cognition is almost always impaired. Concentration in particular is diminished, as is problem-solving ability. Sensation is usually not affected, except in the presence of hallucinations, but psychomotor activity is often altered, either slowed or speeded. Social function is often poor, largely because of lethargy or anhedonia. Individuals who become depressed have poor premorbid interpersonal skills, including level and latency of activity, interpersonal range, and positive reactions (Libet & Lewinsohn, 1973). Silence and negative comments are typical (Howe & Hokanson, 1979). These problems occur in depressed adolescents as well (Puig-Antich et al., 1985). While they may not cause the disorder, they may increase vulnerability (Vanger, 1987).

Poor social skills are problematic because of the reaction of others (Coyne, 1976). Those around the individual may become more hostile, anxious, and rejecting in response to the behavior of the depressed individual. Thus the behavior of the depressed individual sets a cycle of disturbed interaction.

Another area of function likely to be impaired is avocation. Depressed individuals take little pleasure in activity, thus avoid hobbies, social activities, and other activities which they formerly enjoyed. They may be unable to concentrate enough to read or to enjoy television, movies, or other performances. They typically lack energy and motivation to engage in physical activities. Vocational function is also affected. Individuals who have creative jobs, or jobs that require high degrees of motivation, such as sales, may find that they lack the energy and drive necessary to complete their required functions. In addition, cognitive and social impairment may interfere with their completion of tasks.

ADL and IADL may also be affected. In some individuals, this is primarily a matter of "not caring" about appearance or hygiene. In others, irritability, psychomotor retardation, lethargy, and loss of appetite may combine to result in greatly diminished function, sometimes to the extent that the individual takes no care at all of him or herself, and may not even get out of bed.

Coping skills of depressed individuals appear to be worse than those of non-depressed individuals (Billings, Cronkite, & Moos, 1983; Coyne, Aldwin, & Lazarus, 1981). Thus their function may be impaired as they are unable to problem solve for everyday events. There has been some speculation that perceived lack of control over life events is an important factor, though this "learned helplessness" hypothesis is the subject of much controversy (Baucom, 1983).

While depression is the most common of psychiatric diagnoses, it is also one of the most readily treatable (Karasu et al., 1993). There is a vast array of psychotropic medications which may be quite useful in resolving a depressive episode. Many of them have undesirable side effects which make them unappealing over long periods of time, but they can shorten individual episodes and reduce their severity. Some of these medications may be taken on a maintenance basis to prevent recurrence, and in general, medications to treat depression have been improved over the last two decades. For some individuals, electroconvulsive treatments (ECT) may be quite effective (Karasu et al., 1993). Generally speaking, when such treatment is applied, it is done for brief periods in the presence of specific sets of symptoms. This is quite unlike earlier forms of ECT which were given for a wide array of psychiatric disorders, and often for courses of dozens (or even hundreds) of treatments. ECT is particularly helpful for older adults who experience major depressive episodes (Rosenvinge, 1991).

In addition, psychotherapy of various forms is helpful for depression (Beutler, Machado, Engle, & Mohr, 1993). Cognitive therapy has also gained popularity as an intervention with depressed individuals. This therapy is based on the notion that depressed individuals inaccurately interpret events around them, and that they can learn new and more helpful interpretations. Behavior modification and psychoanalysis, as well as a variety of group and family approaches, have all been reported to be successful with depressed individuals.

Failure of treatment has been attributed to several factors. The first of these is the possibility of misdiagnosis (Potter & Manji, 1992). Some nonresponsive individuals may actually have a schizoaffective disorder which would require a different set of interventions (see Chapter 6). Individual reactions to various antidepressant medications vary considerably. In those instances, a change to a different class of medications, or even to a different medication within a class may improve response (Malizia & Bridges, 1992). Finally, individuals with problematic family histories and poor premorbid function tend to be more difficult to treat (Eccleston & Scott, 1991).

Special note should be made about depression in children/youth. While there is much debate on the subject, it appears that depression is quite common in children and adolescents (Fasko & Fasko, 1990-91). Symptoms may differ somewhat from those described for adults, and usually reflect developmental stage. Anxiety, school refusal or school problems, and negative behavior are all common. As with adults, low self-esteem is common.

In children, school and social function are likely to be impaired. It may be difficult for the child to articulate the problem (or even to state that a problem exists). Teens often become sullen and withdrawn, behavior which should not be written off as "just a phase," as adolescents are at considerable risk for depression (McIntosh, 1991). Intervention must be sensitive to the age and stage of the individual child.

Implications for Occupational Therapy

Occupational therapists may focus on assisting the individual to find gratifying activities that improve self-esteem and increase motivation. In addition, activities that provide opportunities for self-expression are valuable since individuals who are depressed may be reluctant or unable to put their feelings into words. Art or other creative activities can provide a valuable outlet for such emotions. One very timid woman was asked to work on a woodworking project. After a few timid taps, she began to pound with the hammer, shouting with great enthusiasm "This is for my husband, this is for my boss, this is for the dog..." She was then better able to express her rage about feeling taken advantage of by those around her. Neville (1986) has suggested four major goals of treatment would be of value: 1) reengagement in valued activities, 2) setting realistic goals for the future, 3) reestablishment of routines and habits, and 4) experiencing success and feelings of competence.

Since most individuals who are depressed do not lack the skills to do a variety of activities, motivation is often the key to improvement. These individuals may be extremely reluctant to engage in activity, and sit passively throughout the day. Behavioral programs which reinforce desired behaviors can be valuable (Johnston, 1986). The exception with regard to skills is in the area of socializing. As has been mentioned, social skills training may be helpful to individuals who are depressed. In addition, activities which ensure positive reinforcement from others can be of great value. One woman spent a week baking cookies every day for the other patients. She thoroughly enjoyed their appreciation. At the end of the week, she was able to say, "Now I think I'll do something for *me*," and she began to knit a scarf for herself. She chose a bright cheery yellow that was in marked contrast to the drab browns and grays she had been wearing.

Manic Episode

These episodes are severe, usually of abrupt onset, and are characterized by major changes in attitude and behavior. Most prominent is an elevated or irritated mood, with at least three of a list of characteristic behaviors. These include grandiosity, decreased need for sleep, talkativeness, flight of ideas, distractibility, increased activity, and excessive involvement in pleasurable activities with disregard for the consequences. For example, individuals experiencing a manic episode may spend money wildly, become involved in inappropriate sexual activities, and so on. Functioning is impaired in all spheres with marked deficits in occupational and social functioning. Hospitalization is often required.

As with all psychiatric disorders, part of the diagnostic process is the exclusion of other possible disorders. If hallucinations and delusions are present, they must be accompanied by alterations in mood. In the face of such symptoms, schizophrenia or other psychotic disorders must be ruled out. While thought disorders may be present in individuals experiencing manic episodes, mood alterations are the most prominent feature of the symptom constellation. Organic factors such as intoxication must also be ruled out.

Other characteristics include emotional lability. The individual may be expansive and grandiose one minute, angry and hostile the next. There are frequent rapid shifts from mania to depression, and occasionally, the symptoms of the two appear together. Furthermore, the individual may be oblivious to his or her behavior, totally unaware that there is a problem.

According to Carlson and Goodwin (1973) three stages can be identified in manic episodes. During the first, prodromal stage, speech is pressured and tangential, mood is happy, and hyperactivity is evident. During the second stage, grandiosity and paranoia appear, and hyperactivity and pressured speech worsen. The third stage is characterized by incoherence, severe delusional content, and even more obvious hyperactivity. Disorientation to time and place is common. Recovery is evidenced by a reversal of stages. Not all patients reach stage three; some go only to the second and then reverse. Similarly, rate of progression is quite variable, from hours to days. In the prodromal phase, the individual might volunteer for a large number of projects at work, buy expensive presents for friends and family, and flit from topic to topic during conversation. This might progress to developing "new ideas" for work which are grandiose and strange, such as developing a space station to protect the country from invasion of aliens. The individual might sleep very little, talk and move constantly, and become extremely irritable. As the manic episode abates, symptoms will diminish.

Etiology and Incidence

Mania most often appears in individuals in their twenties, though it may have later onset (Mirchandani & Young, 1993). The most characteristic pattern of appearance is a rapid, abrupt onset. It is not clear precisely what causes the disorder, though family studies have established that there is a familial pattern (Faraone et al., 1990). This pattern has appeared even when family members have been raised in different environments, and is thus a strong argument for some sort of genetic component to the disorder. It has also been noted that manic disorders may follow severe psychosocial stressors (Dunner & Hall, 1980). For example, mania sometimes first appears following childbirth. Another documented cause of mania is head trauma (Shukla, Cook, Mukherjee, Goodwin, & Miller, 1987).

Pure manic episodes without accompanying depression are rare. Bipolar disorders (mania and depression in combination) are discussed below.

Prognosis

Prognosis for specific manic episodes is good. Duration of episodes is variable, although untreated they may last for a month or more. However, often there is a pattern of recurring episodes, meaning that without maintenance treatment, it is probable that the individual will have manic episodes on a periodic basis. In some individuals, the episodes follow a particular pattern, appearing each spring, for example (Faedda et al., 1993), while in others, they may appear unpredictably. In still others, there may be a single episode, with no recurrence.

Effective long-term treatment involves use of medication (Janicak, Newman, & Davis, 1992). In individuals who are willing to take medication as prescribed, it can be quite useful, and can further improve prognosis. In order to prevent recurrence, however, it must be continued in maintenance doses for long periods of time. As will be discussed in Chapter 11, this presents a set of problems related to the potential for toxicity from the drug and the possible unwillingness of these individuals to follow the prescribed regimen. Use of maintenance doses of medication is problematic, however, given the nature of the disorder itself, and the tendency to impulsive acts. As a manic episode develops, judgment and self-control are reduced, and the individual may stop taking the medication. Further, there are some individuals who do not respond (Janicak et al., 1992) and even among responders, psychosocial consequences continue after individual episodes resolve (Coryell et al., 1993). About half of individuals who experience manic episodes have repeated episodes (Tohen, Waternaux, Tsuang, & Hunt, 1990)

Because of the severity of manic episodes, hospitalization, often involuntary, is frequently warranted. Manic individuals demonstrate extremely poor judgment, and must often be protected from a tendency to engage in illegal or imprudent acts, or to abuse drugs.

Implications for Function and Treatment

As with schizophrenia, function is severely impaired. This is, in fact, a defining characteristic of the disorder. Judgment is extremely poor, and individuals tend to engage in acting out behaviors. For example, the individual may begin to gamble wildly, to take drugs or abuse alcohol, to argue with colleagues at work, or to become involved in promiscuous sexual activity. At the same time, related impulsiveness and grandiosity interfere with vocational and social activities. There are changes in cognition and perception, although the exact reason for these changes is not well understood. While motor skill does not change, hyperactivity is almost always present. It appears that there are some changes in CNS function which contribute to the characteristic symptom constellation (Klerman, 1988). Social impairment is marked (Coryell et al., 1993).

These individuals may be able to function reasonably normally between episodes. Depending on the frequency and duration of the manic periods, it is possible that they may hold jobs, have families, and carry on other activities most of the time. However, all these functions are impaired during episodes, often resulting in loss of job, family disruption, and so on. In those individuals who have reasonable levels of function between episodes, maintenance treatment with drugs, as well as family therapy to assist others to understand the disorder may be quite effective. Recent research suggests that at least some psychosocial impairment persists even when the disorder is in remission (Coryell et al., 1993).

When hospitalization is part of treatment, it is usually brief. The primary objective is to protect the individual from harm to self or others as a result of poor judgment and impulsivity. Once medications have begun to ameliorate the symptoms, hospitalization is no longer necessary.

Implications for Occupational Therapy

During the acute episode, an important role for the occupational therapist is monitoring behavior changes, and providing a structured environment in which behavior can be managed. A typical manic patient might breeze into the clinic to begin "building a castle," switch to "creating a new Mona Lisa" after the first two nails are in place, then to making a leather coat after the first stroke of paint is on the canvas, etc. Clearly, limit setting is important. Signs of behavior change as medication is introduced are important to decision-making about long-term treatment.

Between episodes, the occupational therapist may assist the individual in coping with the possibility of a chronic illness. The individual needs to learn the signs of an impending episode in order to seek help. In addition, activity patterns may need to be examined to determine whether some stressful activities should be stopped or changed. Function in all areas of performance may be assessed to determine how stress can be managed, and how quality of life can be maximized.

For most individuals who have manic episodes, performance and skills are unimpaired between episodes. However, behavior during episodes may have long-term consequences in terms of lost friends, family disputes, lost jobs, and financial difficulties. Clients need to learn how to avoid or manage these difficulties by altering lifestyle, monitoring symptoms, and getting family members involved. One woman recognized that as soon as the lilacs bloomed each spring she'd begin to have problems. Her husband learned to put away the credit cards then, and she learned to go see her physician immediately.

Hypomanic Episode

Hypomanic episode is the diagnosis made when an individual shows signs similar to those in a manic episode, but when the symptoms are less severe and disabling (APA, 1994). The distinction between major manic episode and hypomanic episode is one of degree. While major episodes are quite striking, hypomanic episodes are less so, and are sometimes written off as excess energy. As with ADHD in children, the disorder is, to some extent, in the eye of the beholder. However, in many instances, judgment is impaired, and irritability leads to fights with spouses, employees, etc. The individual may have rapid mood swings from euphoria to irritability, sleep less than usual, or start a wide variety of projects, none of which are finished. Hallucinations and delusions are not present, and the individual does not become disoriented to time and place.

Depressive Disorders

DSM-IV (APA, 1994) lists two main types of depressive disorders. The first of these is major depressive disorder, which is characterized by one or more major depressive episodes. The diagnosis is made only if there are no manic, mixed, or hypomanic episodes. The second is dysthymic disorder, which is described below. A common pattern is a dysthymic disorder which ultimately develops into a major depressive disorder.

Dysthymia

This is a depressive disorder in which the individual has some symptoms of depression most of the time. For the diagnosis to be made, symptoms must be ongoing for at least 2 years, with periods of no more than 2 months at a time symptom-free. As hypomanic episode is a less severe form of manic episode, this is a less severe (though more chronic) form of major depression. The symptoms are milder, but much more persistent. Dysthymia may precede a major depressive episode, leading to so-called "double depression." These are cases in which a major depressive episode is superimposed on a chronic minor depression (APA, 1994; Keller, Lavori, Endicott, Coryell, & Klerman, 1983). This is a particularly pernicious depression, with poor prognosis.

Dysthymia often coexists with other Axis I or Axis III disorders, in which case it is referred to as secondary. For example, many individuals with anorexia are depressed, as are some individuals with arthritis. Secondary depression occurs when there is a clear precipitating event, but normal bounds of the mourning process have been passed. For example, job loss or physical illness may lead to an ongoing secondary depression.

This is a very common disorder, although diagnosis may be difficult, as the boundary between dysthymia and major depressive episode is not clear. While DSM-IV lists specific criteria, these characteristics are largely a matter of degree, and a moderate depression might be diagnosed by one practitioner as dysthymia, by another as major depressive episode. Dysthymia is notable primarily for its chronicity, and for the absence of some of the more severe depressive symptoms, hallucinations and delusions, for example.

Function is generally impaired to a mild or moderate degree in individuals with dysthymia. While they typically hold jobs, have social relationships and interests, these are not maintained at optimal levels because of the lethargy and lack of interest displayed by these individuals. Their constant depression wears on those around them, and they may lose friends as a result of their inability to enjoy activities and to take pleasure in people. The chronicity of the disorder is a problem, as individuals tend to feel bad for long periods of time without relief.

Dysthymia has apparent biological origins. Changes in rapid eye movement (REM) sleep, thyroid functioning, and electroencephalogram (EEG) readings have all been found (Howland & Thase, 1991). These differences are not the same as those found during major depressive episodes.

Treatment for dysthymia is somewhat more problematic than for major depressive episodes. Medication has been used with some success (Conte & Karasu, 1992), but its use is not as frequently helpful as in major depression. Cognitive therapy (Conte & Karasu, 1992) and psychotherapy (Cameron, 1989) have both been reported as somewhat helpful. A mixture of these therapies may be most effective (Conte & Karasu, 1992). However, dysthymic disorder is more intractable than major depression.

Children are also at risk for dysthymia. They may present with anxiety, school phobias, or difficulty sleeping. School refusal or negative behavior are also common signs of depression. School and social function are likely to be impaired. At the same time it may be difficult for them to articulate the problem (or even state that it exists). Intervention must be sensitive to the age and stage of the individual child. Play therapy may help the child express feelings nonverbally.

Bipolar Disorders

These disorders are characterized by fluctuations in mood, with episodes of both mania and depression. Three main types of bipolar disorder have been included in DSM-IV (APA, 1994). Bipolar disorder I is characterized by intermittent manic and major depressive episodes. Bipolar disorder II is characterized by intermittent hypomanic and major depressive episodes with no occurrence of manic episodes (Dunner, 1992). The third type of bipolar disorder, cyclothymia, is discussed separately on page 119.

Etiology and Incidence

There is a clear familial pattern in the appearance of bipolar disorder. In addition, the most effective treatment is lithium. Thus there is strong evidence of a biological cause for the disorder.

The disorder is not uncommon, with estimates of its occurrence running at roughly 1% to 2% of the adult population of the United States (Klerman, 1988).

Prognosis

While single manic or depressive episodes may resolve relatively quickly, bipolar disorder can be chronic (Werry & McClellan, 1992; Winokur et al., 1993). Premorbid function is a good predictor of outcome. Each recurrence may further damage relationships, work performance, and so on, making functional problems cumulative. Education of the family is extremely important, so that they understand the nature of the disorder and recognize that the individual is not being intentionally disruptive. They can also be encouraged to help monitor symptoms, manage stress, and so on.

Implications for Function and Treatment

For specific episodes, functional decrements are the same as those described above for manic episodes and major depressive episodes. Between episodes, function may be quite normal. The individual will be able to work, engage in social and avocational activities, and perform self-care. This is particularly true for individuals who have long periods between exacerbations. However, as noted, some individuals have chronic problems, either because of the frequency of manic or depressive episodes, or because of the consequences of the dysfunctional behavior which they engage in during the episodes.

Treatment of choice is medication. When taken as advised, lithium can minimize symptoms and prevent recurrences. Group psychotherapy seems to contribute to positive outcomes (Cerbone, Mayo, Cuthbertson, & O'Connell, 1992; Kanas, 1992). Behavioral family treatment is also reported as effective (Miklowitz & Goldstein, 1990).

Implications for Occupational Therapy

Interventions for individual manic and depressed episodes in those with bipolar disorder are identical to those described in previous sections. Manic phase and depressed phase are no different for bipolar disorder than for major episodes. However, bipolar disorder tends to be chronic, and intervention must address this as a concern.

Two important considerations apply. First, self-esteem and self-concept are likely to be damaged by both the chronic nature of the disorder and the enormous fluctuations in personality which characterize it. When an individual is sometimes withdrawn, sad, and lethargic and other times energetic and effervescent, it is difficult to form a clear picture of abilities, or even desires. It is also difficult to feel good about one's performance when it is so unstable. Medication may help the individual reach a more even keel, but cannot repair the damage to self done by these mood swings. The occupational therapist must help the individual identify strengths, weaknesses, likes, and dislikes through exposure to a wide range of activities.

A second consideration is that needed skills may have been lost, or may never have been acquired. One young mother had fluctuated between withdrawal from her two preschool children and extreme irritability with them. She needed a good bit of training in parenting skills to resolve this, and to begin to repair the damage done by her inconsistent and unpredictable behavior. This is fairly typical for individuals with long-standing bipolar disorder, particularly those who have not had adequate diagnosis and treatment.

Cyclothymia

This is a chronic disorder in which episodes of hypomania and depressed mood (but not major depressive episode) are interspersed. It is a less severe form of bipolar disorder. In order for the diagnosis to be made, there must be at least a 2 year period during which the individual is symptom-free for no more than 2 months at a time. Some theorists believe that cyclothymia is simply a less severe form of bipolar disorder, and, in fact, the boundary between the two is indistinct. It is not unusual for cyclothymia to eventually develop into bipolar disorder.

By definition, cyclothymia is less severe than bipolar disorder, and this is evident in functional capacity. In fact, some individuals report that they are unusually productive during hypomanic episodes. Vocational function is, however, impaired during depressive periods. Social function is often impaired as the wide, unpredictable mood swings may cause difficulty for those around the individual. Substance abuse may become a problem as the individual attempts to deal with the depressive episodes, or loses some capacity for good judgment during hypomanic episodes.

Implications for Occupational Therapy

For all the less severe mood disorders—hypomanic episode, dysthymia, and cyclothymia—principles discussed for the more severe disorders can be applied. While the functional impact of these disorders is less, they can be very frustrating because of their chronicity. This alone can enhance the depression and irritability which characterize the disorders. Thus, the individual may benefit from support in coping with chronic illness, education and information, and assistance in clarifying valued goals and activities.

Individuals who tend to be hypomanic often have difficulty with time management. They may be over committed, and create interpersonal friction by being unable to meet their commitments. Effective use of time and realistic self-appraisal are important goals for occupational therapy.

Dysthymia presents an opposite problem, although the consequences are somewhat similar. The individual has extremely low motivation which may be quite irritating to others. These individuals are the "Eeyores" of the world (CF Milne, 1947), constantly seeing the gloomy side of life (Munoz, personal communication, August, 1988). In their interactions with others, nothing is ever enough to help them feel loved and happy. These individuals need to discover activities which will be satisfying and motivating to them.

Cyclothymic disorder requires a combination of approaches, much like those suggested for bipolar disorder. While the functional impairments are less extreme, their impact on self-esteem should not be minimized.

Suicide

Suicide is a particular concern related to mood disorders (Karasu et al., 1993). The rate of suicide attempts is 30% for depressed persons (Klerman, 1988), i.e., almost one in three such individuals will make a serious gesture. Many depressed individuals contemplate suicide, and those who appear to have active suicidal intent may require hospitalization to prevent them from harming themselves (Karasu et al., 1993). The problem is complicated by the fact that some antidepressant medication can be lethal if abused, thus requiring careful monitoring, especially before it has had the opportunity to take effect in elevating mood, a process which may take several weeks.

Professionals who work with depressed individuals must be aware of the potential for suicide, note the presence of suicidal potential in these individuals, and take necessary precautions (Bongar, Maris, Berman, & Litman, 1992). It is helpful to ascertain by asking directly whether an individual is suicidal, and to determine whether a plan of action has been developed. This is ordinarily the responsibility of the individual directing treatment (team leader, psychiatrist, etc.), but other professionals should ascertain that this has been done. Individuals with a clear and feasible plan must be considered at high risk for suicide. In addition, individuals whose depression appears to resolve suddenly are considered high risks, as this may signify that they have reached a decision to act. Depressed individuals are at greatest risk during the period when the depression is just beginning to lift because they have increased energy to act on their suicidal wishes.

Precautions include careful monitoring, often in inpatient settings, and removal of means to cause death until the individual is clearly no longer actively suicidal (Appleby, 1992). While most suicide attempts are made with drugs and guns, other lethal substances and sharp implements, as well as access to carbon monoxide, should be guarded as well. Occupational therapists should be sensitive to use of sharp implements and toxic solvents by suicidal patients in their care. There is a belief that some single car accidents are, in fact, suicide attempts, so it may be necessary to monitor driving, especially when accompanied by drinking, in these individuals.

Children and adolescents who are depressed are at risk of suicide, as well as adults (Fasko & Fasko, 1990-91; Rao, Weissman, Martin, & Hammond, 1993). A wish to reunite with a loved one or to punish an adult are common motivations for suicide attempts in this age group. Teens who become sullen and withdrawn should be carefully monitored (McIntosh, 1991). It should not be assumed that the individual is just "going through a phase."

Suicide risk is also high among individuals with human immunodeficiency virus (HIV) or at high risk of acquiring HIV (e.g., homosexuals and intravenous drug users) (Starace, 1993). Another high risk group is older adults, among whom the rate is almost twice what it is for younger adults (Lester & Yang, 1992). It is hypothesized that stressors such as loss of spouse, retirement, and reduced economic circumstances contribute to this risk. Individuals with physical illnesses which cause significant pain are at high risk for suicide as well (Rao, 1990).

Occupational therapists can also focus on providing reasons to live to individuals who feel hopeless and angry. In addition to protecting the individual, the therapsit can help him or her learn to recognize when he or she is feeling depressed, and alternative strategies for minimizing stress and coping with problems. These strategies may include expressive activities, or activities which require physical exertion to provide an outlet for feelings.

Staff in inpatient settings will need to deal with feelings of other patients, as well as their own, when a suicide attempt or completed suicide occurs on the unit (Little, 1992). While precautions can reduce the incidence, individuals who are determined to complete a suicide are quite difficult to stop.

References

Addonizio, G., & Alexopoulos, G. S. (1993). Affective disorders in the elderly. *International Journal of Geriatric Psychiatry, 8,* 41-47.

Alnaes, R., & Torgersen, S. (1993). Mood disorders: Developmental and precipitating events. *Canadian Journal of Psychiatry, 38,* 217-224

American Psychiatric Association (1994). *Diagnostic and Statistical Manual of Mental Disorders* (4th ed.). Washington, DC: Author.

Amsterdam, J. D., Settle, R. G., Doty, R. L., Abelman, E., & Winokur, A. (1987). Taste and smell perception in depression. *Biological Psychiatry, 22,* 1477-1481.

Appleby, L. (1992). Suicide in psychiatric patients: Risk and prevention. *British Journal of Psychiatry, 161,* 749-758.

Baucom, D. H. (1983). Sex role identity and the decision to regain control among women: A learned helplessness investigation. *Journal of Personality and Social Psychology, 44,* 334-343.

Beats, B. C. (1991). Structural imaging in affective disorder. *International Journal of Geriatric Psychiatry, 6,* 419-422.

Billings, A. G., Cronkite, R. C., & Moos, R. H. (1983). Social-environmental factors in unipolar depression: Comparisons of depressed patients and nondepressed controls. *Journal of Abnormal Psychology, 92,* 119-133.

Beutler, L. E., Machado, P. P. P., Engle, D., & Mohr, D. (1993). Differential patient X treatment maintenance among cognitive, experiential, and self-directed psychotherapies. *Journal of Psychotherapy Integration, 3,* 15-31.

Bolwig, T. G. (1993). Regional cerebral blood flow in affective disorder. *Acta Psychiatrica Scandinavia, 371,* 48-53.

Bongar, B., Maris, R. W., Berman, A. L., & Litman, R. E. (1992). Outpatient standards of care and the suicidal patient. *Suicide and Life-Threatening Behavior, 22,* 453-478.

Brown, G., & Harris, T. (1978). *Social origins of depression: A study of psychiatric disorders in women.* New York: Free Press.

Cameron, P. M. (1989). Psychodynamic psychotherapy for the depressive syndrome. *Psychiatric Journal of the University of Ottowa, 14,* 397-402.

Carlson, G. A., & Goodwin, F. K. (1973). The stages of mania. *Archives of General Psychiatry, 28,* 221-228.

Cerbone, M. J. A., Mayo, J. A., Cuthbertson, B. A., & O'Connell, R. A. (1992). Group therapy as an adjunct to medication in the management of bipolar affective disorder. *Group, 16,* 174-187.

Conte, H. R., & Karasu, T. B. (1992). A review of treatment studies of minor depression: 1980-1991. *American Journal of Psychotherapy, XLVI,* 58-74.

Coryell, W., Scheftner, W., Endicott, J. et al. (1993). The enduring psychosocial consequences of mania and depression. *American Journal of Psychiatry, 150,* 720-727.

Coyne, J. C. (1976). Depression and the response of others. *Journal of Abnormal Psychology, 85,* 186-193.

Coyne, J. C., Aldwin, C., & Lazarus, R. S. (1981). Depression and coping in stressful episodes. *Journal of Abnormal Psychology, 90,* 439-447.

Dunner, D. L. (1992). Differential diagnosis of bipolar disorder. *Journal of Clinical Psychopharmacology, 12,* 7s-12s.

Dunner, D. L., & Hall, K. S. (1980.) Social adjustment and psychological precipitants in mania. In R. H. Belmaker & G. Van Praag (Eds.), *Mania: An evolving concept* (pp. 337-347). Jamaica, NY: SP Medical & Scientific Books.

Eccleston, D., & Scott, J. (1991). Treatment, prediction of relapse and prognosis of chronic primary major depression. *International Clinical Psychopharmacology. 6*, 3-10.

Eysenck, H. J. (1952). The effects of psychotherapy: An evaluation. *Journal of Consulting Psychology, 16*, 219-324.

Faedda, G. L., Tondo, L., Teicher, M. H., et al. (1993). Outcome after rapid vs. gradual discontinuation of lithium treatment in bipolar disorders. *Arch Gen Psychiatry, 50*, 17-23.

Faraone, S. V., Kremen, W. S., & Tsuang, M. T. (1990). Genetic transmission of major affective disorders: Quantitative models and linkage analysis. *Psychological Bulletin, 108*, 109-127.

Fasko, S. N., & Fasko, D. (1990-91). Suicidal behavior in children. *Psychology: A Journal of Human Behavior, 27-28*, 10-16.

Gonzalez, L. R., Lewinsohn, P. M., & Clarke, G. N. (1985). Longitudinal follow-up of unipolar depressives: An investigation of predictors of relapse. *Journal of Consulting and Clinical Psychology, 53*, 461-469.

Grahame-Smith, D. G. (1992). Serotonin in affective disorders. *International Clinical Psychopharmacology, 6*, 5-13.

Hirschfeld, R. M. A., & Cross, C. K. (1982). Epidemiology of affective disorders. *Archives of General Psychiatry, 39*, 35-46.

Hill, M. A. (1992). *Annals of Clinical Psychiatry, 4*, 131-146.

Howe, M. J., & Hokanson, J. E. (1979). Conversational and social responses to depressive interpersonal behavior. *Journal of Abnormal Psychology, 88*, 625-634.

Howland, R. H., & Thase, M. E. (1991). Biological studies of dysthymia. *Biological Psychiatry, 30*, 283-304.

Janicak, P. G., Newman, R. H., & Davis, J. M. (1992). Advances in the treatment of mania and related disorders: A reappraisal. *Psychiatric Annals, 22*, 92-103.

Johnston, M. T. (1986). The use of cognitive-behavioral techniques with depressed patients in day treatment. Depression: Assessment and Treatment Update. Rockville, MD: *American Occupational Therapy Association*, 49-61.

Kanas, N. (1992). Group psychotherapy with bipolar patients: A review and synthesis. *International Journal of Group Psychotherapy, 4*, 321-333.

Karasu, T. B., Docherty, J. P., Gelenberg, A., et al. (1993), *American Journal of Psychiatry, 150*, 1-26.

Keller, M. B., Lavori, P. W., Endicott, J., Coryell, W., & Klerman, G. L. (1983). "Double depression": Two-year follow-up. *American Journal of Psychiatry, 140*, 689-694.

Klerman, G. L. (1988). Depression and related disorders of mood (affective disorders). In A. M. Nicholi (Ed.), *The new Harvard guide to psychiatry* (pp. 309-336). Cambridge, MA: Belknap Press.

Lester, D., & Yang, B. (1992). Social and economic correlates of the elderly suicide rate. *Suicide and Life-Threatening Behavior, 22*, 36-47.

Libet, J. M., & Lewinson, P. M. (1973). Concept of social skill with special reference to the behavior of depressed persons. *Journal of Consulting and Clinical Psychology, 40*, 304-312.

Lipsey, J. R., Spencer, W. C., Rabins, P. V., & Robinson, R. G. (1986). Phenomenological comparison of poststroke depression and functional depression. *American Journal of Psychiatry, 143*, 527-529.

Little, J. D. (1992). Staff response to inpatient and outpatient suicide: What happened and what do we do? *Australian and New Zealand Journal of Psychiatry, 26*, 162-167.

McIntosh, J. L. (1991). Middle-age suicide: A literature review and epidemiological study. *Death Studies, 15*, 21-37.

Malizia, A. L., & Bridges, P. K. (1992). The management of treatment-resistant affective disorder: Clinical perspectives. *Journal of Psychopharmacology, 6*, 145-155.

Miklowitz, D. J., & Goldstein, M. J. (1990). Behavioral family treatment for patients with bipolar affective disorder. *Behavior Modification, 14*, 457-489.

Milne, A. A. (1947). *The world of Pooh*, London: Linder.

Mirchandani, I. C., & Young, R. C. (1993). Management of mania in the elderly: An update. *Annals of Clinical Psychiatry, 5,* 67-77.

Neville, A. (1986). Depression and the model of human occupation: Theory and research. *Depression: Assessment and treatment update.* (pp. 14-21). Rockville, MD: American Occupational Therapy Association.

Potter, W. Z., & Manji, H. K. (1992). Commentary on the management of treatment-resistant affective disorder: Clinical perspectives. *Journal of Psychopharmacology, 6,* 164-166.

Puig-Antich, J., Lukens, E., Davies, M., Goetz, D., Brennan-Quattrock, J., & Todak, G. (1985). Psychosocial functioning in prepubertal major depressive disorders. *Archives of General Psychiatry, 42,* 500-507.

Rao, A. V. (1990). Physical illness, pain, and suicidal behavior. *Crisis, 11,* 48-56.

Rao, U., Weissman, M. M., Martin, J. A., & Hammond, R. W. (1993). Childhood depression and risk of suicide: A preliminary report of a longitudinal study. *Journal of the American Academy of Child and Adolescent Psychiatry, 32,* 21-27.

Rosenvinge, H. (1991). The real value of electroconvulsive therapy in the elderly. *Dementia, 2,* 225-228.

Roy, A. (1985). Early parental separation and adult depression. *Archives of General Psychiatry, 42,* 987-991.

Shukla, S., Cook, B. L., Mukherjee, S., Goodwin, C., & Miller, M. G. (1987). Mania following head trauma. *American Journal of Psychiatry, 144,* 93-95.

Starace, F. (1993). Suicidal behaviour in people infected with human immunodeficiency virus: A literature review. *The International Journal of Social Psychiatry, 39,* 64-70.

Tohen, M., Waternaux, C. M., Tsuang, M. T., & Hunt, A. T. (1990). Four-year follow-up of twenty-four first-episode manic patients. *Journal of Affective Disorders, 19,* 79-86.

Vanger, P. (1987). An assessment of social skills deficiencies in depression. *Comprehensive Psychiatry, 28,* 508-512.

Weissman, M. M., Prusoff, B. A., & Merikangas, K. R. (1984). Is delusional depression related to bipolar disorder? *American Journal of Psychiatry, 141,* 892-893.

Werry, J. S., & McClellan, J. M. (1992). Predicting outcome in child and adolescent (early onset) schizophrenia and bipolar disorder. *Journal of the American Academy of Child and Adolescent Psychiatry, 31,* 147-150.

Winokur, G., Coryell, W., Keller, M., et al. (1993). A prospective follow-up of patients with bipolar and primary unipolar affective disorder. *Archives of General Psychiatry, 50,* 457-465.

Chapter 8

Anxiety Disorders

This group of disorders is characterized by the presence of anxiety and, often, avoidance behavior. Disorders in this category include panic attack, agoraphobia, panic disorder, specific phobia, obsessive compulsive disorder, post-traumatic stress disorder, and acute stress disorder (Figure 8-1). Generalized anxiety disorder, a milder and less disabling disorder, will be described only briefly since it is not frequently seen in occupational therapy settings. Occupational therapy intervention for all the anxiety disorders will be considered at the end of the chapter.

Figure 8-1. Anxiety Disorders.

- Panic attack
- Panic disorder
- Agoraphobia
- Specific phobia
- Obsessive compulsive disorder
- Post-traumatic stress disorder

Panic Attack

A single panic attack is not diagnosed as a psychiatric disorder. Occurrence of panic attacks is characteristic of a number of anxiety disorders, so DSM-IV (APA, 1994) does list the criteria for determining whether one has occurred.

Panic attacks are characterized by presence of at least four symptoms from the following list: palpitations, increased heart rate, sweating, trembling, shortness of breath, a choking sensation, chest pain, nausea, dizziness or faintness, fear of dying, chills, and so on. It has been noted that the symptoms of panic attacks can be provoked in the laboratory through chemical means, including excessive caffeine (Nutt & Lawson, 1992). Hyperventilation can also produce a panic attack. It is not clear whether these exactly mimic panic attacks which occur outside the laboratory. In both cases, the panic attack is accompanied by an intense state of fear (Reiss, 1991).

Panic attacks may be perceived by the individual as heart attacks, so it is not unusual for the individual to present in the emergency room. However, each episode resolves, usually within minutes or hours. A person who has experienced such an episode may well develop anxiety about the potential for other attacks.

Panic Disorder

This diagnosis is made when the primary symptom is recurrent unexpected panic attacks. These may result in agoraphobia, an extreme fear of going into new or unfamiliar situations. Sometimes, however, panic disorder occurs in the absence of agoraphobia, and agoraphobia, as noted below, may occur in the absence of panic attacks.

Each panic attack is characterized by severe anxiety and feelings of panic, which may be accompanied by apprehension, shortness of breath, dizziness, nausea, chest pain, hot flashes, numbness, and fear of doing something uncontrolled. These attacks appear unpredictably, particularly at first, and the individual may develop an ongoing fear about the possibility of having a panic attack (Reiss, 1991). Typically, the individual begins to associate these attacks with specific situations, which are then avoided, or begins to fear being anywhere that help might not be readily available, thus developing avoidance of any new situation (agoraphobia).

The attacks may be relatively frequent, several times a day, for example, or rare. Occasionally, the disorder is limited to one attack, or to a brief period during which the attacks occur, followed by a complete disappearance of symptoms. More typically there is a chronic pattern, with some periods of relative freedom from attacks, others during which the attacks become more frequent or more severe.

Etiology and Incidence

Panic disorder is quite common, but not well explained. It may occur in the presence of some form of depression, although the most common pattern is for depression to occur later (Boulenger & Lavallee, 1993), probably because the panic attacks can be so demoralizing. Panic disorder is often accompanied by a substance use disorder (possibly the result of attempts to self-sedate during panic attacks)(Agras, 1993; Brown & Barlow, 1992).

The disorder may have a biological basis, specifically, noradrenergic dysfunction (Agras, 1993). It may also be a learned response, or some combination of biological and learned (Rapee, 1991). Separation from family or disruption of important relationships during childhood is a predisposing factor (Rapee, 1991) as are presence of avoidance behavior in childhood and stressful life events.

Prognosis

Prognosis is variable, depending on severity, and on unknown and unpredictable factors. Some individuals, as noted, have time limited problems (Rapee, 1991). Others have relatively chronic courses. It appears that suicide is common among individuals with a chronic course (Coryell, Noyes, & Clancy 1982) and that there is a marked excess mortality from other causes, such as heart disease, over time (Agras, 1993).

Implications for Function and Treatment

Function is dependent on the severity of the disorder. In some individuals, functional impairment is minimal. While they experience extreme discomfort during attacks, they may be relatively symptom free between attacks, and may have long periods without problems. In other instances, function is severely impaired, particularly occupational and social function (Agras, 1993). Generally speaking, ADL remains intact, although IADL may be impaired by unwillingness to go out. Some of these individuals, for example, experience panic attacks while driving, and, as a result, begin to refuse to drive.

Treatment is often a combination of anti-anxiety medications and behavior modification (Rapee, 1991). Specifically, systematic desensitization has been found useful. This involves pairing of increasingly anxiety-provoking stimuli with relaxation methods to reduce the incidence of panic and to provide the individual with a sense of control of the symptoms (Nemiah, 1988). Overall, treatment is relatively effective (Rapee, 1991). There is at least some evidence that treatment is effective even in the presence of co-existing depression (Laberge, Gauthier, Cote, Plamondon & Cormier 1992; Maddock & Blacker, 1991).

Agoraphobia

Agoraphobia is diagnosed in the context of panic attacks, fear of having panic attacks, or of being in unfamiliar situations. It is not an independently coded diagnosis. Individuals who are agoraphobic are fearful of leaving a familiar environment, usually the house, or even a specific room in the house. When the fear of panic attacks is based on prior experience of having the attacks, the diagnosis is agoraphobia with panic disorder. Some individuals fear panic attacks but have never had them. In this case, a diagnosis of agoraphobia without panic disorder would be made.

Etiology and Incidence

This can be a very severe disorder, but its origin is not well understood. Incidence is roughly 3% in community populations (Franklin, 1991) and it is somewhat more common in women. Risk factors include early loss experiences, childhood separation or school anxiety, and recent loss experiences. Family history of anxiety disorders is also predictive.

In most cases, prognosis is poor, as agoraphobia tends to represent a long-term pattern of maladaptation. While antianxiety medications and behavior modification have been employed with some degree of success, the disorder tends to be intractable. In particular, comorbidity with other mental disorders is prognostic of poor outcome (Brown & Barlow, 1992).

Implications for Function and Treatment

This disorder is extremely disabling (Hoffart, 1993). While underlying skills (cognitive, sensory, motor) appear to be intact, performance is severely impaired. It should be noted that impact of the disorder on skills is not well understood. It is entirely possible, for example, that some sort of sensory change may contribute to the disorder, but this has not been well documented. What is clear is that these individuals have difficulty with most occupations. They cannot work because they fear leaving the house. Their social lives become quite circumscribed, and they are fearful of any activity that requires them to be in new situations. They may be able to maintain ADL, and those IADL functions which do not require them to go out. Their families may be involved in the condition as well. In one extreme case, the individual's husband reported that no one in the family was allowed to use the upstairs portion of the house, as this would precipitate a panic attack for the individual. Since the bedrooms were all upstairs, the family had to move beds into the living room. In some instances, the individual may be able to go out with one trusted companion, a friend or spouse.

Treatments include behavioral fear reduction and avoidance reduction procedures (Franklin, 1991). Cognitive treatment may be helpful (Hoffart, 1993) but research data are equivocal. Medication may be used to reduce anxiety, but effectiveness of this intervention is not well documented (Mattick, Andrews, Hadzi-Pavlovic, & Christensen, 1990). Overall, treatment is effective in somewhere between 20% and 60% of cases (O'Sullivan & Marks, 1991).

Specific Phobia

This is a condition in which excessive, persistent fear is caused by presence of a specific and limited object. In social phobia (which is separately diagnosed, but typical of specific phobias), for example, it is social situations which evoke the response. Specific phobias are often related to a stimulus which has evoked the panic response in the past, for example snakes, or enclosed spaces, high places, driving, flying, and so on. Unlike panic attack disorder, however, the source of the fear is identifiable, and the individual typically recognizes that it is unreasonable.

Specific phobia diagnoses are not made unless the individual alters his or her behavior in some way as a result. Someone who is afraid of flying but does so regardless would not be diagnosed, while someone who avoided flying at all costs would be given a simple phobia diagnosis. In children, crying or tantrums may occur instead of panic attacks, and children, unlike adults may not recognize that the fear is unreasonable. Childhood phobias are predictive of phobias later in life (Strauss & Last, 1993).

Etiology and Incidence

Phobias seem to develop through conditioning, i.e., an individual will have an experience with the stimulus which is anxiety provoking and then associate other similar experiences with the feeling of fear (Ost, 1985). A child who is frightened by a spider while playing outside may develop a feeling of panic in other circumstances where spiders are present. Alternatively, individuals may be taught their phobias, or model on parent fears. In this case, a parent's fear of spiders might be conveyed to a child who then exhibits the fear as well. These phobias may persist for long periods of time. If they begin in adulthood, they will generally continue unless they are treated. Individuals whose phobias began in childhood and persisted into adulthood tend to have worse outcomes than those whose phobias emerged in adulthood (Keller et al., 1992).

In all the anxiety states, neurotransmitters appear to be disturbed, particularly norepinephrine (Redmond & Huang, 1979). It is not clear whether this is the cause or the result of the anxiety.

Phobias are extremely common, occurring in 10% of the general population (Chapman, Fyer, Mannuzza, & Klein, 1993). Almost all individuals experience fear related to specific stimuli, and while most do not have panic attacks as a result, large numbers of people do.

Implications for Function and Treatment

Function is largely dependent on the nature of the feared stimulus. Social phobias may be relatively disabling, as they lead people to avoid any situation in which new people will be present. However, many feared stimuli can readily be avoided without undue impact on the individual's life. Fear of snakes may be managed by avoiding most outdoor activity, a limitation that some individuals would not consider too great a hardship. Among the individuals most likely to seek treatment are those who have relatively late onset of symptoms which do interfere with function e.g., a traveling salesman who develops fear of flying. Another particularly troubling phobia is school phobia, which is not uncommon in children. The phobia may develop as a result of a frightening or anxiety provoking experience at school, although in some instances it is unexplained. One child became sick every morning for weeks, until it was discovered she was afraid of the computer room at school, a small, windowless, rather dark space. Her symptoms abated when the computers were moved. In some cases the child refuses to go to school, in others he or she is too anxious to perform well while there.

Treatment usually involves some sort of behavior modification. Systematic desensitization has been found to be effective. Occasionally, anti-anxiety medications agents will be used, but this is not common, since the phobias tend to be circumscribed and self-limiting. Many individuals, in fact, find ways to alter their routines to avoid the feared stimulus entirely and never seek other treatment. The most effective treatment appears to be a combination of behavioral and physiological methods (e.g., biofeedback) (Ost, 1985). Treatment is clearly effective (Chapman et al., 1993). At least 60% of individuals treated with behavioral methods have reduced phobic reactions (O'Sullivan & Marks, 1991).

It is noteworthy that there is a familial pattern to anxiety disorders, meaning that children whose parents have anxiety disorders are more likely to develop them as well (Bernstein & Borchardt, 1991). For this reason, family therapy is often recommended when the client is a child (Dadds, Heard, & Rapee, 1992).

Obsessive Compulsive Disorder

Obsessions are thoughts or ideas which are intrusive and anxiety provoking. Most common are obsessions with violence or contamination. The individual may recognize that these ideas are internally derived (not based on any external event), but is unable to control them, and finds that the thoughts intrude while he or she attempting to do something else (Nemiah, 1988).

Compulsions are repetitive, purposeful behaviors performed in response to an obsession with the goal of preventing the discomfort caused by the obsession. The activity is, however, either excessive or not realistically helpful in resolving the obsession. For example, someone with an obsession about contamination may engage in ritual handwashing or laundering of clothing, even though this cannot eliminate all possible contaminants in the environment.

Many obsessive compulsive individuals recognize the nature of the obsession, and the futility of the compulsion, but experience great anxiety or tension when attempting to resist them. Over time, the individual will become increasingly unwilling to experience the anxiety, and thus stop resisting the compulsion.

Depression, anxiety, and avoidance of anxiety-provoking situations are commonly seen. Thus in addition to engaging in ritual handwashing, an individual may begin to avoid unfamiliar situations which they may view as providing further risk of contamination.

Etiology and Incidence

Etiology is not well understood, although some people believe this is learned behavior, while others believe that it is another manifestation of biologically generated anxiety. There is often a history of parental psychiatric disorder. It most often occurs in young adults and may be precipitated by stressful events (Goodwin, Guze, & Robins, 1969).

Welner and colleagues (1976) found several different presenting pictures for obsessive compulsive disorder among hospitalized inpatients. These ranged from uncomplicated obsessive compulsive disorder, sometimes with phobias or anxiety attacks, to obsessive compulsive disorder with depression (the most common picture), to obsessive compulsive disorder with psychosis or anorexia nervosa. This categorization is important to considerations of treatment, prognosis, and function.

The disorder in its most severe form is rare, but it appears that many individuals have mild forms of obsessive compulsive disorder. Rasmussen and Eisen (1992) have suggested that obsessive compulsive disorder is substantially underdiagnosed because of shame on the part of the individual, as well as lack of awareness on the part of health care providers. An example they provide is of an individual presenting to a dermatologist with a skin rash, which is not recognized as being the result of excessive washing in a compulsive effort to remove germs.

Prognosis

Among children, obsessive compulsive disorder seems to be chronic. For adults, the course is variable (Rasmussen & Eisen, 1992). Some do quite well, eventually returning to normal function. In others, it may be constant and chronic. The course of recovery is typically marked by exacerbations and remissions.

Implications for Function and Treatment

Depending on the compulsion, function may not be impaired, or may be severely impaired. Many individuals have some ritualistic, almost superstitious, behavior which is not disruptive (e.g., wearing a particular set of clothing when taking a test, or checking the door lock exactly seven times before leaving home). However, in some cases, the compulsion may become the central focus of life (as in the case of a individual who must wash clothing 13 times before wearing it). Some of these individuals may be unable to maintain jobs, social relationships, or have any activity other than the compulsion. This is true in spite of the individual's recognition of the disabling nature of the compulsion.

Obsessive compulsiveness may lead to social isolation, including a tendency to remain single (Goodwin et al., 1969). Many of the fears of these individuals do not materialize, however. They are, for example, not likely to commit suicide, engage in criminal behavior, or become addicted to drugs even though these are common obsessional worries. While the incidence of suicide and drug abuse is higher in these individuals than in the general population, neither is frequent.

Treatment involves the use of anti-anxiety or antidepressant drugs and behavior therapy (Rasmussen & Eisen, 1992). In some cases, treatment is highly effective, but this is not a consistent outcome. The disorder is considered difficult to treat (Davis & Gelder, 1991), although O'Sullivan and Marks (1991) report at least some improvement in 50% to 75% of cases.

Post-Traumatic Stress Disorder (PTSD)

The emergence of this disorder always follows an event which was a major life stress, one which must be more severe and unusual than those found in everyday life. Distress following a divorce would not be considered PTSD, while distress following a life-threatening fire might. The trauma may involve threat to one's life or the lives of one's family, destruction of one's home, victimization during a crime, or seeing someone else severely injured or killed. The trauma may be something that occurs only to the individual, as in cases of sexual or physical abuse in children, or to groups of individuals, e.g., holocaust survivors. In fact, PTSD was identified following the Vietnam war, as a result of the large numbers of combat veterans who had extreme difficulty readapting to civilian life. It should be noted, however, that the syndrome certainly existed prior to this time, for example, as "shell shock" during World War I. World War II veterans who were prisoners of war showed signs of psychological distress long after the event (Tennant, Goulston, & Dent, 1986).

The trauma is usually accompanied by extreme feelings of terror and helplessness, and a primary characteristic of PTSD is a re-experiencing of both the event and these feelings, which are recurrent and intrusive. The individual may have bad dreams, or find these feelings welling up at unpredictable times and in unpredictable places. As this occurs, the individual begins to avoid the situations which seem to stimulate it, or to develop a diminished ability to respond to the world as a mechanism for avoiding the unpleasant emotions.

Individuals who have this disorder have disturbed sleep, exaggerated startle reflexes, poor concentration, and extreme irritability often accompanied by aggression. It frequently occurs in conjunction with depression or anxiety.

Etiology and Incidence

A traumatically stressful event is a necessary precondition to the emergence of this disorder. It is not clear, however, why some individuals are susceptible while others who have similar experiences may not develop PTSD. Not all war veterans develop PTSD (Murray, 1992), for example (although most report some change in outlook as a result of their experiences). There has been some speculation that individuals who develop the disorder had pre-existing psychopathology (Choy & DeBosset, 1992; Keane & Wolfe, 1990), but this is not well established. PTSD may emerge immediately after the trauma, or after a period of months or years.

As the disorder has gained wider attention, the numbers of individuals diagnosed with PTSD has increased dramatically, and it is now considered relatively common. It is estimated that 85% of holocaust survivors and 30% of auto accident and crime victims have PTSD (Choy & DeBosset, 1992).

Prognosis

Because this disorder has been identified so recently, prognosis is not well known. It appears that some individuals have a relatively time limited disorder, while others develop chronic symptoms. By definition, it must last at least 1 month, but may persist for long periods of time. World War II prisoners of war showed high levels of depression 40 years after the war (Tennant et al., 1986).

Good prognosis is predicted by healthy premorbid function, less severe and briefer trauma, and good social support according to some reports (Choy & DeBosset, 1992). There is some dispute on this subject, though, with other researchers reporting that PTSD emerges unpredictably (Resnick, 1993).

Implications for Function and Treatment

Depending on the severity of the disorder, function may be minimally or severely impaired. Some individuals continue to hold jobs and maintain social and avocational activities. It should be noted that a defining characteristic of PTSD is the avoidance of any stimulus that might cause the individual to remember the event. If it occurred in a place that is difficult to avoid, it may become quite disabling. Similarly, some individuals find that the re-experience of the event is frequent, and that the accompanying fears are severe, leading to significant disability.

Where the trauma has been severe and prolonged, rage, depression, and humiliation may persist for years (Herman, 1992). For example, abused children may show signs of trauma throughout adulthood.

Effective treatment is not well understood, although it appears that group therapy, particularly where the individual can talk with others who have had similar experiences, may be of value. Anti-anxiety or antidepressant medication maybe employed, although one of the concerns related to the disorder is the possible emergence of a substance abuse disorder as the individual seeks to relieve tension.

In children, where cases of sexual or physical abuse may be involved, remediation of the situation that led to the disorder is an important component of treatment. The abuser must be treated or the child removed from his or her presence, sometimes by removal from the family.

Special note must be made of the frequent occurrence of PTSD in cases of abused children (Herman, 1992), child sexual abuse (Cole & Putnam, 1992; Rowan & Foy, 1992), rape (Resnick, 1993), and spousal abuse (Woods & Campbell, 1993). These are common occurrences in our society, and therapists must be sensitive to the possibility that observed psychiatric symptoms are a consequence of these events.

Implications for Occupational Therapy

Occupational therapists employ a variety of approaches in working with individuals with anxiety disorders. Several goals are prominent. First, an effort may be made to encourage relaxation, either by diverting attention or through relaxation training. The therapist might, for example, help the individual identify a pleasurable activity that requires attention (writing a poem, playing chess). This approach requires that the therapist be sensitive to the possibility that such activity could increase anxiety for some people.

Activities which require gross motor action to the point of fatigue may also promote relaxation, as will relaxation training. Once the client is relaxed, it may be possible to draw this to the individual's attention so he or she knows what it feels like.

Alternatively, it may be possible to use this relaxed state as a component of a systematic desensitization program. The relaxing activity can be paired with anxiety-provoking stimuli until relaxation can be maintained.

A more controversial approach is flooding, where the individual is confronted repeatedly with the anxiety-provoking stimulus until the anxiety response is exhausted.

For individuals with PTSD, opportunities to express emotion can be valuable. These individuals often benefit from talking with others who have had the experience, and from nonverbal expressive activities. One such client, a rape victim, progressed over time from drawing horrible monsters in stormy skies to drawing pleasant pastoral scenes. She found the activity both relaxing and cathartic.

As anxiety is resolved, attention must be paid to substituting new activities which are satisfying. An agoraphobic who is increasingly able to leave the house must find new and enjoyable ways to spend time formerly spent worrying. Individuals may need help re-establishing social ties, work activities, or leisure pursuits.

Generalized Anxiety Disorder

This disorder is characterized by a generalized state of anxiety or worry in the absence of specific reason to do so. The individual may worry excessively about the state of his or her health, or about finances, when there is no realistic basis for the concern. The diagnosis is not made if substance abuse or depression might cause the anxiety, although mild depressive symptoms may be present. This is usually a chronic disorder, although any functional impairment is mild. It is not unusual for secondary depression to occur, and individuals with this pair of disorders have a more severe and chronic course (Coryell & Winokur, 1982) (Figure 8-2).

Figure 8-2. Anxiety Disorders: Symptoms and Deficits.

Disorder	Symptoms	Functional Deficits
Panic disorder	1. Panic attacks	Work, leisure, ADL during attacks
	2. Attacks include feelings of panic, sweating, dizziness, nausea, chest pain, intense fear	Fear of attack may impact on any function
Agoraphobia	1. Fear of being in situations in which escape is not possible	May be mild-severe; if mild, often no impairment
	2. Avoidance of such situations	If severe, global impairment

Figure 8-2. Anxiety Disorders (continued).

Disorder	Symptoms	Functional Deficits
Specific phobia	1. Intense fear of specific stimulus 2. Avoidance of stimulus	Dependent on stimulus, may not limit or may limit any sphere
Obsessive compulsive disorder	1. Obsessions—intrusive ideas which may be distressing, cannot be suppressed, but are recognized as only ideas (i.e., *not* delusions) 2. Compulsions—repetitive purposeful actions intended to neutralize upsetting aspects of obsessions 3. Obsessions and compulsions cause distress	May be mild-severe Work, leisure, social ADL/IADL
Post-Traumatic Stress Disorder (PTSD)	1. Experience outside the normal range of experience which is distressing 2. Recurrent distressing recollection/dreams about the event 3. Avoidance of stimuli related to the event 4. Insomnia, irritability 5. Physiological signs of fear 6. Minimum 1 month duration	May be mild-marked/most typical social, work, leisure

References

Agras, W. S. (1993). The diagnosis and treatment of panic disorder. *Annual Review of Medicine, 44,* 39-51.

American Psychiatric Association (1994). *Diagnostic and Statistical Manual of Mental Disorders* (4th ed.). Washington, DC: Author.

Bernstein, G. A., & Borchardt, C. M. (1991). Anxiety disorders of childhood and adolescence: A critical review. *Journal of the American Academy of Child and Adolescent Psychiatry, 30,* 519-532.

Boulenger, J. P., & Lavallee, Y. J. (1993). Mixed anxiety and depression: Diagnostic issues. *Journal of Clinical Psychiatry, 54,* 3-8.

Brown, T. A., & Barlow, D. H. (1992). Comorbidity among anxiety disorders: Implications for treatment and DSM-IV. *Journal of Consulting and Clinical Psychology, 60,* 835-844.

Chapman, T. F., Fyer, A. J., Mannuzza, S., & Klein, D. F. (1993). A comparison of treated and untreated simple phobia. *American Journal of Psychiatry, 150,* 816-818.

Choy, T., & DeBosset, F. (1992). Post-traumatic stress disorder: An overview. *Canadian Journal of Psychiatry, 37,* 578-583.

Cole, P. M., & Putnam, F. W. (1992). Effect of incest on self and social functioning: A developmental psychopathology perspective. *Journal of Consulting and Clinical Psychology, 60,* 174-184.

Coryell, W., Noyes, R., & Clancy, J. (1982). Excess mortality in panic disorders. *Archives of General Psychiatry, 39,* 701-703.

Coryell, W., & Winokur, G. (1982). Course and outcome. In E. S. Paykel (Ed.), *Handbook of affective disorders.* New York: Guilford Press.

Dadds, M. R., Heard, P. M., & Rapee, R. M. (1992). The role of family intervention in the treatment of child anxiety disorders: Some preliminary findings. *Behavior Change, 9,* 171-177.

Davis, J. D. R., & Gelder, M. (1991). Long-term management of anxiety states. *International Review of Psychiatry, 3,* 5-17.

Franklin, J. A. (1991). Agoraphobia. *International Review of Psychiatry, 3,* 151-162.

Goodwin, E. W., Guze, S. B., & Robins, E. (1969). Follow-up studies in obsessional neurosis. *Archives of General Psychiatry, 20,* 182-187.

Herman, J. L. (1992). Complex PTSD: A syndrome in survivors of prolonged and repeated trauma. *Journal of Traumatic Stress, 5,* 377-391.

Hoffart, A. (1993). Cognitive treatments of agoraphobia: A critical evaluation of theoretical basis outcome evidence. *Journal of Anxiety Disorders, 7,* 75-91.

Keane, T. M., & Wolfe, J. (1990). Comorbidity in post-traumatic stress disorder: An analysis of community and clinical studies. *Journal of Applied Social Psychology, 20,* 1776-1788.

Keller, M. B., Lavori, P. W., Wunder, J., Beardslee, W. R., Schwartz, C. E., & Roth, J. (1992). Chronic course of anxiety disorders in children and adolescents. *Journal of the American Academy of Child and Adolescent Psychiatry, 31,* 595-599.

Laberge, B., Gauthier, J., Cote, G., Plamondon, J., & Cormier, H. J. (1992). The treatment of coexisting panic and depression: A review of the literature. *Journal of Anxiety Disorders, 6,* 169-180.

Maddock, R. J., & Blacker, K. H. (1991). Response to treatment in panic disorder with associated depression. *Psychopathology, 24,* 1-6.

Mattick, R. P., Andrews, G., Hadzi-Pavlovic, D., & Christensen, H. (1990). Treatment of panic and agoraphobia: An integrative review. *The Journal of Nervous and Mental Disease, 178,* 567-576.

Murray, J. B. (1992). Posttraumatic stress disorder: A review. *Genetic, Social, and General Psychology Monographs, 118,* 313-338.

Nemiah, J. C. (1988). Psychoneurotic disorders. In A. M. Nicholi (Ed.), *The new Harvard guide to psychiatry* (pp. 234-258). Cambridge, MA: Belknap Press.

Nutt, D., & Lawson, C. (1992). Panic attacks: A neurochemical overview of models and mechanisms. *British Journal of Psychiatry, 160,* 165-178.

Ost, L. (1985). Ways of acquiring phobias and outcome of behavioral treatment. *Behavioral Research and Therapy, 23,* 683-689.

O'Sullivan, G., & Marks, I. (1991). Follow-up studies of behavioral treatment of phobic and obsessive compulsive neuroses. *Psychiatric Annals, 21,* 368-373.

Rapee, R. M. (1991). Panic disorder. *International Review of Psychiatry, 3,* 141-149.

Rasmussen, S. A., & Eisen, J. L. (1992). The epidemiology and differential diagnosis of obsessive compulsive disorder. *Journal of Clinical Psychiatry, 53,* 4-10.

Redmond, D. E., Jr., & Huang, Y. H. (1979). New evidence for a locus coeruleus-norepinephrine connection with anxiety. *Life Sciences, 25,* 2149-2162.

Reiss, S. (1991). Expectancy model of fear, anxiety, and panic. *Clinical Psychology Review, 11,* 141-153.

Resnick, P. A. (1993). The psychological impact of rape. *Journal of Interpersonal Violence, 8,* 223-255.

Rowan, A. B., & Foy, D. W. (1993). Post-traumatic stress disorder in child sexual abuse survivors: A literature review. *Journal of Traumatic Stress, 6,* 3-20.

Strauss, C. C., & Last, C. G. (1993). Social and simple phobias in children. *Journal of Anxiety Disorders, 7,* 141-152.

Tennant, C. C., Goulston, K. J., & Dent, O. F. (1986). The psychological effects of being a prisoner of war: Forty years after release. *American Journal of Psychiatry, 143,* 618-621.

Welner, A., Reich, T., Robins, E., et al., (1976). Obsessive-compulsive neurosis: Record, follow-up, and family studies. I. Inpatient record study. *Comprehensive Psychiatry, 17,* 527-539.

Woods, S. J., & Campbell, J. C. (1993). Posttraumatic stress in battered women: Does the diagnosis fit? *Mental Health Nursing, 14,* 173-186.

Chapter 9
Personality Disorders

These diagnoses are identified as Axis II labels according to the DSM-IV schema. It may be recalled that this axis is specifically for disorders that characterize lifelong patterns of adaptation; this is characteristic of personality disorders. In general they are less severe than Axis I diagnoses (with the exceptions of borderline, antisocial, and possibly schizotypal personality disorders), but they are also generally much longer lasting, with no periods of remission.

The personality disorders are also among the more controversial diagnoses for a number of reasons (Widiger, 1991). First, reliability is a concern. To some extent this is because they represent exaggerations of traits evident in people without psychiatric disturbance. In addition, lifelong patterns are difficult to clearly establish in clinical settings. As Gunderson (1988) points out,

> Traits are identifiable as disorders only when they become so prominent and rigid as to cause dysfunction (p. 337).

Some of the diagnostic criteria for these disorders have been described as unclear or overlapping (Widiger, 1991) and there is inconsistency about labeling of some disorders. For example, schizotypal personality is presumably a mild, nonpsychotic relative of schizophrenia and is found in the personality disorder section. Dysthymic disorder, which seems to be at a similar point on the affective disorder continuum (i.e., a mild, nonpsychotic relative of major depression), is an Axis I diagnosis.

Adding to the dilemma presented by these diagnoses, they are most often self-diagnosing, i.e., they are labeled only if the individual comes for help (or is sent by someone else). Many individuals who would otherwise be diagnosed never feel sufficiently bad or behave peculiarly enough to enter therapy. In some instances, it is the development of a co-existing Axis I disorder, most typically an affective or anxiety disorder, that brings these individuals into treatment.

The personality disorders typify the kinds of issues that were considered in revising the DSM. Several new personality disorders, which appeared in the appendices of DSM-III-R (APA, 1987), were considered for inclusion among the personality disorders. These included self-defeating personality disorder (SDPD) (Fiester, 1991), sadistic personality disorder (SPD), (Fiester & Gay, 1991) and depressive personality disorder (Phillips, Hirschfeld, Shea, & Gunderson, 1993). Arguments for and against each focused on reports of clinicians and research evidence of validity and reliability, particularly issues of overlap with other personality disorders. Some of the arguments for and against reflected concerns about potential for abuse of labels, as well as the scientific data. For example, there was concern that a diagnosis of SDPD might be used to "blame the victim" in abusive relationships (Fiester, 1991) and SPD to excuse the perpetrator (Fiester & Gay, 1991).

In another instance, a personality disorder found in DSM-III-R was considered for elimination (Millon, 1993). Passive-aggressive personality disorder was the most controversial personality disorder in that edition, because of its reliance on a single trait as a diagnostic marker.

Ultimately, depressive personality disorder and passive-aggressive personality disorder were placed in the appendices, among the list of disorders requiring further research. SDPD and SPD were both eliminated entirely.

DSM-IV (APA, 1994) identifies three clusters of personality disorders, grouped according to common symptomatology. Paranoid, Schizoid, and Schizotypal personality disorders (cluster A) are characterized by odd or peculiar behavior. Cluster B, Antisocial, Borderline, Histrionic, and Narcissistic personality disorders, present with flamboyant or dramatic behavior. The third category, cluster C, is characterized primarily by anxiety or fear. The personality disorders will be grouped in this fashion for discussion here (Figure 9-1). It should be recognized, however, that the clusters are somewhat subjective (Frances, 1980). Occupational therapy intervention will be discussed at the end of the chapter.

Figure 9-1. Personality Disorders.

Cluster A	Cluster B	Cluster C
Paranoid Schizoid Schizotypal	Antisocial Borderline Histrionic Narcissistic	Avoidant Dependent Obsessive Compulsive

Paranoid Personality Disorder

This disorder is identified by the individual's tendency to experience a sense of being threatened or persecuted. Associates (friends are few) and coworkers will be suspected of intent to harm the individual, and jealousy and suspicion characterize most relationships. This leads to withdrawn, suspicious, and frequently hostile behavior on the part of the individual (Gunderson, 1988). The personality disorder is less severe than paranoid schizophrenia, and is characterized more by misinterpretation of input rather than by outright delusions. For example, someone who has a paranoid personality disorder may interpret a minor reprimand from a boss as "he's never liked me; he wants to fire me; everyone here hates me." Someone with paranoid schizophrenia might interpret the same reprimand as part of a CIA/Mafia plan to kill him.

Typically such individuals are argumentative, withdrawn, with little sense of humor and a "chip on their shoulders." They look for slights and frequently find them, tend to bear grudges, and may be litigious. They are hypercritical of others, while accepting criticism of themselves poorly. They tend to be excessively self-sufficient and quite egocentric. One such individual had constant trouble at work because he routinely violated company rules, reasoning that they had been instituted only to harass him.

Etiology and Incidence

The etiology of this personality disorder is not clear (Widiger, 1991). Incidence is estimated at .5% to 2.5% of the general population (APA, 1994). One explanation that has been advanced about its origin is that this is a learned pattern of behavior. Others feel that it is the result of some sort of CNS disturbance. No clear risk factors have been identified (Bernstein, Useda, & Siever, 1993), and there is little evidence of a familial link (Dahl, 1993).

Implications for Function and Treatment

As can be imagined, this behavior pattern creates considerable difficulty for these individuals. The primary problem area is interpersonal relationships, both social and work. The suspiciousness and irritability of these individuals, coupled with their tendency to believe others are plotting against them makes for troubled interactions, often resulting in lost jobs, divorce, and so on. In particular, relationships with authority figures tend to be problematic.

Other skills and functions remain largely intact. Motor and sensory skills, sensory integration, and cognition are, for the most part unaffected, except in those situations where the individual may believe he or she hears others talking about him or her. ADL, IADL, and work functions other than relationships with coworkers are maintained at acceptable levels, and these individuals may certainly maintain some leisure activities, mostly solitary. Treatment, through behavior modification, medication, education, or psychotherapy is not notably successful with these individuals. Their personality pattern tends to be intractable, although some individuals can be taught how to interact more effectively with others.

Schizoid Personality Disorder

This is the oldest and best established of the personality disorder categories (Gunderson, 1988). It is defined by an absence or indifference to social activity and a restricted range of emotion (Kalus, Bernstein, & Siever, 1993). These are individuals often identified as "loners" who have no interest in friendships, appear aloof and withdrawn, and demonstrate little emotion. They may seem self absorbed and vague. One such woman rarely spoke to coworkers, but often had what others described as a "peculiar smile" on her face.

Etiology and Incidence

The cause of schizoid personality disorder is not well established. As with paranoid personality, the major theories about its emergence are 1) that it is a learned pattern of behavior, or 2) that it is due to some sort of CNS dysfunction. The latter explanation seems more likely. The disorder is more common in men, and incidence is estimated at 1% to 2% of the general population (Widiger, 1991). This is a rough estimate at best, since these individuals are unlikely to seek treatment (Kalus et al., 1993).

Implications for Function and Treatment

Again, the primary functional impairment is in the area of social relationships. Unlike paranoid personalities, however, these individuals tend to display little aggression, making work situations easier to maintain. Such people do well in jobs which require little social interaction (Gunderson, 1988). They have few social relationships, however, and rarely marry or have close friends. Akhtar (1987) identifies deficits in six areas of psychosocial functioning: self-concept, interpersonal relations, social adaptation, ethics, standards and ideals, love and sexuality, and cognitive style. Other skills and functions are unimpaired, meaning that these individuals are functional, but lead lives restricted by the absence of meaningful friendships. The disorder persists throughout life, though some changes in specific characteristics may occur (e.g., the symptoms may come to more closely mirror narcissistic personality) (Akhtar, 1987).

When such individuals come into treatment, it is often because they are depressed about their isolation. Social skills training may provide a mechanism for helping them to establish relationships, although their interactions tend to remain stilted, awkward, or distant. Psychotherapy is sometimes attempted.

Schizotypal Personality Disorder

Schizotypal personalities have peculiar thought patterns, behaviors, and appearance (Siever, Bernstein, & Silverman, 1991). This may include bizarre fantasies, beliefs about special senses or powers, or odd patterns of speaking. Typically, odd perceptual experiences are present as well. Affect is either inappropriate or flat and social isolation is common. It is differentiated from schizophrenia largely by matter of degree; the symptoms are not severe enough to fit the criteria for schizophrenia, although the disorders are related (McGlashan, 1986). Such individuals are often described by neighbors as strange and as loners. If they have friends, their friends are often rather odd, too.

Etiology and Incidence

As with the other personality disorders in this cluster, etiology is unclear, but suspected to be the result of either CNS dysfunction or learning. Incidence is unknown, although the disorder is more common in family members of individuals who are schizophrenic (Siever et al., 1991). The diagnostic category is relatively new, so data are sparse, but there is speculation that this disorder may be an attenuated form of schizophrenia (Kotsaftis & Neale, 1993).

Implications for Function and Treatment

It is unclear whether there is some dysfunction at the skill level. It is possible that CNS function is impaired, particularly ability to accurately process sensory input. Research has identified, for example, that smooth pursuit eye movement is impaired in these individuals (Siever, Coursey, Alterman, Buchsbaum, & Murphy, 1984). In addition, identification of characteristic cognitive-perceptual deficits have been helpful in making the diagnosis (Widiger, Frances, & Trull, 1987). These deficits may be the cause of some of the peculiar ideas held by these individuals.

At the performance level, function is distinctly impaired. Social function, in particular, is poor. Odd ideas held by these individuals make it difficult for others to understand them. The individual may avoid others because of discomfort in social situations. They appear to misperceive the social environment (Raulin & Henderson, 1987). Vocational function is impaired to the extent that social skills are required to do a job. As with schizoid personalities, these individuals may do best at jobs which require little social interaction. Actual work performance may also be poor, however, lending credence to the speculation that there is some underlying CNS or cognitive dysfunction. ADL performance is impaired; these individuals tend to be unkempt or to dress peculiarly.

Efforts at intervention are similar to those used for other disorders in this cluster, including medication, skill training, behavioral interventions, and verbal therapies.

Antisocial Personality

Of all the personality disorders, this is most likely to be brought to the attention of health care professionals by someone other than the individual. The individual himself (this diagnosis is much more common in males) tends not to be concerned about the behavior problems which create serious problems for others. This is also the personality disorder with the clearest (and most cumbersome) diagnostic criteria (Widiger, 1992), making its diagnosis more clear-cut than many of the others.

The diagnosis is made in individuals who are at least 18 years old prior to this a conduct disorder would be diagnosed, since antisocial personality is characterized by a lengthy pattern of behavior. The individual will have a pattern of antisocial behavior prior to age 15, e.g., truancy, fighting, cruelty to animals or people, stealing, and so on. In addition this behavior will continue after age 15, with the addition of problems in work settings (loss of jobs, unemployment, absence from work), illegal activity, aggressiveness, impulsivity, lying, recklessness, and inability to function responsibly in significant relationships, e.g., parenting. A significant characteristic is the lack of remorse for any of these behaviors.

It is important to distinguish antisocial personality from other disorders, especially mania, since many behaviors typical of antisocial personality also occur during manic episodes. The long standing pattern of antisocial behavior makes it noticeably different, as does the absence of periods of remission. It should also be recognized that while these individuals are prone to criminal behavior, this is a unique characteristic among psychiatric diagnoses. There is a common misperception that individuals with psychiatric disorders are prone to criminal behavior. In reality this is untrue except for those with antisocial personality disorders (Tepelin, 1985).

Etiology and Incidence

Among the beliefs about the origin of antisocial personality is the theory that it is learned behavior, the result of overprotective or inconsistent parenting which does not allow the individual to learn that actions have consequences.

Another theory is that cognitive and moral development are arrested at the 7 to 11-year-old age level, as these individuals show moral reasoning of this developmental level (Reid, 1985). There is also speculation about a biochemical etiology, supported by research showing neurotransmitter alterations, and by family research suggesting genetic links (Dahl, 1993). None of the research is definitive. This disorder is more common in men, and is found in 2% to 3% of the general population (APA, 1994). There is some concern that the disorder is overdiagnosed in criminal justice settings and underdiagnosed elsewhere (Widiger, 1992). In addition, this disorder has an extremely high rate of comorbidity with substance abuse (Widiger & Corbitt, 1993).

Implications for Function and Treatment

There has been some speculation that antisocial individuals have sensory impairments. Some research suggests that a large percentage of the prison population shows signs of learning disabilities linked to sensory processing problems, but this remains unproven. Other research is conflicting: Gorenstein (1982) found evidence of deficits in cognitive tasks, specifically frontal lobe, however Hare's (1984) findings refute this.

Performance is impaired primarily in social and work spheres. ADL is intact with the exception of management of finances. Typically money is a serious problem, with stealing a common solution. Social relationships are impaired by the lack of depth and conscience displayed by these individuals. They are unable, for example, to maintain monogamous relationships, and are unable to consider the feelings of others. Frances (1980) suggested that this personality disorder would be better clarified if ability to experience loyalty, anxiety, and guilt were identified as factors to rule out the diagnosis, since prognosis is more favorable for those who have these emotions. One individual who was imprisoned for armed robbery and murder explained that he had to kill the security guard because the guard got in the way and therefore deserved to die. The prognosis for this individual, clearly, was poor.

In work situations, the belligerence and aggressiveness of these individuals is problematic. They may be quite able to perform the tasks required, but are not able to maintain acceptable relationships with coworkers and supervisors. They misinterpret some social situations, responding with excessive anxiety or anger (Sterling & Edelman, 1988). One man, during his short tenure on a construction job, routinely punched new employees just to "let them know who the real boss is!"

In general, these individuals do not respond well to treatment. Those who have a diagnosis of depression as well do better (Woody, McLellan, Luborsky, & O'Brien, 1985), lending support to Frances's (1980) assertion that individuals who experience guilt represent a specific subset. Psychotherapy and inpatient and outpatient milieu therapy have all been shown to have some value. Milieu settings are usually structured to assure that actions do have consequences, thereby, at least theoretically, remediating previous faulty learning. Psychotropic medications do not seem beneficial (Reid, 1985).

Borderline Personality

The diagnosis of borderline personality disorder (BPD) has become increasingly common in the last decade, a source of dispute, since some do not believe it exists as a clinical entity (Gunderson, Zanarini, & Kisiel, 1991). Recent research suggests a significant overlap with other personality disorders, especially histrionic personality disorder (Gunderson, Zanarini et al., 1991). BPD is marked by instability of mood, relationships, and self-image, usually appearing during early adulthood. Relationships and affect tend to be unstable. Affect may also be inappropriate, in particular reflected by poor control of anger. Suicidal ideation and self-mutilation may also occur, and these individuals tend to be quite impulsive. They fear abandonment and have self-image problems characterized by uncertainty about sexual orientation, long-term goals, or values. It is common to find depression and/or substance abuse co-existing in these individuals, and to find a family history of alcoholism (Loranger & Tullis, 1985). A distinguishing characteristic, added in DSM-IV (APA, 1994) to help clarify diagnosis, is the occurrence of transient psychotic-like or dissociative episodes (Gunderson, Zanarini et al., 1991).

One borderline client had achieved a relatively stable work situation, but found herself in great difficulty with social life. Her boyfriends, all short term, routinely abandoned her and her roommates moved out. Much of this was due to the extreme instability of her behavior toward them. She would be quite enamored and invested, bring daily gifts, and write long letters about how close she felt to them. Within hours or days of this behavior she would write angry spiteful letters, splatter their clothes with ink, and scream obscenities at them.

Etiology and Incidence

Since the disorder is more common in families in which there is a history of alcoholism (Loranger & Tullis, 1985), it is possible that a genetic component exists. However, it is also possible that borderline behaviors are learned from these dysfunctional relatives. The contribution of CNS dysfunction to the emergence of the disorder is not known, although individuals with BPD do have cognitive-perceptual problems (Gunderson, Zanarini et al., 1991). It occurs in about 2% of the population (APA-, 1994).

Implications for Function and Treatment

As with other personality disorders, function seems to be impaired at the level of performance of self-care, work, and leisure tasks as opposed to motor, sensory, and other skills. There is no persuasive evidence to suggest abnormalities in sensory processing or other CNS function. However, vocational and social function are markedly impaired. Relationships tend to be unstable with these individuals fluctuating wildly between excessive involvement with others and devaluation of friends. These relationship difficulties are the most consistent diagnostic criteria (Modestin, 1987). Difficulty handling anger, and impulsiveness magnify interpersonal difficulties, as does a feeling of depersonalization which arises for many individuals with borderline personality disorder. Similar problems affect work. However, work problems are not solely the result of interpersonal difficulties. Since these individuals have problems identifying and maintaining a set of values and goals, they are unable to select and pursue career goals. Work history is unstable as they move from job to job, or miss work because of substance abuse or suicide gestures.

ADL is unimpaired at a basic level, i.e., these individuals are able to dress, maintain hygiene, cook, eat, and so on. However, their impulsivity may lead them to ignore their ADL needs, to manage money poorly, drive recklessly, and so on. A particular issue with borderline personality is the tendency to "split," to see him or herself and others as "all good" or "all bad" and to fluctuate rapidly between these poles (Goodman, 1983). These rapid shifts in attitude impact both on self-concept and on relationships with others.

Treatments recommended include long-term psychotherapy (Walding & Gunderson, 1987). In addition, a combination of short-term hospitalization, family education, and low dose neuroleptics seems effective. Long-term milieu hospitalization has been reported effective, as well (Tucker, Bauer, Wagner, Harlam, & Shey, 1987). Prognosis is fair. In one study, 75% of borderline personality disorder patients followed for an average of 15 years were no longer diagnosable and showed functional improvement (Paris, Brown, & Nowlis, 1987). However, there was also a high risk for completed suicide.

Histrionic Personality Disorder

Individuals with histrionic personality disorder (HPD) demonstrate excessive emotionality or theatricality and attention-seeking behavior. They tend to need a great deal of approval or reassurance, which they may seek by being sexually seductive, excessively concerned with physical attractiveness, and attempting to be the center of attention in all situations. Self-centeredness is extreme, and emotions are exaggerated. At the same time, emotions shift rapidly and are quite shallow. These individuals have low thresholds for frustration, and are unable to delay gratification. It has been suggested that they fear being unlovable and seek attention to reassure themselves that this is not so (Gunderson, 1988).

Etiology and Incidence

This is almost certainly a learned pattern of behavior, although some weak support for a family link for women with HPD has been reported (Goodwin & Guze, 1989). Problem relationships with family members have been implicated as fostering the insecurity which is notable in these individuals. Prevalence is unknown.

Implications for Function and Treatment

Skills do not appear impaired in histrionic personalities. Cognition, sensory, and perceptual skills are intact. This disorder impairs function at the performance level, specifically in social situations. Friendships are superficial and focused on the individual. People with HPD are unable to respond with genuine emotion to the needs of others. They romanticize relationships, and respond with excessive disappointment to disagreements. One such young woman arrived at work to announce loudly and tearfully that she would have to "end it all" because her boyfriend had to cancel a date because he had the flu.

Such individuals are unpleasant to be around, but they are typically able to function at work. They may, however, have problems with coworkers or supervisors, and are prone to quit unpredictably in fits of pique, or when they become bored. ADL is usually not impaired; in fact such individuals may spend a great deal of time on hygiene and grooming in order to be attractive to others. They often dress quite seductively, then act puzzled when others respond to the apparent seduction.

Some of these individuals are able to learn new behaviors, often through behavior modification, and to develop insight into their behavior through psychotherapy. Making the changes tends to be quite difficult, however, and most often, when they seek treatment, these individuals want a "quick fix" for an immediate crisis, rather than any major change in their attitudes or behaviors. One woman came into therapy because her father had "disowned" her and she was "now an orphan." It turned out he had stopped her allowance when, at age 25, she got a job. Her wish for therapy was that the therapist call her father and tell him to resume the allowance.

Narcissistic Personality Disorder

Grandiosity is the defining feature of this disorder (APA, 1994). This is accompanied by a lack of empathy for others and excessive need for attention. Individuals with narcissistic personality disorder (NPD) identify themselves as special, exaggerate accomplishments, and feel entitled to recognition and special attention. However, these feelings fluctuate with feelings of insecurity and unworthiness. Self-esteem is poor, but masked by expressions of superiority. There is focus on fantasies of power and success, accompanied by feelings of envy for those who have accomplished more.

Etiology and Incidence

Like histrionic personality disorder, this appears to be a learned pattern of adaptation, the result of a disordered family life. These individuals may get conflicting messages from parents, feel undervalued, and, as a result, come to undervalue themselves. At the same time, their grandiosity is an attempt to win approval that may not have been forthcoming in their homes. Incidence is unknown.

NPD is not well researched, given that it was added to the diagnostic list only in DSM-III (Gunderson, Ronningstam, & Smith, 1991). Incidence is estimated at less than 1% of the general population (APA, 1994).

Implications for Function and Treatment

This disorder does not appear to cause dysfunction at the skill level. Sensation, cognition, and motor function are intact. Primary dysfunction is noted in interpersonal relationships. These individuals are self-centered and unable to display empathy for others, making friendships difficult for them. They charm others briefly, until their disregard for others' feelings becomes obvious. Thus, any relationships tend to be brief and often contentious. This pattern of relationships is also problematic in work situations where relationships with supervisors may be difficult. In some situations, vocational performance may be unusually good as the individual strives for great success, while in others, performance is poor as the individual becomes resentful of expectations of others. Good performance rarely lasts. One man had a long work history of jobs which lasted 6 months at a stretch. As each began he had "great new plans to save the company." As each ended, he excoriated his coworkers for failing to recognize his "genius." ADL is usually unimpaired, although money management may become an issue. In an attempt to impress others, these individuals may spend to excess.

When these individuals present for treatment, it is usually for depression as a result of their social isolation. It is rare that they are able to develop insight or to change behaviors, as they tend to blame others for their problems and to be impatient with the therapeutic process. In most instances, the depression rather than the personality disorder is the focus of treatment.

Avoidant Personality Disorder

Social discomfort and avoidance of interpersonal relationships is the primary characteristic of this disorder (APA, 1994). Individuals with avoidant personality disorder fear that others will disapprove of them, and, as a result, avoid interaction (Frances & Widiger, 1986).

Etiology and Incidence

This is probably a learned pattern of behavior. It appears to result from poor early experiences with relationships. Incidence is estimated at .5% to 1% of the general population (APA, 1994).

Implications for Function and Treatment

Most function is intact in these individuals at the level of performance, but affected by the inability to form relationships. These individuals work and care for themselves, but have emotionally and socially restricted lives. Skills are unimpaired, with the exception of social skills. Even in this sphere, superficial relationships may be adequate. One client was a university professor who managed brief casual interactions with students, as well as the more formalized classroom relationships. His personal life, however was barren of friends or close family ties; four marriages had ended in divorce because of his inability to sustain close relationships.

As with narcissistic personality disorder, these individuals often seek treatment as a result of depression. Treatment may focus on insight or behavior change, or a combination of the two. Unlike individuals with narcissistic personality disorders, these individuals may be able to make a commitment to treatment and benefit from it.

Dependent Personality Disorder

Individuals with avoidant personality disorder avoid relationships; individuals with dependent personality disorder feel they cannot survive without them. They are dependent and submissive in an attempt to win approval and to avoid abandonment. They have difficulty making decisions and look to others to tell them what to do. As a result, they are unable to successfully initiate activity. They fear being alone.

Etiology and Incidence

As with other disorders in this cluster, this is probably a learned behavioral pattern (Hirschfeld, Shea, & Weise, 1991). It is the most commonly reported personality disorder in clinical settings (APA, 1994). This may be an artifact, given that these individuals may be more likely to seek treatment than others with personality disorders.

Implications for Function and Treatment

Performance is intact in these individuals, although they are limited by their need for approval and advice from others. In social situations, friends are granted excessive control, and in work situations, they are unable to progress because of their inability to take initiative and function independently. One woman refused to buy new clothes without approval from her husband and her mother. Work performance can be compromised by inability to make decisions independently or by excessive need for approval.

Individuals with dependent personality disorder often come into treatment as a result of depression or anxiety which results from fears of abandonment. In some instances, the abandonment is real, as dependent personalities are quite draining to others. This is a difficult disorder to treat, although psychotherapy and behavior modification can be of value in some instances.

Obsessive Compulsive Personality Disorder

This is potentially the most disabling of the cluster C personality disorders, as these individuals are perfectionistic, rigid, and engage in ritualistic behavior. They never feel they have done well enough, and they focus on minor detail, wasting time which could be better spent. Decision making is difficult as these individuals are unable to evaluate choices and act. They are judgmental and moralistic, often quite stingy and have difficulty expressing warmth. It has been theorized that these individuals have an extreme need for acceptance, causing conflicts about autonomy (Salzman, 1980).

Etiology and Incidence

Etiology is not well established. It is possible that the same CNS dysfunction that seems to contribute to obsessive compulsive disorder may also contribute to obsessive compulsive personality disorder, making it simply a less severe manifestation of the same problem. It is also possible that this is a learned problem, or evidence of developmental delay, as many young children demonstrate obsessive compulsive behavior (e.g., "step on a crack, break your mother's back" leads to careful avoidance of cracks in the sidewalk in many 8-year-olds). Most children outgrow these compulsions rather quickly, but there is speculation that these individuals do not for some reason. Prevalence is estimated at 2% in the adult population (APA, 1994).

Implications for Function and Treatment

Primary impairments which result from this disorder are social and vocational. The rigidity and moralistic nature of these individuals makes it difficult for them to form warm relationships. Their perfectionism, difficulty making decisions, and inability to use time well make work performance less than optimal. Task completion, in particular, is problematic. One individual, a bookkeeper, was unable to complete any page that had an erasure, and as a result was unable to complete assigned tasks.

Treatment of the personality disorder is difficult, although most often intervention focuses on depression. These individuals tend to be aware of their behavior and the problems it causes. In some instances, this leads to considerable depression or anxiety.

Implications for Occupational Therapy

Although the manifestations of various personality disorders differ, the underlying issues are similar: 1) inaccurate perceptions of self and others, 2) inadequate social skills, 3) poorly developed personal values and goals, and 4) poor self-esteem. For some, particularly the cluster A disorders, inaccurate perceptions extend to many situations. This cluster may also be characterized by subtle neurological deficits in addition to the faulty learning which has been implicated as an etiological factor for all the personality disorders.

Because of the commonality of issues, some general approaches may be taken by the occupational therapist. Opportunities for group interaction with clear, consistent feedback may be quite valuable. A variety of group/cooperative activities may be helpful, from planning a social event to social skills training. A particular goal for feedback is interpreting accurately what others say and developing empathy. It is fairly characteristic that individuals with personality disorders show little regard for or understanding of the feelings of others, and they must learn to make an active effort to do so. One histrionic client, a young female college student, was quite astonished to learn that other females resented her tendency to flirt with their boyfriends. It had never occurred to her to consider their feelings, even though she felt unhappy about her lack of girlfriends.

Realistic appraisal of self is similarly problematic. Provisions of a range of activities may be useful as a mechanism for exploration and for learning strengths and weaknesses. Both successes and failures must be analyzed. This not only enhances self-awareness, but also is a way to explore values and goals. Activity that builds self-esteem through experiences of success and the appreciation of others may help convince these individuals of their worth. The insecurity tends to be so deep, however, that it is quite problematic to provide them with all the reassurance they need.

The three clusters present with somewhat differing characteristics which must also be addressed (Figure 9-2). Cluster A personality disorders, because of the suspected neurological component, may respond to sensory integrative/ sensory-motor interventions. Cluster B, because of the probability that they reflect deficits in early learning, may benefit from behavioral approaches. For example, a work experience might be structured in the clinic, with reinforcement for desired behaviors.

Cluster C personality disorders may be particularly amenable to social skills training since this is the predominant deficit for these individuals. Behavior modification may be helpful in reducing anxiety for these individuals.

All the personality disorders are, however, somewhat intractable. While change is possible, it requires considerable motivation which is often lacking in these individuals. Even those who are motivated may find change frightening, and will certainly find ingrained habits hard to alter.

Figure 9-2. Personality Disorders: Symptoms and Deficits.

Disorder	Symptoms	Functional Deficits
CLUSTER A Paranoid Personality Disorder	1. Tendency to suspect others, to interpret their actions as hostile	Work, leisure, social
Schizoid	1. Lack of interest in social relationships 2. Restricted emotional range.	Work, leisure, social
Schizotypal	1. Poor relationships 2. Restricted emotional range 3. Odd perceptual experiences 4. Odd appearance, speech 5. Inappropriate effect	Work, leisure, social, ADL/IADL

Figure 9-2. Personality Disorders (continued).

Disorder	Symptoms	Functional Deficits
CLUSTER B Antisocial	1. At least 18 years old 2. Previous conduct disorder 3. At least four types of antisocial behavior (theft, lying, child abuse, etc.) which occur in a persistent pattern 4. Lacks remorse/guilt 5. Inability to sustain relationships	Work, leisure, social, IADL (especially financial)
Borderline	1. Relationships fluctuate between intense involvement and devaluation 2. Impulsiveness, instability 3. Lack of control of anger 4. Suicide gestures or self-mutilation	Work, leisure, social, ADL/IADL
Histrionic	1. Excessive concern with appearance; seductive 2. Excessive need for praise reassurance 3. Self-centered; lack of empathy for others 4. Exaggerated expression of emotion, with rapid mood shifts, shallow emotion 5. Need for constant attention	Work, leisure, social
CLUSTER C Avoidant	1. Discomfort with social relationships 2. Avoidance of social relationships and activities	Social, possibly work and leisure
Dependent	1. Excessively dependent and submissive behavior 2. Fear of abandonment 3. Easily hurt by criticism	Social, possibly work and leisure

References

Akhtar, S. (1987). Schizoid personality disorder: A synthesis of developmental, dynamic, and descriptive features. *American Journal of Psychotherapy, 41,* 449-518.

American Psychiatric Association (1987). *Diagnostic and Statistical Manual on Mental Disorders* (3rd ed. rev.). Washington, DC: Author.

American Psychiatric Association (1994). *Diagnostic and Statistical Manual of Mental Disorders* (4th ed.). Washington, DC: Author.

Bernstein, D. P., Useda, D., & Siever, L.J. (1993). Paranoid personality disorder: Review of the literature and recommendations for DSM-IV. *Journal of Personality Disorders, 7,* 53-62.

Dahl, A. A. (1993). The personality disorders: A critical review of family twin, and adoption studies. *Journal of Personality Disorders, 7,* 86-99.

Fiester, S. J. (1991). Self-defeating personality disorder: A review of data and recommendations for DSM-IV. *Journal of Personality Disorders, 5,* 194-209.

Fiester, S. J., & Gay, M. (1991). Sadistic personality disorder: A review of data and recommendations for DSM-IV. *Journal of Personality Disorders, 5,* 376-385.

Frances, A. (1980). The DSM-III personality disorders section: A commentary. *American Journal of Psychiatry, 137,* 1050-1054.

Frances, A., & Widiger, T. (1986). Avoidant personality. In B. Karasu (Ed.), *Treatment of psychiatric disorders.* Washington, DC: American Psychiatric Press.

Goodman, G. B. (1983). Occupational therapy treatment: Interventions with borderline patients. *Occupational Therapy in Mental Health, 3,* 19-32.

Goodwin, D., & Guze, S. (1989). *Psychiatric diagnosis.* New York: Oxford University Press.

Gorenstein, E. E. (1982). Frontal lobe functions in psychopath. *Journal of Abnormal Psychology, 91,* 368-379.

Gunderson, J. C. (1988). Personality disorders. In A. M. Nicholi (Ed.), *The new Harvard guide to psychiatry* (pp. 337-357). Cambridge, MA: Belknap Press.

Gunderson, J. G., Ronningstam, E., & Smith, L. E. (1991). Narcissistic personality disorder: A review of data on DSM-III-R descriptions. *Journal of Personality Disorders, 5,* 167-177.

Gunderson, J. G., Zanarini, M. C., & Kisiel, C. L. (1991). Borderline personality disorder: A review of data on DSM-III-R descriptions. *Journal of Personality Disorders, 5,* 340-352.

Hare, R. D. (1984). Performance of psychopaths on cognitive tasks related to frontal lobe function. *Journal of Abnormal Psychology, 93,* 133-140.

Hirschfeld, R. M. A., Shea, M. T., & Weise, R. (1991). Dependent personality disorder: Perspectives for DSM-IV. *Journal of Personality Disorders, 5,* 135-149.

Kalus, O., Bernstein, D. P., & Siever, L. J. (1993). Schizoid personality disorder: A review of current status and implications for DSM-IV. *Journal of Personality Disorders, 7,* 43-52.

Kotsaftis, A., & Neale, J. M. (1993). Schizotypal personality disorder I: The clinical syndrome. *Clinical Psychology Review, 13,* 451-472.

Loranger, A. W., & Tullis, E. H. (1985). Family history of alcoholism in borderline personality disorder. *Archives of General Psychiatry, 42,* 153-157.

McGlashan, T. H. (1986). Schizotypal personality disorder. *Archives of General Psychiatry, 43,* 329-334.

Millon, T. (1993). Negativistic (passive-aggressive) personality disorder. *Journal of Personality Disorders, 7,* 78-85.

Modestin, J. (1987). Quality of interpersonal relationships: the most characteristic DSM-III BPD criterion. *Comprehensive Psychiatry, 28,* 397-402.

Paris, J., Brown, R., & Nowlis, D. (1987). Long-term follow-up of borderline patients in a general hospital. *Comprehensive Psychiatry, 28,* 530-535.

Phillips, K. A., Hirschfeld, M. A., Shea, M. T., & Gunderson, J. G. (1993). Depressive personality disorder: Perspectives of DSM-IV. *Journal of Personality Disorders, 7,* 30-42.

Raulin, M. J., & Henderson, C. A. (1987). Perception of implicit relationships between personality traits by schizotypic college subjects. A pilot study. *Journal of Clinical Psychology, 43,* 463-467.

Reid, W. H. (1985). The antisocial personality: A review. *Hospital and Community Psychiatry, 36*, 831-837.

Salzman, L. (1980). *Psychotherapy of the obsessive personality.* New York: Aronson.

Siever, L. J., Bernstein, D. P., & Silverman, J. M. (1991). Schizotypal personality disorder: A review of its current status. *Journal of Personality Disorders, 5*, 178-193.

Siever, L. J., Coursey, D., Alterman, I. S., Buchsbaum, M. S., & Murphy, D. L. (1984). Impaired smooth pursuit eye movement: Vulnerability marker for schizotypal personality in a normal volunteer population. *American Journal of Psychiatry, 141*, 1560-1565.

Sterling, S., & Edelman, R. J. (1988). Reactions to anger and anxiety-provoking events: Psychopathic and nonpsychopathic groups compared. *Journal of Clinical Psychology, 44*, 96-100.

Tepelin, L. A. (1985). The criminality of the mentally ill: A dangerous misconception. *American Journal of Psychiatry, 142*, 593-599.

Tucker, L., Bauer, S. F., Wagner, S., Harlam, D., & Sher, I. (1987). Long-term hospital treatment of borderline patients: A descriptive outcome study. *American Journal of Psychiatry, 144*, 1443-1448.

Walding, R., & Gunderson, J. (1987). *Effective psychotherapy with borderline patents.* New York: MacMillan.

Widiger, T. A. (1991). DSM-IV reviews of the personality disorders: Introduction to special series. *Journal of Personality Disorders, 5*, 122-134.

Widiger, T. A. (1992). Antisocial personality disorder. *Hospital and Community Psychiatry, 43*, 6-8.

Widiger, T. A., & Corbitt, E. M. (1993). Antisocial personality disorder: Proposals for DSM-IV. *Journal of Personality Disorders, 7*, 63-77.

Widiger, T. A., Frances, A., & Trull, T. J. (1987). A psychometric analysis of the social-interpersonal and cognitive-perceptual items for the schizotypal personality disorder. *Archives of General Psychiatry, 44*, 741-745.

Woody, G. E., McLellan, A. T., Luborsky, L., & O'Brien, C. P. (1985). Sociopathy and psychotherapy outcome. *Archives of General Psychiatry, 42*, 1081-1086.

Chapter 10

Other Disorders

There are a large number of disorders that have not been discussed in previous chapters either because they are uncommon, or because they are seen infrequently by occupational therapists. However, it is useful to be familiar with their fundamental characteristics, as they do appear not only in mental health facilities but also in other health care settings.

All the categories of diagnosis previously discussed include a "not otherwise specified" (NOS) label. These may be considered residual categories, used in situations in which the individual fits most but not all of the criteria, or when presentation is in some way atypical (Figure 10-1). There are also labels for deferred diagnoses, or for those situations in which there is an Axis I but not Axis II disorder, or Axis II without Axis I. For example, an individual may present with clear symptoms of schizophrenia, but not fit precisely in one of the subgroups. In this case, NOS would be applied. If someone is diagnosed as having dysthymia, the therapist might defer Axis II diagnosis rather than say none, if he or she is uncertain whether or not a personality disorder co-exists.

In addition, many of the categories have subheadings which allow for greater specificity where it is possible to make more concrete identification of the symptom constellation. For example, panic disorder may be with agoraphobia or without agoraphobia, major depression may be identified as single episode or recurrent, and so on. Causes of the disorder may be reflected in the diagnostic label, as in the case of dementia due to head trauma. These subheadings, which can be seen in Appendix A, provide clarifying information to assist with treatment decisions.

There are also several groups of disorders that are useful to recognize, as they may well be represented in psychiatric populations. Because the disorders described in this section are not frequently seen in occupational therapy, description of each will be brief. When individuals with these disorders are

Figure 10-1. Other Psychiatric Disorders.

- Feeding and Eating Disorders of Infancy or Early Childhood
- Tic Disorders
- Elimination Disorders
- Other Disorders of Infancy, Childhood or Adolescence
- Amnestic Disorders
- Mental Disorders Due to a General Medical Condition Not Elsewhere Classified
- Somatoform Disorders
- Factitious Disorders
- Dissociative Disorders
- Sexual and Gender Identity Disorders
- Eating Disorders
- Sleep Disorders
- Impulse Control Disorders Not Elsewhere Classified
- Adjustment Disorders
- Other Conditions That May Be a Focus of Clinical Attention

referred to occupational therapy, treatment must be based on a theoretical framework which can guide assessment and intervention.

Feeding and Eating Disorders of Infancy or Early Childhood

Occupational therapists frequently treat infants with feeding problems (Pratt & Allen, 1989). They are well aware that psychological problems often co-exist, sometimes as precursors of the problem, sometimes as a consequence. DSM-IV (APA, 1994) reflects the psychological content of feeding disorders, and includes pica (persistent eating of non-nutritive substances), rumination (long-term chewing of food that is regurgitated by the child), and a more general "feeding disorder" category. The last of these is used in situations of failure to thrive, when no medical cause can be identified.

Tic Disorders

These include Tourette's Disorder, Chronic Motor or Vocal Tic Disorder, and Transient Tic Disorder. Tics are involuntary, sudden, stereotyped motor or vocal movements. They may be simple, as an involuntary eye-blinking or neck jerking movement, or grunting or snorting. Complex tics include stereotyped facial gestures, hitting self, touching, or echolalia.

Tourette's Disorder is characterized by numerous motor and vocal tics occur at varying frequencies, and which change over time. Frequently the head is involved, along with other parts of the body, and these are almost always accompanied by vocal tics, such as barking, grunting, and coprolalia (uttering obscenities). This disorder usually appears in childhood, and is apparently the result of CNS dysfunction, possibly genetic. It has been associated with obsessive compulsive disorder (Cohen, Riddle, & Leckman, 1992) and with learning disabilities (Lerer, 1987). This finding raises the possibility that all three disorders are the result of similar CNS dysfunction.

Tourette's is a chronic condition, with periods of exacerbation and remission. Severity of the disorder varies. As can be imagined, function in all performance spheres is impaired to a great extent in the most severe cases. However, medication (neuroleptics) in combination with education, psychological counseling, and other support can be valuable (Cohen et al., 1992; Lerer, 1987). Chronic Motor or Vocal Tic is much more limited, usually to a single motor or vocal tic. Severity of symptoms, and of occupational impairment is much less than with Tourette's Disorder.

Transient Tic Disorder is most often a single tic such as eye-blinking or another facial tic. Tics appear during childhood or adolescence, but disappear within a year. Tics may be precursors to Tourette's, or disappear completely, or they may be intermittent throughout life. Tics are common among children, and many seem to resolve themselves in time (Lerer, 1987).

Elimination Disorders

This category includes encopresis (inability to control feces), and enuresis (inability to control urine). The lack of control may be voluntary or involuntary. In order for the diagnosis to be made, the child must be at least 4 (encopresis) or 5 years old (enuresis), with correlating mental age. Thus it will not be diagnosed in retarded individuals who may lack both motor control and intelligence to be readily trained. For both disorders, the problem may be transient (e.g., caused by the stress of a new sibling or hospitalization), or may become chronic. In making this diagnosis, it is vital to rule out possible physical problems, such as urinary tract infections.

Other Disorders of Infancy, Childhood, and Adolescence

This category includes five disorders. They are separation anxiety disorder, selective mutism, reactive attachment disorder of infancy or early childhood, stereotypic movement disorder, and disorder of infancy, childhood, or adolescence NOS.

Separation anxiety, a form of anxiety disorder, is discussed in Chapters 3 and 8. Selective mutism is a refusal to talk in one or more specific social situations, after it is clear that the child can speak. While it is rare, it can be quite disabling.

Disturbance of social relatedness in early childhood is characteristic of reactive attachment disorder. It is believed to be the result of severely inadequate care during infancy and early childhood (Lyons-Ruth, Repacholi, McLeod, & Silva, 1992; Tibbits-Kleber & Howell, 1985). Symptoms include failure to initiate or respond in social interaction, diffuse attachments to adults, and pathogenic care by caregivers, such as disregard for emotional and physical needs. Failure to thrive may be related to this disorder.

Stereotypic movement disorder is demonstrated by repetitive non-functional behaviors such as head banging. The activities are usually intentional, and may cause injury to the child or interfere with activity.

Amnestic Disorders

These disorders are listed along with the dementias and delirium. Unlike these two disorders, amnestic disorders are focal cognitive disorders (Caine, 1993). This means that only memory is affected, rather than cognition more globally. Amnestic disorder may be due to substance abuse (Jacobson & Lishman, 1987), or to a variety of medical conditions.

These conditions are characterized by inability to learn new material or to recall previously learned material, to an extent that impairs function (APA, 1994).

Mental Disorders Due to a General Medical Condition Not Elsewhere Classified

When a mental disorder is known to be caused by a medical condition, this diagnostic grouping would be used. In particular, catatonia and personality change that resulted from a medical condition would be noted using this set of diagnoses.

Somatoform Disorders

These include body dysmorphic disorder, conversion disorder, hypochondriasis, somatization disorder, and somatoform pain disorder. These disorders are important to understand, as they frequently present in settings other than mental health facilities.

Body dysmorphic disorder reflects an obsessive dissatisfaction with a portion of the body (Hollander, et al., 1992). The individual may, for example, believe that his or her nose is ugly or face too wrinkled. There may actually be some minor anomaly with regard to the feature in question, but this disorder appears in normal looking individuals. The result is often frequent visits to plastic surgeons, with dissatisfaction with surgical outcomes. Extreme functional impairment is rare, but may occur when the individual becomes so fixated on the "disfigurement" that other activities are excluded.

Conversion disorder is characterized by a loss of body function or physical impairment which suggests a physical disorder, in the absence of physical findings. The individual does not intentionally produce the physical symptom, but it will lack some features of the true physical condition. Baker and Silver (1987), in discussing hysterical paraplegia, note that accompanying sensory deficits do not fit an anatomical pattern, and that reflexes remain normal. Conversion reactions appear suddenly, and often as a result of identifiable psychosocial stressors. They tend to occur in individuals with histrionic personality disorder. In some instances there is also a lack of concern about the condition, "la belle indifference" (Nemiah, 1988). This attitude is quite striking, as the individual is apparently unworried by a sudden paralysis, loss of hearing, and so on. Furthermore, sudden, rapid recovery may occur. Suggestion (e.g., hypnosis) appears to be an effective treatment (Hafeiz, 1980).

Obsessive worry about physical condition is the defining feature of hypochondriasis. The fears are unwarranted by any physical finding, though in the absence of physical findings the individual is likely to assume the physician has not done enough. The individual makes frequent visits to the physician, and changes doctors often as he or she assumes that care is inadequate or improper. This is usually a chronic condition, and impairs performance in all spheres to some extent. Those around the individual become annoyed by the obsession with physical worries, and the individual misses work because of physical concerns. In severe cases the individual may decide to become an invalid and refuse to function for fear of "further harm" to physical condition.

An initial diagnosis of hypochondriasis may result in one of four different outcomes (Idzorek, 1975): 1) a warning of future psychiatric or physical dysfunction, 2) a symptom of psychosis, 3) a symptom of depression, and 4) a "true" hypochondriasis. Obviously, making these distinctions can be difficult, but vital to treatment. Hypochondriasis has been linked to depression, anxiety, and paranoid reactions (Hyer, Gouveia, Harrison, Warsa, & Coutsouridis, 1987).

While hypochondriasis appears to respond well to anti-anxiety medication (Kellner, 1983), particularly in individuals with disorder of short duration and without accompanying personality disorders, these patients can be very frustrating to care providers (Idzorek, 1975). Recognition that these are individuals who typically lack self-esteem and social skills, and need inordinate amounts of attention can help shift focus to needs and away from annoying behaviors.

Somatization disorder is characterized by multiple physical complaints over a period of years with no accompanying physical disorder (Bucholz, Reich, et al., 1993). The individual seeks care for the specific disorder, presenting complaints in a vague or dramatic way. There is usually a pattern of intensive investigation of these complaints, with no positive findings. As with hypochondriacs, physician switching is common. Unlike hypochondriasis, where there is simply generalized fear that "something" may be wrong or go wrong, these individuals have specific, though unwarranted, physical complaints. The disorder is more common in women (Guze, Cloninger, Martin, & Clayton 1986), and has been thought to parallel antisocial personality which is much more common in men. Prognosis for Briquet's syndrome, the most common somatization disorder, is poor (Guze et al., 1986) with 80% having the same diagnosis 6 to 12 years later.

Somatoform pain disorder is the preoccupation with pain when there is no physical reason for such pain. It often occurs in individuals with a history of conversion reactions, and, like other disorders in this group, occurs in the absence of any positive physical findings. In some cases, it may develop following a physical trauma, but continue once the physical problem is resolved.

Factitious Disorders

These are physical or psychological disorders that are intentionally produced, and under the voluntary control of the individual. The concept of voluntary control is somewhat problematic here, however. While the individual may actively induce a symptom (e.g., through ingestion of drugs), they are not able to control the impulse to do so. This group does not include malingering, in which the individual both produces the symptom voluntarily and wishes to do so at a conscious level.

The best known factitious disorder is Munchausen syndrome (Gattaz, Dressing, & Hewer, 1990). This syndrome is characterized by numerous hospitalizations for a variety of symptoms, with accompanying physical signs, such as nausea and vomiting, rashes, and bleeding, all of which have been induced by the individual. Their symptoms are dramatic, but vague, and they have extensive knowledge of hospital routines. They are difficult to manage once hospitalized, because they are both noncompliant and demanding. It appears that these individuals are socially isolated and derive most of their social satisfaction by being taken care of in an inpatient setting. When confronted with the real nature of their symptoms, they often leave against medical advice, often to seek re-admission elsewhere.

Gattaz and colleagues (1990) have noted that the somatoform and factitious disorders fit along several continua. One is the degree to which the symptoms emerge as a result of voluntary action on the part of the individual as opposed to involuntary emergence of symptoms. The second continuum relates to the degree to which the individual has conscious awareness of the source of the problem. These researchers note that somatoform disorders are the result of unconscious motivation producing involuntary physical symptoms, while factitious disorders are the result of unconscious motivation but voluntary production of symptoms. They compare these to malingering, which is both under voluntary control and a conscious effort to appear ill.

An additional interesting condition is factitious disorder by proxy, in which one individual, typically a parent, induces physical illness in another, typically a child, to get attention from the health care system (Gattaz, 1990).

There is much to suggest that these disorders may be prodromal to psychosis, particularly when the disorder feigned is a psychosis (Hay, 1983; Pope, Jonas, & Jones, 1982). Long-term outcomes are poor, particularly since many of these individuals have accompanying personality disorders.

Dissociative Disorders

Dissociative Identity Disorder (formerly Multiple Personality Disorder) (DID), Dissociative Fugue, Dissociative Amnesia, and Depersonalization Disorder are included in this group. Interest in this category of diagnoses has clearly escalated (Spiegel & Cardena, 1991). They are striking, and have frequently been portrayed in movies and television programs as "mental illness" in a global sense.

Rate of occurrence is not well established. Some researchers believe dissociative identity disorder is quite rare, while others believe it is common but frequently misdiagnosed (Kluft, 1986).

A common thread in dissociative identity disorder is a history of psychological trauma (Spiegel & Cardena, 1991). The analytic explanation of the phenomenon is that the individual develops different personas as a defense mechanism (Kluft, 1988). For example, one personality may not remember an anxiety-provoking event which is "managed" by another, or one may express anger which is frightening to the dominant persona. Personalities tend to be separate from each other and may be very highly developed. They seem to reflect different facets of the individual which are split or dissociated from the primary personality. This primary personality is often amnestic for the other personalities.

Function depends on the extent and frequency with which dissociative reactions occur in the individual. Some individuals with dissociative identity disorder are quite functional (Kluft, 1986) while others are incapacitated.

The goal of treatment is most often unification, i.e., reintegration of the separate personalities into one functional whole (Kluft, 1988). Hypnotherapy and cognitive therapy are among those reported effective (Ross & Gahan, 1988). Expressive therapy, psychoeducation (Richert & Bergland, 1992), and group therapy (Angel, 1989) have been used with success. Occupational therapists who work with individuals with DID may want to emphasize sensorimotor activities that allow the person to experience a sense of control which might otherwise be absent (Waid, 1993).

Sexual and Gender Identity Disorders

There are two main groups of sexual disorders: paraphilias and sexual dysfunctions. Paraphilias are characterized by sexual arousal in response to objects or situations which are not normally part of sexual activity, with accompanying problems relating in normal sexual activity. These include pedophilia, sexual sadism and masochism, transvestic fetishism, and others. Sexual dysfunctions represent problems in engaging in sexual relationships, including sexual aversion, inhibited orgasm, dyspareunia, premature ejaculation, and so on. Functional impairment is primarily in the area of sexual relationships, but may extend to heterosexual relationships more generally if the sexual problem begins to generalize to feelings of low self-esteem or anxiety.

Gender identity disorders reflect conflict between assigned sex and gender identity. Specifically, they reflect extreme discomfort with assignment as male or female, and a conviction that the individual should be the other sex. In the most extreme form, this is reflected as transsexualism, in which the individual may simply choose to live as if the other sex, and possibly to have hormonal and surgical treatment to allow reassignment. Transsexualism is quite rare, and is not to be confused with tomboyishness in girls, "feminine" behavior in boys, or anxiety about living up to sex role expectations. It reflects a profound belief that the individual was born in the wrong body. This belief is most often present in childhood, where the child is distressed about his or her sex, insisting that he or she is really the opposite sex. The cause of these disorders is unknown, with speculation ranging from prenatal hormonal exposure to genetic flaws to learned behaviors. Research is inconclusive about the roots of the problem, but it does seem to appear early in childhood in most cases.

Treatment provides two primary alternatives (Edelman, 1986). One involves sex reassignment, including hormonal treatment and sometimes surgery, to make the body more consistent with gender assumed by the individual. This approach also requires extensive therapy to work through psychological difficulties associated with this kind of dramatic change, and to provide training about appropriate gender behavior. The other treatment is to help the individual feel more comfortable with existing sex assignment. This second alternative is facilitated through skill training, behavior therapy, psychotherapy, and occupational therapy to teach appropriate sex role behavior (Khanna, Desai, & Channabasavanna, 1987). Both approaches report success with some individuals (Edelman, 1986; Khanna et al., 1987).

There is a group of individuals who present the greatest treatment problem. This is the group who choose not to have surgery, but are uncertain about the decision (Kockott & Fahrner, 1987). These individuals have the poorest long-term adaptation, and are most likely to need psychotherapy. They are typically older, and have made an effort to live within their biological sex role by marrying, having children, and so on.

Eating Disorders

In DSM-III-R (APA, 1987), eating disorders were listed with the disorders of infancy, childhood, and adolescence. Their move to a separate section reflects the fact that while they may occur in children (Hodes, 1993), these disorders may occur at any time during the life span, and are most likely to emerge in adolescents and young adults. It is quite possible for them to emerge in older adults as well (Cosford & Arnold, 1992). Unlike other diagnostic categories in this chapter, individuals with eating disorders are often seen by occupational therapists. Moreover, because they have become so common, they are frequently seen in patients presenting with physical problems in general medical, school, or rehabilitation settings.

Anorexia Nervosa
Anorexia nervosa is characterized by a refusal to gain weight, fear of gaining weight, and belief that one is overweight in individuals who refuse to maintain minimally normal body weight (APA, 1994). In women, amenorrhea is also present.

Bulimia Nervosa

Bulimia is characterized by a binge/purge cycle in individuals who are more likely to be of normal weight or overweight. The purging is accomplished through induced vomiting or the use of laxatives, and the entire cycle is accompanied by a sense of loss of control of eating. Binging and purging occurs frequently, at least twice a week, and must persist over at least 3 months before the diagnosis is made. Bulimics are excessively concerned about weight.

Etiology and Incidence

To some extent, these disorders are cultural, as thinness is considered desirable. Vocation also correlates with eating disorders. Ballet dancers, for example, are very likely to suffer from bulimia or anorexia (Herzog, Kelly & Lavori, 1988), as are gymnasts and wrestlers. Bruch (1973) hypothesized that obesity and anorexia stemmed from issues of maternal control. The family has been implicated as the source of the disorder by others, as well (Steiger, Leung, Puentes-Neuman, & Gattheil, 1992). Some suggest that anorexia is likely to occur in families where expectations are high for performance (Waller, 1992).

It has also been suggested that these disorders are related to sexual abuse (Connors & Morse, 1992). Approximately 30% of individuals with eating disorders report earlier sexual abuse.

A variety of biological changes occur in individuals with anorexia and bulimia, leading some to suggest that the cause is biological (Herzog, Kelly & Lavori, 1988; Kaye, Ebert, Gwirtsman, et al., 1984). It is difficult to know which change occurs first, however. Menstruation is affected in anorexics, and abnormal brain serotonergic metabolism has been found in both anorexics and bulimics (Kaye et al., 1984).

Anorexics' disturbed body image, absence of concern about the problem, overactivity, and inability to recognize hunger led Bruch (1962) to speculate that these individuals have a perceptual disorder.

Examination of bulimics has identified similarities between this disorder and substance abuse on Minnesota Multiphasic Personality Inventory profiles (Hatsukami, Owen, Pyle, & Mitchell 1982) suggesting that this is another form of addictive behavior or impulse control difficulty. Binging may cause a short term "high," encouraging the behavior (Kaye, Gwirtsman, George, Weiss & Jimerson al., 1984). Individuals with bulimia nervosa are highly impulsive (Fahy & Eisler, 1993).

It now appears that approximately 5% of American women have anorexia nervosa (Patton, 1992), 1% bulimia nervosa, and another 3% subclinical cases of one of these disorders. Approximately 90% to 95% of cases occur in women.

Prognosis

It has been estimated that between 5% and 18% of anorexics ultimately die of the disorder (Herzog, 1992). The death rate goes up with duration of the disorder. Physical consequences include cyanosis, difficulty tolerating cold temperatures, bradycardia, hypotension, dental enamel and skin changes, gastrointestinal problems, and heart, thyroid, and renal problems (Herzog, 1992). Severe depression is also common and is a poor prognostic sign (Maddocks & Kaplan, 1991).

In some cases, only one period of anorexia or bulimia occurs, after which weight and eating return to normal (Cosford & Arnold, 1992). In others, however, the disorder may be chronic, persisting into late life.

Hsu, Crisp, and Harding (1979) reported that approximately 50% of anorexics had good long-term outcomes. Outcome appeared related to age at onset and severity of symptoms, with earlier onset having worse prognosis, and milder symptoms better prognosis. Morgan and Russell (1975) found that their subjects could be divided roughly by thirds into those with good, fair, and poor outcomes. Norman and Herzog (1984) found persistent functional difficulties particularly related to social interaction and activity related to food in a 1 year follow-up of 40 patients.

Implications for Function and Treatment

Anorexics often have good vocational function. A follow-up study of 100 women found 80 employed 4 to 8 years after diagnosis (Hsu et al., 1979). Social functioning, however, tends to be poor, as these individuals are often isolated and asexual. It has been estimated that between 22% and 73% have satisfactory social functioning on a long-term basis. One study reported 60% to have good sexual adjustment 50% good socioeconomic adjustment (Morgan & Russell, 1975) The figures are quite variable, leading to some confusion about the exact nature of long-term function in anorexics (Herzog, Kelly, & Lavori, 1988).

ADL and IADL are generally not affected, except in the area of eating and cooking. The term anorexia is somewhat misleading, as these individuals are often obsessed with food and plan their lives around it.

Bulimia appears to be a much more chronic and episodic disorder, often continuing for a lifetime (Herzog, 1982). While it is not as likely to cause death, a number of serious health problems may result, including digestive disorders heart and kidney problems. Bulimics are more likely to recognize the need for help and to accept it, but the disease is relatively intractable (Herzog, 1982). Predictors of outcome are not clear (Herzog, Kelly & Lavori, 1988).

An obsession with food is the key factor interfering with function in bulimics (Herzog, 1982). They are so preoccupied with food and eating that their work may suffer and social activities are often badly affected. These problems are the result of the time taken with obsessing about food, as well as the fear that they will be rejected by anyone who learns of the obsession. As with anorexics, ADL and IADL are not affected, except as they relate to food and its preparation.

A variety of treatments has been employed for both anorexics and bulimics. In some cases, anorexics require hospitalization, often as the result of life-threatening weight loss, while bulimics are almost always treated in outpatient settings. Behavioral techniques are used both in inpatient and outpatient settings (Garner & Bennis, 1982). In addition, group therapy has been advocated (Brotman, Alonso, & Herzog, 1985), as has family therapy (Schwartz, Barrett, & Saba, 1985). The use of antidepressant medications shows promise, particularly in treating anorexics (Pope, Hudson, Jonas, & Yurgelon-Todd, 1985).

Other recommended approaches include individual psychotherapy, cognitive therapies, education, and self-help groups (Herzog, Kelly & Lavori, 1988). For bulimia, cognitive-behavioral therapy can be helpful (Wilson & Fairburn, 1993).

Implications for Occupational Therapy

Occupational therapists may contribute to behavioral programs for anorexics and bulimics (Rockwell, 1990). The occupational therapist may, for example, assist the client in developing acceptable leisure pursuits which de-emphasize food. In addition, the therapist may provide social skills training to remediate difficulties these individuals have in developing and maintaining satisfying relationships. Therapists also offer stress management techniques, and opportunities for self-expression through the expressive arts.

Bridgett (1993) recommends that occupational therapists focus on body self-image, time management, and development of a greater sense of internal control through use of activity.

Sleep Disorders

Sleep disorders will not be diagnosed in situations where the duration of the problem is brief. Many individuals have periods of sleep disturbance when stressed or ill, but for most people these are brief and transient. In some cases, though, the problem persists, either in the form of dyssomnia (difficulty sleeping) or hypersomnia (excessive sleeping). The DSM-IV listing does not include physical disorders such as narcolepsy, but only those which are thought to be psychogenic.

Also included in this category are sleep-wake disturbances, in which the normal diurnal cycle of sleep is disturbed, and parasomnias, which are characterized by abnormal events during sleep (e.g., nightmares and sleepwalking.) Again, the problem must be of several months duration for a diagnosis to be made, as occasional problems are not unusual.

Impulse Control Disorders Not Elsewhere Classified

These include intermittent explosive disorder, kleptomania, pathological gambling, pyromania, and trichotillomania. In each, the individual is driven to engage in a behavior which is damaging to self or others, which he or she is unable to control (Lesieur & Rosenthal, 1991). Origin of the disorders is not well understood, but interference with function is common. Explosive disorder, kleptomania, and pyromania may ultimately result in imprisonment, while pathological gambling is damaging to social and work relationships. Trichotillomania (pulling out one's own hair) is the least damaging of these disorders, although it may indicate poor self-esteem which is reflected in other performance.

Pathological gambling is often compared to substance abuse, and is, in fact, often comorbid with alcoholism (Lesieur & Rosenthal, 1991). Individuals who are pathological gamblers often suffer from vocational and social difficulties, particularly marital difficulties, as gambling takes increasing amounts of their time and financial resources. Treatment reflects a belief that it is an addictive behavior, as 12 step programs such as Gamblers Anonymous are often suggested (Murray, 1993; Shaffer & Gambino, 1989).

Adjustment Disorders

These disorders may appear at any time in life, but occur within 3 months of a stressful event. By definition, function is impaired, as the individual has difficulty with social, vocational, school, or leisure activities. Stressors include such things as divorce, loss of a job, physical illness, or natural disaster. The severity of the disorder is not necessarily in proportion to the severity of the stressor, but rather a reflection of the individual's ability to cope. Anxiety, depression, and physical complaints may accompany the disorder. These symptoms are self-limiting, occurring within 3 months of the stressor, with a duration of no more than 6 months following the stressor.

In most instances, these disorders can be resolved through supportive therapy and intervention to teach new coping skills. However, in adjustment disorders which reoccur, or are accompanied by behavioral symptoms such as conduct disorder, outcome is worse (Andreasen & Hoenk, 1982). In children, outcomes also tend to be worse (Newcorn & Strain, 1992).

Studies of the validity of the category provide evidence of face, descriptive, and predictive validity among adults (Andreasen & Hoenk, 1982). It is clear, for example, that the majority of adults improve in the absence of continued stress.

Other Conditions That May Be a Focus of Clinical Attention

There are times when individuals enter treatment for specific problems that are not directly tied to psychiatric disorders. Academic problems, marital problems, uncomplicated bereavement, occupational (vocational) problems, and parent-child problems are among those on this list. While individuals seeking treatment for these problems may have accompanying disorders, the difficulty may not have resulted from the mental disorder. As an example, an individual who has had anxiety problems may still experience uncomplicated bereavement as a result of loss of a spouse.

Implications for Occupational Therapy

For each of these disorders occupational therapy may be warranted if: 1) the disorder impacts negatively on function, 2) the disorder impacts negatively on self-esteem, or 3) remediation requires learning a new set of performance skills.

As an example, transsexual individuals may have performed quite adequately in both work and social spheres, but have suffered severe difficulty in terms of self-esteem and self-concept. Should they opt for sex reassignment, a whole set of new skills will be needed. The well-publicized case of Renee Richards is an example. She was a successful male physician, married with several children. Because she believed she was a woman wrongly born into a male body, and because life was not comfortable to her, she ultimately opted for sex reassignment. This necessitated, among many other concerns, considerable learning about how to behave as a female.

A more commonly encountered example would be individuals with hypochondriasis. Function is typically impaired as the individual worries about health, and takes to bed with every real or imagined ailment.

Self-esteem is likely to be impaired, either as a precursor to the disorder or as a consequence of the inability to function and the inevitable annoyance of others. These individuals clearly need a new set of behaviors which can provide a source of satisfaction and improved self-esteem. In the absence of such learning, remediation of symptoms is difficult. This is because hypochondriasis is so often a plea for attention from individuals who have very low self regard.

Review of disorders in this chapter provides an opportunity to restate the occupational therapy view of dysfunction. This view cuts across lines drawn by medical diagnosis. Issues of self-esteem, self-concept, and performance appear almost regardless of diagnosis. While the degree of impairment and the specific nature of the impairment differ, these themes are consistent and primary to the occupational therapist.

References

American Psychological Association (1987). *Diagnostic and Statistical Manual of Mental Disorders* (3rd ed. rev.). Washington, DC: Author.

American Psychological Association (1994). *Diagnostic and Statistical Manual of Mental Disorders* (4th ed.). Washington, DC: Author.

Andreasen, N. C., & Hoenk, P. R. (1982). The predictive value of adjustment disorders: A follow-up study. *American Journal of Psychiatry, 139,* 584-590.

Angel, S. L. (1989). Toward becoming one self. *The American Journal of Occupational Therapy, 11,* 1037-1043.

Baker, S., & Silver, J. R. (1987). Hysterical paraplegia. *Journal of Neurology, Neurosurgery, and Psychiatry, 50,* 375-382.

Bridgett, B. (1993). Occupational therapy evaluation for patients with eating disorders. *Occupational Therapy in Mental Health, 12,* 79-89.

Brotman, A. W., Alonso, A., & Herzog, D. B. (1985). Group therapy for bulimics: Clinical experience and practice recommendations. *Group, 9,* 15-23.

Bruch, H. (1962). Perceptual and conceptual disturbances in anorexia nervosa. *Psychosomatic Medicine, 24,* 187-194

Bruch, H. (1973). *Eating disorders: Obesity, anorexia nervosa, and the person within.* New York: Basic Books.

Bucholz, K. K., Dinwiddie, S. H., Reich, T., et.al. (1993). Comparison of screening proposals for somatization disorder empirical analyses. *Comprehensive Psychiatry, 34,* 49-64.

Caine, E. D. (1993). Amnesic disorders. *The Journal of Neuropsychiatry and Clinical Neurosciences, 5,* 6-8.

Cohen, D. J., Riddle, M. A., & Leckman, J. F. (1992). Pharmacotherapy of Tourette's syndrome and associated disorders. *Pediatric Psychopharmacology, 15,* 109-129.

Connors, M. E., & Morse, W. (1992). Sexual abuse and eating disorders: A review. *International Journal of Eating Disorders, 13,* 1-11.

Cosford, P., & Arnold, E. (1992). Eating disorders in later life: A review. *International Journal of Geriatric Psychiatry, 7,* 491-498.

Edelman, R. J. (1986). Adaptive training for existing male transsexual gender role: A case history. *Journal of Sex Research, 22,* 514-531.

Fahy, T., & Eisler, I. (1993). Impulsivity and eating disorders. *British Journal of Psychiatry, 162,* 193-197.

Garner, D. M., & Bennis, K. M. (1982) A cognitive-behavioral approach to anorexia nervosa. *Cognitive Therapy Research, 6,* 123-150.

Gattaz, W. F., Dressing, P., & Hewer, R. (1990). Munchausen syndrome. *Psychopathology, 23,* 33-39.

Guze, S. B., Cloninger, C. R., Martin. R. L., & Clayton, P. J. (1986). A follow-up and family study of Briquet's syndrome. *British Journal of Psychiatry, 149,* 17-23.

Hafeiz, H. B. (1980). Hysterical conversion: A prognostic study. *British Journal of Psychiatry, 136,* 548-551.

Hatsukami, D., Owen, P., Pyle, R., & Mitchell, J. (1982). Similarities and differences in the MMPI between women with bulimia and women with alcohol or drug abuse problems. *Addictive Behaviors, 7,* 435-439.

Hay, G. G. (1983). Feigned psychosis—A review of the simulation of mental illness. *British Journal of Psychiatry, 143,* 8-10.

Herzog, D. B. (1982). Bulimia: The secretive syndrome. *Psychosomatics, 23,* 481-487.

Herzog, D. B. (1992). Eating disorders. *Psychosomatics, 33,* 10-15.

Herzog, D. B., Kelly, M. B., & Lavori, P. W. (1988). Outcome in anorexia nervosa and bulimia nervosa: A review of the literature. *Journal of Nervous and Mental Diseases, 176,* 131-143.

Hodes, M. (1993). Anorexia nervosa and bulimia nervosa in children. *International Review of Psychiatry, 5,* 101-108.

Hollander, E., Neville, D., Frenkel, M., et al. (1992). Body dysmorphic disorder: Diagnostic issues and related disorders. *The Academy of Psychosomatic Medicine, 33,* 156-165.

Hsu, L. K., Crisp, A. H., & Harding, B. (1979). Outcome of anorexia nervosa. *The Lancet,* Jan. 13, 61-65.

Hyer, L., Gouveia, I., Harrison, W. R., Warsa, J., & Coutsouridis, D. (1987). Depression, anxiety, paranoid reactions, hypochondriasis, and cognitive decline of later-life inpatients. *Journal of Gerontology, 42,* 92-94.

Idzorek, S. (1975). A functional classification of hypochondriasis with specific recommendations for treatment. *Southern Medical Journal, 68,* 1326-1332.

Jacobson, R. R., & Lishman, W. A. (1987). Selective memory loss and global intellectual deficits in alcoholic Korsakoff's syndrome. *Psychological Medicine, 17,* 649-655.

Kaye, W. H., Gwirtsman, H. E., George, D. T., Weiss, S. R., & Jimerson, D. C. (1984). Relationship of mood alterations to bingeing behavior in bulimia. *British Journal of Psychiatry, 149,* 479-485.

Kellner, R. (1983). Prognosis of treated hypochondriasis: a clinical study. *Acta Psychiatrica Scandinavia, 67,* 69-79.

Khanna, S., Desai, N. G., & Channabasavanna, S. M. (1987). Case study: A treatment package for transsexualism. *Behavior Therapy, 2,* 193-199.

Kluft, R. P. (1986). High-functioning multiple personality patients: Three cases. *The Journal of Nervous and Mental Disease, 174,* 802-803.

Kluft, R. P. (1988). The postunification treatment of multiple personality disorder: First findings. *American Journal of Psychotherapy, 42,* 212-227.

Kockott, G., & Fahrner, E. M. (1987). Transsexuals who have not undergone surgery: A follow-up study. *Archives of Sexual Behavior, 16,* 511-522.

Lerer, R. J. (1987). Motor tics, Tourette syndrome, and learning disabilities. *Journal of Learning Disabilities, 20,* 266-267.

Lesieur, H. R., & Rosenthal, R. J. (1991). Pathological gambling: A review of the literature (prepared for the American Psychiatric Association Task Force on DSM-IV Committee on Disorders of Impulse Control not Elsewhere Classified). *Journal of Gambling Studies, 7,* 5-37.

Lyons-Ruth, K., Repacholi, B., McLeod, S., & Silva, E. (1992). Disorganized attachment behavior in infancy: Short-term stability, maternal and infant correlates, and risk-related subtypes. *Development and Psychopathology, 3,* 377-396.

Maddocks, S. E. & Kaplan, A. S. (1991). The prediction of treatment response in bulimia nervosa: A study of patient variables. *British Journal of Psychiatry, 159,* 846-849.

Morgan, H. G., & Russell, G. F. M. (1975). Value of family background and clinical features as predictors of long-term outcome in anorexia nervosa: Four-year follow-up study of 41 patients. *Psychological Medicine, 5,* 355-371.

Murray, J. B. (1993). Review of research on pathological gambling. *Psychological Reports, 72,* 791-810.

Nemiah, J. C. (1988). Psychoneurotic disorders. In A. M. Nicholi (Ed.), *The new Harvard guide to psychiatry* (pp. 234-258). Cambridge, MA: Belknap Press.

Newcorn, J. H., & Strain, J. (1992). Adjustment disorder in children and adolescents. *Journal of the American Academy of Child and Adolescent Psychiatry, 31,* 318-326.

Norman, D. K., & Herzog, D. B. (1984). Persistent social maladjustment in bulimia: A 1 year follow-up. *American Journal of Psychiatry, 141,* 444-446.

Patton, G. C. (1992). Eating disorders: Antecedents, evolution and course. *Annals of Medicine, 24,* 281-285.

Pope, H. S., Hudson, J. L., Jonas, T. M., & Yurgelun-Todd, D. (1985). Antidepressant treatment of bulimia: A 2-year follow-up study. *Journal of Clinical Psychopharmacology, 5,* 320-327.

Pope, H. S., Jonas, T. M., & Jones, B. (1982). Factitious psychosis: Phenomenology, family history, and long-term outcome of nine patients. *American Journal of Psychiatry, 139,* 1480-1483.

Pratt, P. N., & Allen, A. S. (1989). *Occupational therapy for children* (2nd ed.), St. Louis: C.V. Mosby.

Richert, G. Z., & Bergland, C. (1992). Treatment choices: Rehabilitation services used by patients with multiple personality disorder. *American Journal of Occupational Therapy, 46,* 634-638.

Rockwell, L. E. (1990). Frames of reference and modalities used by occupational therapists in the treatment of patients with eating disorders. *Occupational Therapy in Mental Health, 10,* 47-64.

Ross, C. A., & Gahan, P. (1988). Cognitive analysis of multiple personality disorder. *American Journal of Psychotherapy, 42,* 229-239.

Schwartz, R., Barrett, M. J., & Saba, G. (1985). Family therapy for bulimia. In D. M. Garner & P. E. Garfinkel (Eds.), *Handbook of psychotherapy for anorexia nervosa and bulimia.* New York: Guilford Press.

Shaffer, H. J., & Gambino, B. (1989). The epistemology of "addictive disease": Gambling as predicament. *Journal of Gambling Behavior, 5,* 211-227.

Spiegel, D., & Cardena, E. (1991). Disintegrated experience: The dissociative disorders revisited. *Journal of Abnormal Psychology, 100,* 366-378.

Steiger, H., Leung, F. Y. K., Puentes-Neuman, G., & Gottheil, N. (1992). Psychosocial profiles of adolescent girls with varying degrees of eating and mood disturbances. *International Journal of Eating Disorders, 11,* 121-131.

Tibbits-Kleber, A. L., & Howell, R. J. (1985). Reactive attachment disorder of infancy (RAD). *Journal of Clinical Child Psychology, 14,* 304-310.

Waid, K. M. (1993). An occupational therapy perspective in the treatment of multiple personality disorder. *American Journal of Occupational Therapy, 47,* 872-876.

Waller, G. (1992). Sexual abuse and bulimic symptoms in eating disorders: Do family interaction and self-esteem explain the links? *International Journal of Eating Disorders, 12,* 235-240.

Wilson, G. T., & Fairburn, C. G. (1993). Cognitive treatments for eating disorders. *Journal of Consulting and Clinical Psychology, 61,* 261-269.

Chapter 11

Psychopharmacotherapy

Philip J. Fischer, MD
Director, Medical Education
and Recovery Programs
Laurelwood Hospital
Willoughby, OH

Introduction

For more than four decades, research on mental disorders has followed several parallel tracks. Once such track has led to a literal explosion of information about brain functions and behavior. Beginning in the late 1950s, specific and dramatic improvement of major mental disorders to medications led to theories and research about the possible biological influences of these illnesses. This illness model has led to a change in the way mental health professionals, and the general public, have come to understand these disorders. Thus, the idea that these illnesses are solely due to personal weakness or improper parenting has given way to the biopsychosocial approach to diagnosis and treatment. One result of this paradigm shift has been a careful re-analysis of the diagnostic categories we use. In order for our new tools to be used appropriately, reliable diagnostic systems and rating scales became essential.

Research diagnostic criteria were developed and used in multidisciplinary field trials leading to the American Psychiatric Association's *Diagnostic and Statistical Manual of Mental Disorders*, Fourth Edition (DSM-IV) (1994). The careful application of this diagnostic system based on observable symptoms and behaviors not only serves to improve the specificity of treatment but has led to advances in epidemiologic research. This, in turn, has decreased somewhat, the degree of stigma psychiatric patients experience and will hopefully influence society to include mental illness equally in the health care reform efforts.

The efficacy of psychotropic medications has led to economic pressure in the new world of managed care delivery of treatment because medications are cheaper to administer than psychosocial treatments. They can often be prescribed by primary care physicians, who are perceived as being less expensive than specialists. However, medications should never be perceived as the singular solution to the complex problems related to human emotion and behavior. Furthermore, primary care physicians usually do not have the training or the time to perform a thorough pretreatment assessment of people with overlapping biological, social, environmental, and characterologic syndromes.

There are many unanswered questions and many clinical and social controversies around the use of psychotropic medications and these discussions are outside the scope of this chapter. Hopefully, the reader will develop a balanced perspective through critical analysis of the clinical literature and the popular press. The purpose of this chapter is to introduce some general principles for using psychopharmacology so that all the members of the multidisciplinary treatment team can recognize adverse reactions and side effects, reinforce gains, and communicate problems that interfere with the patient's maximal functioning.

History

Mankind has been searching for ways to reduce the pain and suffering of psychic distress throughout history. Each culture has had its armamentarium of treatments. Ancient peoples bored holes in the skull to let out evil spirits (trephination). The use of alcohol to reduce dysphoria, herbal remedies, opiates, cocaine, marijuana, coffee, tobacco, and many other plant-derived psychotropic agents have been used as folk remedies. The effects of some of these compounds have been studied and many found their way into traditional medicine.

The chance discoveries of the anti-manic effect of lithium and of chlorpromazine's (Thorazine) antipsychotic properties signaled the beginning of modern psychopharmacology. In the ensuing 40 years many new drugs have been developed that have improved the quality of life in patients afflicted with a variety of psychiatric disorders. The discovery and development of these compounds started with unexpected clinical findings of efficacy. Ongoing research has improved understanding of basic psychopharmacology and drug side effects, leading to the ongoing development of better drugs and suggesting biologic theories of causation for some psychiatric illnesses.

Chlorpromazine (Thorazine) was synthesized as an antihistamine in 1952 and was found to produce an easily arousable sedation that was useful as a pre-anesthetic (Davis, 1985). The observation that it produced behavioral changes led to experimental trials of the drug in psychotic patients. Many of these "hopeless cases" experienced dramatic improvement. Since that time the further development of newer antipsychotic drugs has permitted many individuals to function outside of psychiatric hospitals instead of being institutionalized for life.

The first two major classes of antidepressants, tricyclics and monoamine oxidase inhibitors (MAOI), were also discovered accidentally. Imipramine (Tofranil), the first of the tricyclic antidepressants, was discovered while researchers were looking for a better chlorpromazine-like drug (Davis, 1985). It was found that though imipramine was ineffective in schizophrenics, it did produce improvement in depressed patients. The first MAOI, ipronozid, was used to treat tuberculosis and was observed to produce an elevated mood in tuberculosis patients (Davis, 1985).

Many of the psychotropic drugs were discovered by chance when they were given to see what would happen, or were given for one condition and were observed to be helpful in a different disorder. In 1949, Cade, an Australian state hospital superintendent, tried lithium experimentally and found that it reduced mania. The history of the development of antidepressant and antipsychotic drugs points up the fact that major scientific discoveries can evolve as consequences of clinical investigation rather than deductions from animal models (Davis, 1985). More recently, however, the development of new drugs has been due to specific engineering for selective actions leading to increasing more effective and "cleaner" agents.

General Principles of Psychopharmacotherapy

When considering, initiating, and maintaining drug treatment of major mental disorders, the following principles should be followed:

1. A thorough diagnostic assessment is the foundation of treatment. When a patient presents with symptoms, the clinician's goal is to formulate these problems based upon objective and subjective signs and symptoms, keeping in mind that multiple causes can produce very similar syndromes.

2. Pharmacotherapy alone is generally insufficient to complete recovery. While drug therapy may be the cornerstone of recovery, there is always a need for some type of educational and psychosocial intervention, as well as psychotherapy.

3. The phase of an illness, whether acute or chronic, is of critical importance in terms of the initial treatment as well as treatment duration. Some patients may need short-term care, while others may need lifetime

maintenance and/or prophylaxis.

4. The risk to benefit ratio must always be considered. Physical and psychiatric conditions must be kept in mind. The presence of medical conditions, pregnancy, addictive disorders, etc., must be evaluated so that the treatment is not worse than the disease. Another important consideration is cost; a treatment the patient cannot afford will not be useful.

5. Prior personal and family history of a good or bad response to a specific treatment modality usually provides guidance for treatment.

6. It is important to target specific symptoms that serve as markers for the underlying psychopathology and monitor their presence or absence over an entire course of treatment. Certain symptoms may respond differently at different times. For example, the neurovegetative symptoms of depression may improve weeks before the mood actually improves.

7. It is necessary to monitor for the development of adverse effects throughout the entire course of treatment, often using the laboratory to ensure safety and optimal efficacy.

Role of Laboratory Testing in Diagnosis and Medication Use

Regardless of the type of medication, practitioners are increasingly better able to make decisions because of expanding knowledge about drug actions. When psychotropic medications were first discovered, they were used largely on a trial and error basis. Now, however, laboratory tests are routinely being used to rule in or out other medical conditions that can mimic or complicate psychiatric illnesses. Increasingly, the laboratory results are used to aid in diagnosis and to monitor the safety and efficacy of drug treatment. The ability to monitor blood levels of psychotropic drugs can help the clinician know if the proper dosage is being prescribed to get the patient to a therapeutic level. This has taken some of the guesswork out of prescribing.

In the past, a psychiatrist might select an antidepressant, for example, and adjust the dose based on clinical response, side effects, and published data on the acceptable dosage range. This sometimes led to improper dosing and subsequent treatment failure. For example, under earlier guidelines the dosage range for the antidepressant imipramine (Tofranil) was considered to be between 50 mg to 350 mg per day. It was thought that at doses below 50 mg per day there would be no response and more than 350 mg per day was thought to be toxic and unlikely to yield further significant improvement. The former practice was to start the drug at a low dose and increase it every few days until one of three outcomes was observed, namely:

1. A clear and clinical improvement was noted, in which case the drug would be maintained at this level for 3 to 9 months.
2. Intolerable side effects occurred, in which case the drug would be discontinued and another drug tried; or
3. The dose was increased to what was believed to be the maximum allowed. If there was no improvement in 4 to 6 weeks, another drug was tried. Sometimes, what might have been considered treatment resistant depression was really the result of undertreatment.

Now it is possible to tailor treatment with more precision. It is now known that therapeutic blood levels can be seen at what was previously thought to be extremely low doses, 25 mg to 50 mg of imipramine, for example, with good clinical improvement. In principle, it is always best to use the lowest effective dose possible, especially in children, the elderly, and persons with medical illnesses. However, using laboratory results to guide dosage, the clinician now has the flexibility to exceed the upper limits of dosage, turning many "failed drug trials" into positive outcomes and in shorter time.

The laboratory can also be used to detect medication noncompliance, drug abuse, and to monitor blood levels for relapse prevention. In addition to blood and urine parameters, there are several other diagnostic tools available to the clinician today, including EEG and polysomnography, computerized axial tomography (CAT scan), magnetic resonance imaging (MRI), position emission tomography (PET scan), topical brain mapping, and psychological tests (psychometrics) (Gold, Potash, & Extein, 1984).

The laboratory, then, is an increasingly vital part of modern psychiatric treatment and as refinements and new technology develop, will be even more important.

The psychotropic drugs to be discussed in this chapter have proved efficacy as well as the potential to cause serious adverse effects. When prescribing any medication, a careful judgment has to be based on consideration of the risk versus benefit ratio.

Antidepressants

Pathophysiology of Depressive Illness

Before discussing specific agents, it is important to have an overview of what is believed about "biological" depression. As a diagnosis, depression implies an underlying chemical imbalance of the CNS. The most commonly accepted hypothesis today is that a functional deficiency of two neurotransmitters (norepinephrine and serotonin) is important in depressive illness. These two substances, also called monoamines, are contained in vesicles and stored in the presynaptic neuron (Figure 11-1a). These monamines are discharged into the interneuronal space (synaptic cleft) and become carriers of impulse transmission to the postsynaptic neuron (Figure 11-1b) (Hackett & Cassem, 1978). Transmission occurs when these monoamines bind to the postsynaptic neuron. The binding is brief and the molecule is released back into the synaptic cleft to be reabsorbed or metabolized (Figure 11-1c). For norepinephrine, about 50% of that stored comes from re-uptake. Destruction of the unstored monoamine occurs within the cell by the monoamine oxidase enzymes and in the extracellular space by the enzymes called methyltransferases (Hackett & Cassem, 1978).

The complexity of the electrochemical processes necessary for normal brain function makes the possibility of dysfunction readily understandable. Failure to terminate the action of a released neurotransmitter would be likely to prolong, inhibit, or exaggerate its action. Likewise, the production and release of excess monoamines or excessive sensitivity of the receptor site at the action of these neurotransmitters would produce an exaggerated effect at the cellular level, which might be seen as a clinical abnormality. Deficient synthesis or release of neurotransmitter molecules, or decreased sensitivity of the receptor site, also would likely produce a physiologic abnormality that again could be

Figure 11-1a	Figure 11-1b	Figure 11-1c
	Stored Monoamines (seratonin, epinephrine) discharged in neurotransmission	Reception by binding neurotransmitters
seratonin epinephrine		

manifested clinically in abnormalities of thought process, mood, or behavior (Hackett & Cassem, 1978). The antidepressant drugs work at the level of neurotransmission to "normalize" transmission of impulses.

Tricyclic Antidepressants

The tricyclic antidepressant drugs (TCA) such as amitryptyline (Elavil), imipramine (Tofranil), and doxepin (Sinequan, Adapin) were, for many years, the mainstay of the pharmacologic treatment of depression. There are a variety of tricyclic drugs that are more or less equally effective in the treatment of depression (Table 11-1). These compounds probably work by blocking neuronal re-uptake of norepinephrine and serotonin. The TCAs mainly differ in the extent and severity of their side effects. To varying degrees, all available tricyclic antidepressants block acetylcholine and consequently inhibit the parasympathetic nervous system. This cholinergic blockade by TCAs is responsible for commonly reported side effects which include blurred vision, dry mouth, reduced sweating, constipation, urinary retention, and tachycardia (Bassuk & Schoonover, 1977). Patients with cardiac diseases or other medical

Table 11-1. Summary of Antidepressant Drugs Currently Used in the United States.

Name			Avail. Preps (mgs) Oral		Comments, Advantages/ Disadvantages
Class	Generic	Trade	Tablet	Capsule	
Tricyclic Type Norepinephrine (NE) Seratonin (SHT) Inhibitors	Imipramine	Tofranil SK-Pramine Imavate Janamine	10, 25, 30	75, 100, 125, 150	
	Amitriptyline	Elavil Endep	10, 25, 50 75, 100, 150		
	Doxepin	Sinequan Adapin		10, 25, 50 75, 100, 150	
	Amoxapine	Asendin	25, 50, 100, 150		
	Trazadone	Desyrel	50, 100, 150		
	Trimipramine	Surmontil		25, 50, 100	

(continued)

Table 11-1. Summary of Antidepressant Drugs Currently Used in the United States (continued).

Class	Generic	Trade	Tablet	Capsule	Comments, Advantages/ Disadvantages
Tricyclic Type					
Norepinephrine (NE) Seratonin (SHT) Inhibitors	Chlorimipra-mine	Anafranil	25, 50		Tricyclic-like, drug of choice for OCD, effective antidepressant
Norepinephrine (NE) Uptake Inhibitors	Desipramine	Norpramin Pertofrane	10, 25, 50, 75, 100, 150	25, 50	Metabolite of Imipramine Less sedative Frequently used as research standard
	Nortriptyline	Aventyl Pamelor		10,25,75	Amitriptyline Metabolite Less sedative Less hypotension May have adv. in elderly
Tricyclic Type					
NE Uptake Inhibitors	Protriptyline	Vivactil	5,10 mg	15-60 mg/d	
	Mapratoline	Ludiomil	20, 50, 75 mg	75-225 mg/d	
Norepinephrine Synthesis Enhancer	Miansedin				An experimental tetracyclic not yet available in the U.S.
Norepinephrine Potentiator	Bupropion	Wellbutrin	100 mg	225-450 mg/d	Reported advantages are: • No NE or SHT reuptake block • Non-sedative • No weight gain • Non-stimulant • Not cardiotoxic • Minimal anti-cholinergic effects • Overdose safe

Column headers: Name (Class, Generic, Trade); Avail. Preps (mgs) Oral (Tablet, Capsule)

Table 11-1. Summary of Antidepressant Drugs Currently Used in the United States (continued).

Name			How supplied	Dosing Range*	Comments, Advantages, Disadvantages
Class	Generic	Trade			
(NE) Uptake Inhibitors	Alprazolan	Xanax	.25, .5, 1 mg	1-4 mg/d	Developed as an anti-anxiety drug. Few side effects. Addiction potential with prolonged use.
Serotonin Uptake Inhibitors	Fluoxetine	Prozac	10,20 mg	20-60 mg/d	Unique structure, No anticholinergic effect
	Paroxetine	Paxil	20,30 mg	20-50 mg/d	
	Sertraline	Zoloft	50,100 mg	50-200 mg/d	
	Venlafaxine	Effexor	37.5-75 mg	150-375 mg/d	
Monoamine Oxidase Inhibitors	Phenelzine	Nardil	15 mg	30-90 mg/d	Good in resistant atypical depression. Avoid tyramine.
	Tramycypromine	Parnate	10 mg	10-40 mg/d	Stimulant, Avoid Tyramine

problems that would make them particularly vulnerable to anticholinergic drugs should be treated cautiously with TCAs. [For such patients it would be preferable to use doxepin (Sinequan) or desipramine (Norpramin) because of their lower anticholinergic potency (Roose & Glassman, 1989)].

Sedation is probably the most common side effect associated with TCAs. This effect may be inconvenient or unpleasant in that it may interfere with the life functions of the patient during the day. However, this sedative side effect can be beneficial since insomnia and anxiety are frequently among the most troublesome symptoms of depression. Usually the sedation lessens over a 2 to 4 week period as the patient "adjusts" to the medication. Interestingly, this same 2 to 4 week period is when the properly dosed patient notices a subjective sense of improvement.

It should be kept in mind that TCAs may interact with a variety of other medications. The sedative effect of TCAs may be increased when they are used with a variety of CNS depressant drugs. Alcohol should be avoided since its effects will be increased and because alcohol, a CNS depressant, can worsen depression itself. Patients should be cautioned about driving or working around hazardous machinery until a functional assessment can be made (Smiley, 1987). The selection of the least sedative TCA is prudent in the patient who must be alert during the day. Frequently, giving the medication as a single evening dose can minimize this problem. Although the sedative effect is usually transient, a trial of a different class of drug may be needed to identify the drug with the least sedative side effects. TCAs interfere with the antihypertensive effect of several types of blood pressure medications, specifically, guanethidine and clonodine (Bassuk & Schoonover, 1977). If a TCA is indicated, the antihypertensive drug can be changed in cooperation with the patient's primary care specialist.

TCAs can produce orthostatic (postural) hypotension (the transient and precipitous lowering of blood pressure as the patient arises from a supine to standing position). This can lead to blackouts, which can further lead to falls and serious injury (Smiley, 1987). The elderly are particularly prone to this side effect, which can lead to devastating injuries, particularly fractured hips and wrists. Therefore, it is extremely important to discuss this and the other side effects carefully with the patient and, if possible, with a significant family member or friend.

The anticholinergic effects tricyclic drugs can be additive with anticholinergic effects of other agents that medical patients may be receiving (e.g., antiparkinsonian drugs). TCAs can also produce or worsen cardiac arrhythmias. Therefore, it is a good idea to obtain baseline and follow up EKGs, especially in the elderly (Roose & Glassman, 1989).

Some patients receiving tricyclic antidepressants may become confused or agitated. This effect is linked either to their anticholinergic effect or to the ability of these drugs to uncover a previously unrecognized psychotic disturbance.

Larger doses of tricyclic drugs may cause toxic psychosis with auditory and visual hallucinations (Davis, 1985). Visual hallucinations are assumed to be organically based until proven otherwise so drugs must be considered as a possible cause. Some patients with an unrecognized underlying bipolar disorder may experience a "manic switch" or acute manic psychosis after treatment for depressive illness with tricyclic drugs (Davis, 1985). Occasional confusion and less well-defined memory deficits have been associated with tricyclic antidepressants. Table 11-2 summarizes side effects.

The antidepressant drugs do not markedly influence the normal organism in a baseline state but rather correct an abnormal condition. The action may be similar to aspirin, which will lower a fever but does not lower normal temperatures (Davis, 1985). The TCAs and MAOIs are antidepressants, not

Table 11-2. Summary of Antidepressant Side Effects.

Dry mouth	Vomiting	Aggravation of narrow
Palpitations	Constipation	angle glaucoma
Tachycardia	Sedation	Urinary retention
Heart block	Agitation	Paralytic ileus
Myocardial infarction		
Loss of accomodation	Hallucinations, delusions	Peculiar taste
(blurred vision)	in latent psychosis	Skin rash
Orthostatic hypotension	Diarrhea	Galactorrhea
Fainting	Black tongue	Gynecomastria
Nausea	Edema	Bone marrow depression

general euphoriants or stimulants. Thus, although imipramine has marked antidepressant action on depressed psychiatric patients, good evidence indicates that it has little euphoriant action on normal persons (Hackett & Cassem, 1978). It is known that when the MAOIs are used to treat high blood pressure, most patients do not experience marked mental effects. In contrast, amphetamine is a euphoriant and a stimulant, but is not an antidepressant in the precise sense of the word (Hackett & Cassem, 1978).

The TCAs—imipramine (Tofranil), amitriptyline (Elavil), desipramine (Norpramin), nortriptyline (Pamelor), and protriptyline (Vivactil)—are structurally similar to the phenothiazines. That similarity emphasizes the importance of minor structural differences in drugs in the production of critical changes in pharmacological activity. The great majority of the TCAs block the re-uptake of norepinephrine or serotonin (5-hydroxytryptomine, 5HT), down-regulate GLB-NE receptors, and produce the same range of effects. The pharmacology of the tricyclic-type is complex because those drugs also affect histamine-2 receptors (Kalinowsky, Hippius, & Helmfried, 1982). As a result of these properties there is a compensatory decrease of norepinephrine synthesis, presumably as a result of noradrenergic potentiation.

The TCAs are readily absorbed from the gastrointestinal tract. In humans, imipramine (Tofranil), amitriptyline (Elavil), chlorimipramine (Anafranil), and doxepin (Sinequan, Adapin), are partially metabolized to their respective desmethyl derivation. These metabolites are therapeutically active and have fewer side effects (Davis, 1985).

Clinical Effects
In normal persons, tricyclic drugs produce slight sedation; however, in severely depressed psychotic patients they produce a striking improvement in

behavior and marked lessening of depression, often 3 to 10 days after the start of treatment. Using the drug doubles the chance of recovery after 3 to 4 weeks of treatment. Patients who do not respond after receiving an adequate dose of the drug for 3 weeks probably will not respond at all. Furthermore, the degree of response in the first week predicts the ultimate therapeutic response (Bassuk & Schoonover, 1977).

Monoamine Oxidase Inhibitors

This group of psychoactive agents is frequently effective in the treatment of severe endogenous depression, panic disorders, and in the atypical depression associated with borderline personality disorder (Par, 1987). These agents are divided into two categories: hydrazines and non-hydrazines. The hydrazines include isocarboxazid and phenylzine (Nardil). The only non-hydrazine in use is tranylcypromine (Parnate). The structural difference is clinically important. Tranylcypromine has somewhat stimulant amphetamine-like qualities that often produce clinical improvement in about 10 days. Tranylcypromine, however, has a greater degree of side effects, particularly of the cardiovascular system. The hydrazines are effective within 3 to 4 weeks and have a lower incidence of side effects (Bassuk & Schoonover, 1977).

The MAOIs inhibit many enzyme systems. They elevate body levels of epinephrine, norepinephrine, 5HT, and dopamine by irreversibly binding to the degradation enzymes of these substances. This process greatly increases the body's available biogenic amines. It is hypothesized that this CNS effect is responsible for the antidepressant activity. The MAOIs can produce many serious side effects and should be prescribed only by experienced practitioners (Bassuk & Schoonover, 1977).

Cardiovascular side effects of the MAOIs, including orthostatic hypotension, tachycardia, and palpitations, can be life-threatening. In cardiac patients, these agents can eliminate or delay the onset of angina pectoris by blocking the response of the cardiovascular system to exercise (Jefferson, 1989). This effect can promote conditions that predispose to myocardial infarction (Jefferson, 1989). The most worrisome cardiovascular side effect is hypertension. This can occur at therapeutic doses, but usually occurs when high doses of the MAOIs are taken, when the drug is combined with a tricyclic antidepressant or sympathomimetic agents (such as cough and cold preparations), or when tyramine (found in a variety of foods) is consumed. The hypertension is caused by the release of catecholamines in the peripheral nervous system. A severe, atypical headache is usually the first sign and may foretell an impending hypertensive crisis that can lead to a cerebrovascular accident (stroke) and death.

Eating foods with a high tyramine content is a major concern. Tyramine is a fermentation by-product, so foods with aged protein should be avoided. Aged cheeses, meats, and fish, most alcoholic beverages, especially beer and red wine, and overripe fruits and vegetables should be avoided. Consumption of chocolate and coffee should be limited.

MAOIs and many pharmacologic agents are synergistic and can result in hypertensive crisis. These include amphetamines, ephedrine, procaine preparations, such as Novocain, epinephrine, methyldopa, meperidine (Demerol), and phenylpropanolamine, which is found in many over-the-counter cold preparations. Patients must be informed to check with their psychiatrist before taking any other medication while on MAOIs. An instruction sheet is usually provided to the patient as part of the informed consent.

Tricyclic antidepressants should be discontinued at least 7 days before a trial of MAOIs and vice versa. Fluoxetine (Prozac) should be discontinued 5 to 6 weeks before starting a MAOI. MAOIs and TCAs are occasionally combined for severe, treatment-resistant depressions under special and controlled circumstances. Fortunately, hypertensive reaction is very rare and can be reversed with prompt administration of an antidote, phentolamine.

The drug can precipitate hypomania or mania. The overall side effect profile is similar to the TCAs and is summarized in Table 11-1.

Overall, the MAOIs are safe and effective in experienced hands, with proper precautions, and in patients able and willing to comply with restrictions. Newer MAOI Type A, which are "reversible" MAOIs are being developed. The first of these, Meclobimide, is available in Europe and Canada, and is scheduled for release in the United States in 1995. These reportedly have fewer side effects and are less likely to cause drug-drug and drug-food interactions.

Selective Serotonin Inhibitors

Over the past 15 years there has been increasing evidence that serotonin neurotransmission is decreased in depression. Fluoxetine (Prozac), introduced in 1988, represents the first of a new class of antidepressants that selectively inhibits neuronal uptake of serotonin. Recent literature suggests that serotonin may be the most important neurotransmitter implicated in depression. Prozac has now been used in the United States for more than a year and is becoming one of the most prescribed antidepressants because of its relative safety (Cooper, 1988), favorable side effects to main effect profile, and patient acceptance. In addition to its antidepressant effects, this agent has shown promising results in the treatment of obsessive compulsive disorder and bulimia.

Prozac has very little anticholinergic activity, therefore there is a low incidence of drowsiness, dry mouth, cognitive impairment, constipation, or weight gain. The most common side effects are transient nausea, nervousness, and insomnia. In comparison studies, Prozac is as effective as the TCAs (Schuckit, 1988).

Sertraline (Zoloft) was put on the United States market in 1992. Several studies have found this drug superior to placebo and comparable in efficacy to the TCAs. It is effective in patients with moderate to severe depression, with or without melancholia, with low or high anxiety, with or without insomnia, with psychomotor agitation or psychomotor retardation. The dosage range is 50 to 200 mg per day.

Paroxetine (Paxil) became available in 1993. It too has been shown to be superior to placebo and equally effective to other SSRIs, TCAs, and MAOIs. Dosage range is 20 to 50 mg per day.

Effexor (Venlafaxine) is a novel compound with demonstrated antidepressant properties that has a neuropharmacologic profile distinct from that of other current agents. It significantly inhibits the uptake of serotonin and epinephrine, and to a lesser extent, dopamine. It has no significant affinity for serotonergic, adrenergic, dopaminergic, cholinergic, or histaminergic receptor sites. The dosage range is 75 mg to 375 mg per day in 2 or 3 divided doses. It may have a more rapid onset of action than other antidepressants. The drug is well tolerated, the main side effects being nausea, somnolence, dizziness, dry mouth, sweating, and headaches. The side effects are generally mild and transient. The risk of suicide by overdose is very small.

In general, all the SSRIs are effective, well-tolerated, and represent a major breakthrough in treating depression and OCD. Furthermore, they can be administered once a day which increases the compliance rate. Also, it is generally believed that overdosing on these medications is much less likely to produce fatality. The most common side effects of SSRIs are shown in Table 11-2A. These are usually mild and transient, often clearing in 10 to 14 days.

A rare sequela to SSRI is termed the Central Serotonergic Syndrome. This is a toxic hyperserotonergic event that is thought to result from hyperstimula-

Table 11-2A. Common Side Effects of SSRI.

• Nausea	• Diarrhea
• Anorexia	• Drowsiness
• Insomnia	• Dry mouth
• Nervousness	• Loss of libido
• Tremor	• Sexual dysfunction

Table 11-2B. Central Serotonergic Syndrome.

Gastrointestinal	Neurological	Cardiovascular	Psychiatric	Other
Abdominal cramping	Tremulousness	Tachycardia	Hypomania	Diaphoressis
Bloating	Myoclonus	Hypotension	Racing thoughts	Elevated temp
Diarrhea	Dysarthia	Hypertension	Pressure speech	Hyperthermia
	Uncoordination	Cardiovascular collapse (death)	Confusion	Hyperreflexes
	Severe headache		Disorientation	

tion of brainstem and spinal cord 5-ht 1A receptors. This syndrome is characterized by gastrointestinal, neurological, cardiovascular, and psychiatric symptoms. (Sternback, 1991) (Table 11-2B).

Buproprion (Wellbutrin) is the only marketed aminoketone antidepressant. It is neither an uptake inhibitor, an MAOI, nor TCA, but does produce down regulation of post-synaptic beta-noradrenergic receptors (Golden, DeVane, Laizure, et al, 1988). The possible advantages of Wellbutrin are that it is non-sedating, has low incidence of weight gain, low toxicity with overdose, little effect on sexual function, and little effect on EKG. The potential disadvantages are overstimulation, tremor, and/or lower seizure threshold (Mahta, 1983). Buproprion (Wellbutrin) is an antidepressant of the aminodetone class and is chemically unrelated to other known antidepressant agents. The exact neurochemical mechanism of the antidepressant effect is unknown. It exerts minimal receptor blockage (i.e., it does not block reception of impulses of the synapse). Buproprion's efficacy is equal to the TCAs, with most patients responding in 3 weeks. The adverse effects most frequently observed are agitation, dry mouth, insomnia, nausea, constipation, and tremor. In 1985, this drug was voluntarily withdrawn from the United States market because of concern about the potential for seizures. Subsequent studies have shown this to be a safe drug but it is not recommended for use in anyone with a seizure potential nor in those with a history of bulimia or anorexia nervosa (Mahta, 1983).

Antianxiety Agents

Anxiety is a universal response to stress and is necessary for effective functioning and coping. It is experienced as a state of tension accompanied by feelings of dread and potential danger. However, in some individuals, the symptom complex is so severe that the patient is immobilized and

Table 11-3. Antianxiety Drugs.

Class	Chemical Name	Trade Name	Dosage
Benzodiazepine	Chlordiazepoxide Diazepam Oxazepam Flurazepam Alprazolam Clorazepate	Librium Valium Serax Dalmane Xanax Tranzene	10-100 mg/d 2-40 mg/d 15-90 mg/d 15-30 mg/d .1254 mg/d 15-60 mg/d
Antihistamines	Cyclizine Hydroxyzine Diphenhydramine	Maverzine Atarax, Visteril Benedryl	 75-400 mg/d 25-100 mg/d
Barbituates		Amytal Seconal Nembutal	
Carbamate	Meprobamate		400 mg

dysfunctional. The decision whether to medicate for anxiety is complex, and clearly, medication is one modality that should be integrated into a more comprehensive plan.

Antianxiety drugs produce symptomatic relief of anxiety. Even if the anxiety is adaptive, an antianxiety agent may improve the patient's ability to cope, or enhance the effectiveness of other types of treatment. Antianxiety drugs are useful in only a few situations and always in the context of an ongoing relationship between the patient, the prescribing physician, and the interdisciplinary treatment team. Generally, they should be used for short-term administration. Major types of antianxiety agents are listed in Table 11-3.

Benzodiazepines

The benzodiazepines have been the most prescribed of all psychotropic drugs for the past 20 years. The currently marketed benzodiazepines are listed in Table 11-3. In 1985, six of the 25 most prescribed drugs were benzodiazepines (Sussman & Chou, 1988). In that year, they accounted for one in every two prescriptions among adults. Such extensive use is associated with considerable controversy. Critics of benzodiazepines cite two properties of the drugs that make them susceptible to abuse: they produce euphoriant effects and have a rapid onset of action. Others argue that abuse and habituation is relatively infrequent and limited primarily to those with histories of substance abuse (Shader & Greenblatt, 1984). The negative publicity surrounding the benzodiazepines has produced a number of problems, foremost among them a hesitancy to prescribe the medications in cases in which their benefits clearly outweigh their potential harm. Sensation-alized accounts of diazepam (Valium) abuse have served to deflect attention from the therapeutically useful role benzodiazepines can play (Sussman & Chou, 1988). They have also obscured awareness of some important liabilities

Table 11-4. Therapeutic Effects of Benzodiazepines.

• Anxiety reduction	• Anesthesia
• Sedation	• Amnesia
• Anticonvulsant activity	• Antipanic activity
• Muscle relaxation	• Antidepressant
• Antistress effect	• Alcohol withdrawal

associated with the class as a whole, some of which are more prevalent and clinically significant than abuse per se.

The widespread use of benzodiazepines derives from their therapeutic usefulness for a broad range of indications (Table 11-4). Most reviews emphasize their effectiveness as antianxiety agents. Specific effects include reduction in worry, shakiness, physiologic symptoms, and panic attacks (Sussman & Chou, 1988). They appear to be more effective in people suffering from severe anxiety and appear to have little impact on those with low anxiety levels. There is conflicting evidence about the efficacy of long-term benzodiazepine therapy. Some studies do not demonstrate continued effects beyond 6 months, although others suggest some anxious patients benefit from lifelong treatment (Haskell, Cole, & Schneibolk, 1986).

The inability to dissociate the sedative from the anxiolytic effects of benzodiazepines leaves unanswered the degree to which these drugs specifi-cally reduce anxiety, rather than reducing overall CNS arousal. Some evidence suggests that the initial effects of benzodiazepines are sedative with anxiolytic action appearing after about a week of treatment. Tolerance of the sedative effect appears about this time (File & Pellow, 1987).

Panic attacks have long been known to respond to treatments with antidepressants and beta-blockers, but not to treatment with standard benzodiazepines (File & Pellow, 1987). However, recent experience has shown that alprazolam (Xanax) produces significant improvement in panic disorder. Full therapeutic effects are generally achieved within the first week of treatment. Another benzodiazepine, clonazepam (Klonopin), normally used as an anticonvulsant, has been found to be an effective antipanic drug (Tesar & Rosenbaum, 1986).

Benzodiazepines also produce an anti-stress effect, blocking stress induced increases in corticosteroid concentration and plasma catecholamines (Sussman & Chou, 1988). Therefore, these drugs are often used for patients with medical disorders. Especially in coronary heart disease, the administration of antianxiety drugs may reduce the incidence of subsequent myocardial infarction.

Benzodiazepines are widely employed to help ease alcoholic withdrawal syndrome. Since these agents attach to the same receptor sites in the brain as alcohol, these agents can be substituted and then tapered off over a 5 to 7 day period.

All the benzodiazepines produce similar pharmacologic effects. The differences among the drugs involve pharmacokinetics, such as rates of absorption, elimination of half-life, pathways of metabolism and lipid solubility, factors that contribute to the overall effect by influencing the onset and duration of action. The single most important difference is elimination half-life (Sussman & Chou, 1988). Slowly eliminated drugs accumulate and lead to an increased risk of accidents and cognitive impairment. Problems of accumulation are even more problematic in the elderly because of slowed metabolic activity of the liver and kidneys, which is part of the normal aging

Table 11-5. Side Effects of Benzodiazepines.

• Sedation	• Impaired concentration
• Psychomotor impairment	• Weakness
• Depression	• Impaired sexual function
• Amnesia	• Agitation (rare)
• Dependence	

progress. Short half-life drugs also have special risks such as a more intense withdrawal syndrome, as well as interdose rebound anxiety.

Although comparatively safe, benzodiazepines can produce a wide array of adverse effects. Psychomotor impairment may be the most lethal of all benzodiazepine-related side effects (Table 11-5). Impairment of driving skills put drivers at nearly five times more risk of involvement in a serious accident than those not taking benzodiazepines (Linnoila, Erwin, & Brende, 1983). Global cognitive impairment in the elderly is a significant problem with long half-life anxiolytics and hypnotics accounting for the greatest incidence. The onset of impairment is often insidious, with signs of cognitive impairment becoming evident after years of treatment. Thinking ability improves once the drug is discontinued (Fang, Hinrich, & Ghonheim, 1987).

While benzodiazepine-induced amnesia is an unwanted effect when these agents are used as anxiolytics, it is a necessary property in anesthesia as it helps the patient forget the more traumatic aspects of diagnostic and surgical procedures (O'Boyle et al., 1982).

Other side effects include treatment-emergent depression and paradoxical aggression or mania (Lydiard et al., 1987). Benzodiazepines can cause ventilatory impairment and thus should be used with extreme caution in patients with chronic obstructive lung disease.

About 40% of those who use benzodiazepines for 6 months or more show definite withdrawal on discontinuation. Some may develop dependence after only 6 weeks. Nevertheless, many patients who have been taking benzodiazepines for years do not experience withdrawal symptoms (Busto et al., 1986).

Some commonly reported withdrawal symptoms are anxiety and insomnia. Withdrawal symptoms also include tinnitus (ringing in the ears), involuntary movements, perceptual changes (increased sensitivity to environmental stimuli), confusion, and depersonalization (Busto et al., 1986).

Abrupt discontinuation of high dose therapy with diazepam produces the most severe withdrawal syndrome with disorientation, delirium, seizures, and psychotic reactions. General strategies for minimizing the clinical impact of withdrawal include stopping the drug as soon as the reason for taking it has ceased, and avoidance of abrupt withdrawal by tapering the dose gradually (Busto et al., 1986).

Buspirone (Buspar) is a more recent antianxiety agent distinct from the benzodiazepines. Studies suggest that it is as effective as benzodiazepines in the treatment of generalized anxiety disorder. There is no evidence suggesting it is an effective antipanic agent. Buspirone shows a consistently low incidence of sedation, psychomotor impairment, interaction with alcohol, dependency, and does not impair memory (Davis, 1985). There is preliminary information that buspirone does not cause ventilatory impairment. Buspirone does not block benzodiazepine withdrawal symptoms, creating a problem in switching over to buspirone. The major limitations of buspirone include efficacy in patients recently treated with benzodiazepines, the need for multiple doses and a lag period of 1 to 2 weeks for full anxiolytic effects to appear. These latter features limit patient acceptance (Davis, 1985).

Propranolol and Related Drugs

Anxiety is characterized by a number of autonomic symptoms such as palpitations, rapid heartbeat, tremor, tingling, cold sweats, chest tightness, etc. These symptoms could, in part, be caused by the secretion of epinephrine during stress. Many of the symptoms can be blocked by a beta adrenergic receptor blocker. Propranolol (Inderal), as well as other beta blockers, have been used for general anxiety and for anxiety provoking situations such as public speaking. Ongoing research has verified their usefulness in situational anxiety and less impressive results in panic disorders. These drugs are generally prescribed for a variety of medical conditions such as hypertension and angina pectoris. Their side effects include hypotension and depression. They are contraindicated in asthma and cardiac conditions for which slowing of the heart would be detrimental (Cole, Altesman, & Weingarten, 1979).

Sedatives/Hypnotics

Drugs used to facilitate sleep are known as hypnotics. They are CNS depressants that, in large doses, can produce anesthesia and death. Most of the hypnotic agents effectively induce and maintain sleep the first few days, but this effect diminishes after several days. These agents should only be used for very brief periods because of the addiction and abuse potential. The side effects have already been discussed under the section on benzodiazepines and include hangover, memory impairment, and paradoxical combativeness.

Psychostimulants

Psychostimulants have been studied for the treatment of hyperactivity and attention deficit disorder since 1936. These agents are moderately to significantly effective in 75% of affected children and adults (Tables 11-5A and 11-5B). They have also been used to augment therapy in patients with treatment resistant depression, especially in the elderly and the severely medically compromised patient. It is also found that these agents may improve the quality of life in the terminally ill who can get energized to put their affairs in order and to stay awake and alert to interact with their loved ones.

Psychostimulants are controlled substances that can only be prescribed in limited quantities and for the specific indication of Attention Deficit Hyperactivity Disorder, Narcolepsy, and treatment resistant depression. They can not legally be prescribed for weight control or to help people remain awake at work. The calming effect is actually a response to the improvement in attention, concentration, and overall cognitive functioning. These effects can be demonstrated in nearly anyone who takes these medications in low to moderate doses. At higher doses these can cause distractibility and increased psychomotor activity (see Table 11-5B). When used appropriately these agents are safe, well tolerated, and have a much lower addiction potential than the general public thinks. The belief that "speed kills" is due to the street abuse of amphetamines.

Table 11-5A. Psychostimulants Used to Treat ADHD in Children and Adults.

Feature	Methylphenidate (Ritalin)	Pemoline (Cylert)	Dextroamphetamine
Elimination half-life	2-3 hours	2-12 hours	6-7 hours
Time to peak plasma concentration	1-3 hours	1-5 hours	3-4 hours
Onset of behavioral effect	1 hour	3-4 weeks	1 hour
Duration of behavioral effect	3-4 hours	not available	4 hours
Daily dose range			
mg/kg/day	0.6 - 1.7	0.5 - 3.0	0.3 - 1.25
mg/day	10 - 60	37.5 - 112.5	5 - 40

(Janicak, Davis, Preskorn, & Ayd, 1993)

Table 11-5B. Summary of Psychostimulant Adverse Effects.

Common and Time Limited	Less Common, More Serious
Anorexia	Increased blood pressure
Weight loss	Tachycardia
Irritability	Precipitation of tic-like movement disorder
Abdominal pain	Nightmares
	Hepatotoxicity
	Psychotic symptoms
	Rash

The main drawbacks and side effects of these drugs are jitteriness, palpitations, insomnia, sexual dysfunction, rebound depression, and psychic dependence. Florid psychosis, resembling acute paranoid psychosis, can be precipitated or unmasked by these drugs (Chiarello & Cole, 1987). Anorexia is the most troublesome side effect but can be managed by giving the drug after meals. Tolerance to anorexia and insomnia usually develops after a few weeks. Increased motor activity, abdominal pain, tearfulness, social withdrawal, and tachycardia are frequently encountered. The seizure threshold may be lowered. Again, habituation to CNS stimulants in children has not been reported and, as stated previously, there is no evidence suggesting that these drugs predispose to later addictive diseases (Chairello & Cole, 1987). In fact, the rate of comorbidity of drug addiction and antisocial behavior in later life is much higher in untreated ADHD patients (Hechtman, Weiss, & Perlman, 1984).

Methylphenidate (Ritalin) is the most widely used and best studied medication for ADHD. It is generally given in divided doses since the elimination half-life is short. A sustained release preparation is also available but its pharmacokinetics are inconsistent (Pelham, Bender, Caddell, Booth & Moorer, 1985).

Pemoline (Cylert) has a longer half-life, which further increases with chronic administration. It therefore may be given once a day and is generally reserved for cases where the effects of methylphenidate do not persist long enough for optimal control of hyperactivity and distractibility. Because of a long onset of action it is believed that it has less abuse potential than methylphenidate or dextroamphetamine. It has not been shown to be as efficacious as methylphenidate or amphetamines (Connors & Taylor, 1980).

Amphetamines also have a longer half-life than methylphenidate but not as long as pemoline. Because of the rapid onset of action and longer half-life, proponents think that amphetamines are better agents for the treatment of ADHD. It is clearly a useful alternative, since up to 20% of children who respond poorly to one psychostimulant will respond well to another. Dextroamphetamine is also less expensive but there is more concern about these agents being diverted to the illicit drug market (Janicak, Davis, Preskorn, & Ayd, 1993).

In summary, these agents are very effective in the treatment of ADHD, narcolepsy, and depression. They are relatively safe and well tolerated. Research has shown improvement in task and off task behavior, increase in positive social behavior, improved parent-child and teacher-child relationships leading to improved self-esteem (Loney, Kramer & Milich, 1981).

Antipsychotic Drugs

Psychoses are among the least understood and most devastating illnesses to affect mankind. Psychotic illnesses cause serious disruption in the lives of individuals and their loved ones and have a major impact on society by incapacitating significant numbers of people. The discovery of chlorpromazine (Thorazine) a scant 34 years ago was one of the significant advances in the understanding and treatment of psychotic illness. Since chlorpromazine became available in clinical practice, there have been significant advances in understanding the mechanisms and etiologies of psychosis. It is unlikely that a single cause will explain what appears to be a varied group of illnesses. Over 300,000 Americans alone are afflicted with schizophrenias, bipolar disorders, and other psychotic illnesses. Many others will develop transient psychotic conditions for a multitude of reasons. This section will discuss the drugs useful in treating these conditions.

To avoid confusion, these drugs are best referred to as antipsychotic drugs.

The agents have also been called "neuroleptics" and "major tranquilizers." There are now about 20 antipsychotic drugs on the market, divided among five distinct chemical classes. Only eight or nine of these products are in widespread clinical use by practitioners. These antipsychotic drugs appear to act by the mechanism of dopamine blockage, suggesting the possibility that in schizophrenia, the underlying disease mechanism may involve an abnormality of dopamine release or receptor sensitivity (Farde, 1989).

Unfortunately, all available therapeutic agents in this class produce some degree of extrapyramidal effects (EPS) (e.g., tremor, shuffling gait) that must be managed when these drugs are administered to the patient. The connection between the beneficial effects and the side effects has become better understood as dopamine receptor blockage has been recognized as the most likely mechanism of antipsychotic drug action.

One experimental antipsychotic compound, clozapine, appears to exert its action in another way. This drug was released early in 1990 and could herald a new direction in the treatment of these disorders, and most of the current antipsychotics may become obsolete in the next 10 years (Meltzer, 1989).

The clinical use of antipsychotic drugs is primarily directed toward syndrome and symptoms. The main target symptoms are disturbed psychomotor behavior, abnormal affect, psychotic perceptual disturbances (hallucinations), delusional thinking, catatonic behavior, autistic withdrawal, and others (Schultz & Pata, 1989).

Most experts agree that the various agents do not differ in their antipsychotic effects if equivalent doses are given. Although there is little evidence that any of these drugs is clearly superior to another in antipsychotic effect, they do have different side effect profiles. Since specific side effects maybe more or less problematic in particular patients, this is one basis for the choice of a particular drug. Although there are no clear indications for specific antipsychotic drugs, clinicians observe that patients who fail to respond to one antipsychotic drug may respond to another, even though it belongs to the same chemical group.

As plasma levels of antipsychotics reveal, there are extreme individual variations in absorption, metabolism, and excretion of psychoactive drugs which may explain why a certain person may respond to one drug but not another (Kane, 1989). A basic pharmacotherapeutic requirement is that these drugs be given in a generally accepted dosage range and over a certain time. There is little to be gained in changing hastily from one drug to another without an adequate clinical trial.

Therapy with antipsychotic drugs can be divided into three phases. The initial phase of treatment is generally aimed at providing behavioral control and reducing agitation, fear, delusions, and hallucinations. This can take from hours to weeks (Kane, 1989).

The next phase of antipsychotic chemotherapy involves stabilization and gradual reduction of the medication dosage to receive the best possible control using the lowest possible dose, thereby reducing the patient's vulnerability to drug side effects.

The third phase of treatment of the psychotic patient may be referred to as maintenance therapy and involves long-term continuous administration of the lowest possible dose of effective medication to prevent recurrence of the illness. Clearly, a great deal of emotional support to patients and their families, rehabilitation services, and community networking are essential to maximize the patient's recovery and reintegration. Specific psychotherapeutic intervention is beyond the scope of this chapter. It has been repeatedly shown, however, that psychotherapeutic interventions in the absence of adequate drug treatment of psychotic disorders lead to suboptimal outcomes.

In the schizophrenic patient, treatment is generally best accomplished by starting and continuing treatment with a single antipsychotic agent, provided the patient can tolerate this medication without incapacitating side effects. If side effects do develop, they can usually be managed by dosage adjustment, addition of an antiparkinsonism medication, or changing to a different medication.

In the treatment of the acutely manic patient, treatment is usually initiated with an antipsychotic drug in conjunction with lithium carbonate. The antipsychotics can usually be withdrawn gradually and the patient maintained on lithium.

Treatment of the psychotically depressed patient is usually initiated by using antipsychotic drugs to manage the delusions, along with an antidepressant. The patient with psychosis should generally receive maintenance medication consisting either of antidepressant drugs alone or in combination with antipsychotic drugs or lithium. The duration for maintenance therapy varies. About 70% of psychotically depressed patients who respond to pharmacologic treatment are off all medication within 1 year. The majority of schizophrenic patients may require maintenance medication for many years, possibly for life.

Side Effects
The side effects of antipsychotic drugs can be classified as follows: autonomic effects, extrapyramidal effects, other CNS effects, behavioral toxicity, allergic reactions, agranulocytosis, skin and eye effects, and endocrine effects.

The autonomic side effects that can occur include dry mouth, blurred vision, skin flushing, constipation, paralytic ileus, mental confusion, and postural hypotension. Dry mouth is one of the most often complained about side effect and can be managed by advising the patient to rinse the mouth frequently with water. The use of sugarless chewing gum can be helpful. Regular sugared gum and candy should be avoided since the sugar added to the dry mouth can predispose to fungal infections and dental caries. Patients usually develop tolerance to blurred vision, which is often problematic only in the first few weeks of treatment. The blurred vision can be managed with reassurance that this is temporary and by the use of magnifying lenses. Inexpensive premade glasses are readily available in drug stores in various strengths of magnification.

Orthostatic hypotension may occur in the first few days of treatment. The main danger of this is that patients may fall and injure themselves. Instructing the patient to arise slowly from a lying to standing position is important. Support hose may help by preventing blood pooling in the lower extremities. The most dramatic and the most theoretically important group of side effects shown by all the antipsychotic drug agents are the extrapyramidal reactions (EPS) (Kane, 1989). These side effects are classified into three categories: parkinsonian syndrome, dystonias, and akathesia. The parkinsonian syndrome consists of a mask-like face, tremor at rest, rigidity, shuffling gait, and motor retardation (bradykinesia) (Kane, 1989). This syndrome is symptomatically identical to idiopathic parkinsonism (Parkinson's disease). The dystonias consist of a broad range of bizarre movements of the tongue, face, and neck. The patient may experience severe muscle spasms of the neck. The tongue may protrude and partially obstruct the airway. The patient's eyes may roll upward (oculogyric crisis). Akithesia is a motor restlessness in which the patient has a great urge to move about and may not be able to sit or stand still.

These side effects are fairly common, vary in intensity, and are easily reversible. They are very distressing to the patient and if not properly managed, can lead to medication noncompliance, thereby compromising the patient's chances for recovery.

Younger patients tend to experience dystonic reactions more often than middle-aged patients, possibly because they have higher levels of dopamine. The acute dystonias typically occur early in the course of treatment even with small doses of antipsychotic drugs. They usually resolve within minutes of intramuscular administration of one of the antiparkisonian drugs such as benztropine (Cogentin), diphenhydramine (Benedryl), or trihexphenidryl (Artane). Amantadine (Symmetrel) is helpful with parkinsonian symptoms and akithesia.

There is controversy in psychiatry about whether one should prophylactically administer an antiparkinsonian medication to all patients being treated with antipsychotic drugs or give it only if side effects occur. Common practice is to co-administer antiparkinsonian drugs and then attempt to discontinue them gradually after about 3 months.

A rare syndrome, described as the neuroleptic malignant syndrome (NMS), characterized by muscular rigidity, hyperthermia, altered consciousness, and autonomic dysregulation has been recognized (Kane, 1989). This is a potentially fatal complication that must be diagnosed and treated early. Discontinuance of the drug, supportive measures such as lowering body temperature, using muscle relaxants such as dantrolene, IV fluids, and possible, emergency electroconvulsive therapy, are life saving. Antipsychotics can usually be safely restarted if needed when the crisis is over. There is little evidence implicating one class of antipsychotic drug over another. There may be a greater likelihood of NMS when multiple psychotropic drugs are used together.

Tardive dyskinesia (TD) is an extrapyramidal syndrome that emerges relatively late in the course of antipsychotic treatment. Long-term, high-dose treatment increases the incidence of TD. TD may also appear days or weeks after antipsychotics are discontinued. This syndrome is sometimes irreversible and no consistently effective treatment has been identified. TD presents with facial grimaces, bucco-lingual movements such as lip smacking, lateral jaw movements, flicking of the tongue, jerking movements of the arms (chorea), and athetoid movements of arms and fingers. Neck and trunk movements can also be found. Symptoms are absent during sleep. The overall incidence of TD is about 15% and is correlated with length of exposure to the drug and total lifetime dose (Glazer, 1989).

As with all forms of treatment, careful decisions have to be made considering the risks of a drug versus its potential benefits. Psychosis is a frightening, debilitating affliction and usually renders patients dysfunctional. The antipsychotic drugs, despite their liabilities, have helped hundreds of thousands to live outside of psychiatric institutions, and, in conjunction with psychotherapies, social and occupational rehabilitation, to lead relatively normal lives.

The various antipsychotic drugs and their side effects are shown in Table 11-6.

Lithium

Lithium has been extensively studied for a variety of clinical conditions. Its widest and best known application is in the treatment of mania and bipolar disorders. The main use of lithium today is for prophylaxis in recurrent affective

Table 11-6. Antipsychotic Drugs.

Name				Name		
Class	Generic	Trade	Side Effects of Antipsychotics	Class	Generic	Trade
Aliphatic	Chlorpromazine	Thorazine	Dry mouth and throat	Piperidine	Thioridazine	Mellaril
	Trifluoproaine	Vesprin	Blurred vision Cutaneous flushing		Mescridazine Piperacelazine	Berentil Quide
Piperazine	Prochlorperazine	Compazine	Constipation Uninary retention Paralytic ileus	Butyrophe-nones	Haloperidol	Haldol
	Perphenazine	Trilafon	Mental Confusion Miosis		Pimozide	Orap
	Trifluoperazine	Stelazine	Myariasis	Thioxanthines	Chlorpre-thizene	Taractan
	Fluphenazine	Prolixin	Orthostatic hypotension		Thiothixene	Navane
		Permitil	Parkinsonian syndrome: Tremor at rest Drooling Mask-like face Rigidity Shuffling gait Motor Retardation			
	Acetophenazine	Tindal	Dyskinesias: Tardive dyskinesia	Dibenzoxaz-epines	Loxapine	Loxitane
	Butaperazine Carphenazine	Repoise Proketazine	Sedation Bizarre dreams Uncoordination Confusion Dermatitis Photosensitivity Deposits in the cornea and lens breast engorge-ment and lactation Weight gain Delayed ejaculation Jaundice Blood dyscrasias	Dihydroin-doline	Molindone	Moban

disorders. It has been shown to be highly effective in preventing both depressive and manic episodes of affective disorder and schizoaffective disorders. The prophylactic effect does not differ in unipolar and bipolar patients. Lithium prevents, or at least reduces, intensity and duration of affective episodes in the majority of these patients. A patient with an atypical affective or cyclic psychosis responding to prophylactic lithium treatment should be maintained on it (Schou, 1989). Other indications, such as therapy for schizophrenia, alcoholism, and some types of personality disorders, are less clearly established (Ortiz, Dabbagh & Gershon, 1984). Its use as adjunctive therapy for depression is becoming more popular as is its use in treatment resistant migraine headaches, thyrotoxicosis, and premenstrual syndrome.

Because of its slower effect and lack of sedation, lithium alone often cannot adequately control acute manic symptoms. Therefore, lithium and antipsychotic drugs are often combined during acute phases of the disorder (Abou & Cooper, 1987).

Numerous trials have shown that the prophylactic effect of lithium in affective disorders is obtained in only 70% to 80% of cases. Because of this, along with the fact that a significant number of patients are lithium intolerant, other bipolar drugs are being tried, particularly the anticonvulsants carbamazepin (Tegretol) and sodium valproate (Depakote).

Lithium is contraindicated in patients with severe cardiovascular disease, in diseases in which dietary sodium is restricted, in Addison's disease, and the first 4 months of pregnancy. Women on lithium should be counseled against breastfeeding. The use of lithium with diuretics is a relative contraindication since urinary sodium loss and volume depletion can produce toxic lithium blood levels. Lithium is relatively contraindicated in certain kidney diseases (Ortiz, Dabbagh & Gershon, 1984).

Side effects occurring in the initial period of lithium therapy tend to disappear with continued treatment. They include polydipsia (excessive thirst), polyuria (excessive urination), fine hand tremor, and diarrhea. Less often found are nausea, sedation, dizziness, fatigue, and abdominal discomfort. Side effects occurring days or weeks later include edema, weight gain, and myxedema (hypothyroidism). It is rarely necessary to discontinue lithium because of its side effects.

Lithium produces a generally benign lowering in the concentration of circulatory thyroid hormones. In most cases the effects of lithium on thyroid function are not of sufficient magnitude to require treatment. If necessary, thyroid supplementation may be administered. Underlying thyroid disorder is not a contraindication to lithium therapy per se.

Lithium produces two distinct categories of renal effects. The most frequent and benign effect is a nephrogenic diabetes insipidus. The other more serious effect, is damage to kidney morphology (structure) (Ortiz, Dabbagh & Gershon, 1984). Several contradictory studies raise doubt whether these lesions are due to lithium alone. With appropriate patient selection, careful renal evaluation, and close clinical and lab follow up, the risk of kidney disease is remote.

The effects of lithium on the CNS range from commonly observed mild effects to irreversible life threatening brain damage in rare instances of severe toxicity. The neurotoxic reaction is characterized by symptoms of organic brain syndrome such as disorientation, confusion, dysarthria (slurred speech), ataxia, reduced concentration, somnolence, lethargy, and extrapyramidal signs

(Ortiz, Dabbagh & Gershon, 1984). Although neurotoxicity has been reported with lithium alone, the extreme neurotoxic syndrome is more often associated with the combination of lithium and an antipsychotic drug (Abou & Cooper, 1987). This neuroleptic malignant syndrome may be caused by the antipsychotic drug itself, whether the addition of lithium causes a greater vulnerability is still not clear (Schou, 1989).

Prior to lithium therapy, a general medical workup should be done including physical examination, EKG, complete blood count, kidney function tests, urinalysis, and thyroid functions. Renal and thyroid functions should be rechecked at least once a year. Treatment is usually started at a dose expected to produce plasma levels within the therapeutic range. After 1 week of continued treatment with a constant dose, the blood level is checked and dosage is adjusted accordingly until effective serum levels of 0.5 to 0.8 mg/L are attained. In manic states, higher levels may be necessary. Once the lithium level is established it should be checked monthly the first half year and then every 3 months thereafter.

Lithium is available as lithium carbonate (Eskalith, Lithonate, Lithane) in capsules and liquid (as citrate). It is also available in sustained release form (Lithobid, Eskalith CR) in various doses (300 mg, 450 mg), and as lithium citrate, lithium acetate, and lithium sulphate. The sustained release forms may be preferable because they might avoid peaks in blood levels and are apt to cause fewer side effects. These medications are administered in divided doses, two or three times per day, although single doses may be as effective with fewer renal effects (Schou, 1989).

Alternative Treatment Strategies for Mood Disorders

While lithium has been a major advance in the treatment of bipolar affective disorder and other mood disorders, there are some factors that limit its usefulness, including: slow onset of action, inadequate response (20% to 40%), intolerance to the drug, adverse effects on thyroid and kidney, tremor, edema, and weight gain. Furthermore, certain subgroups of mood disordered patients may be less likely to benefit from lithium, including: rapid cyclers (5% to 20% of all bipolar patients); dysphoric, mixed, or complex mania (up to 40% of all episodes); severe episodes with psychosis; schizoaffective disorder; the elderly manic patient; patients with co-existent alcohol or substance abuse; personality disorders; and/or mental retardation.

As a result, there has been significant research to develop alternative treatments for these patients (Janicak, Newman, & Davis, 1992). One such strategy is the use of electroconvulsive therapy (ECT) which is the only truly bimodal therapy, in that it is equally effective for both the acute depressed and manic phases of mood disorders. A full discussion of ECT is outside the scope of this chapter however.

The drugs that have taken a prominent position in the treatment of mood disorders are the anticonvulsants carbamazepine (Tegretol) and valproic acid (Depakote, Depakene).

Carbamazepine (Tegretol) is labelled for the management of temporal lobe epilepsy and paroxysmal pain disorders (tic doloreaux). Tegretol has a chemical structure similar to imipramine. Research has shown it to be a potential alternative treatment for acute mania when lithium has been unsuccessful. Its spectrum of efficacy appears similar to that of lithium, and it may be superior in mixes of dysphoric mania, rapid cyclers, and more severe episodes (Post, 1990).

If Tegretol is considered in mania, the pretreatment evaluation should include the assessment of baseline hematological and hepatic functions, since these two organ systems may be affected by this agent. The typical starting dose is 400 to 600 mg/d given in divided doses, and the dose is increased by 200 mg every 2 or 3 days until the desired clinical effect is achieved or side effects preclude further increases. Blood levels of 4 to 12 mcg/mL are therapeutic for convulsions, but the ideal blood level for mania is unknown (Chou, 1990). Tegretol has also been tried with variable results in the management of aggression and in chronic self-injurious, self-mutilating behaviors.

The most serious adverse effect is aplastic anemia, occurring in one out of 125,000 patients. Agranulocytosis is more rare, usually occurring within 2 to 3 months of treatment, but may occur at any time. In addition to monitoring blood counts at appropriate intervals, patients should be instructed to look for signs and symptoms of hematological dysfunction such as fever, sore throat, and malaise, and to report such symptoms to their physician immediately. Tegretol may also adversely affect the liver, so liver function tests should be monitored every 6 to 12 months. Other side effects are listed in Table 11-7 (Joffe, 1985).

Reports on the benefit of valproic acid in various formulations date to the mid 1960s. The first work concentrated on maintenance therapy of manic depressive disease with patients stabilized on valproate for up to 10 years. A few researchers studied the drug in acute mania and found it to be beneficial. Valproic acid's anticonvulsant efficacy may be related to its ability to increase CNS levels of GABA (gamma amino butyric acid). It has a rapid onset of action reaching peak plasma levels in 1 to 4 hours and the half-life ranges from 6 to 16 hours. It is highly protein bound and needs to saturate 50% or more of binding sites to reach its psychotropic effect (McElroy et al., 1991).

Valproic acid appears to be at least comparable to lithium and Tegretol for the

Table 11-7. Anticonvulsants: Adverse Effects.

Carbamazedine (Teqdetol)	Valproic Acid (Depakote)
Nausea, anorexia, vomiting Sedation Ataxia, clumsiness Dizziness Blurred vision, diplopia Inappropriate antidiuretic hormone secretion Lethargy Impaired task performance Irritability Dysomnia Depression Confusion Blood dyscrasias	Nausea, anorexia, vomiting Sedation Tremor Weight gain or loss Transient abpecia Edema Impaired task performance Hyperactivity Aggression Depression Psychosis Liver failure

acute manic phase of bipolar disorder (McElroy et al., 1991). Similarly, like lithium and Tegretol, it does not appear to be as beneficial for the depressive phase of the illness. The drug appears to be especially useful in patients with mixed states and rapid cyclers (Calabrese, Woyshville, Kimmel & Rapport, 1993).

Starting doses are 250 to 500 mg twice per day with doses titrated to blood levels in the range of 50 to 120 mg/mL. The average dose to reach these levels is 750 to 1250 mg/d. The most serious adverse effect of valproic acid involves the liver. There have been a few deaths due to liver failure in patients receiving more than one anticonvulsant. There are no reports of deaths due to liver failure in adults receiving valproic acid monotherapy. Baseline liver function tests, repeat testing in the first few weeks, and every 3 to 6 months thereafter is necessary. Signs and symptoms of hepatotoxicity may include decreased appetite, gastrointestinal distress (nausea, vomiting, abdominal pain), dependent edema, malaise, and easy bruising. See also Table 11-7 for the common adverse effects. Woman of child bearing age should be counseled as to possible birth defects. For example there is a 1% to 2% incidence of spina bifida (Jeavons, 1982).

Calcium Channel Blockers

The calcium antagonists (calcium channel blockers) have been used mainly for the treatment of heart disorders such as arrythmias, hypertension, and angina. These calcium ion inhibitors, such as verapamil (Calan), exert their effects by modulating an influx of calcium across the cell membrane, thus interfering with calcium dependent functions. More recently based partly on the common effects of lithium and this class of drugs, they have been studied as a potential treatment for psychiatric illnesses ranging from mania, rapid cycling, and aggression. However, some promising results should at least encourage further research (Barton & Gitlin, 1987; Post & Ketter, 1992).

Verapamil is administered orally in doses ranging from 80 mg twice daily to 160 mg three times daily. The drug is well tolerated and no specific laboratory monitoring is needed. The most common adverse effects are hypotension and bradycardia, which are usually easily managed with dose adjustments.

Novel Antipsychotic Agents

Until very recently, clinicians have had low expectations and little reason for optimism in the treatment of a significant proportion of the population with schizophrenia. Given the limitations of available treatments, the best one could hope for in the management of many patients with schizophrenia was to dampen some of the positive symptoms of psychosis and to bring about some marginal increase in level of functioning. In this, the "decade of the brain," there is increasing evidence that new, atypical antipsychotic agents, can not only ameliorate both positive and negative symptoms of schizophrenia in heretofore treatment resistant patients but can also improve patient's vocational, social, and cognitive functioning (Christison, Kirch & Wyatt, 1991). The next section will discuss clozapine and respiridone, two new agents that represent the most significant developments in the treatment of schizophrenia since chlorpromazine was introduced forty years ago.

The commercial reintroduction of Clozaril (Clozapine) to the United States market in 1989 was heralded as the first truly major advance in antipsychotic drugs since the introduction of chlorpromazine (Thorazine) 35 years earlier. This hope was based on a possibly greater efficacy in treatment resistant schizophrenic patients, a markedly reduced tendency to produce extrapyramidal symptoms (EPS), and improvement in the "negative symptoms" of schizophrenia (Meltzer, 1990).

The pharmacology of clozapine is complex, in part because of the multiplicity of its neurotransmitter interactions. The proposed pharmacologic mechanisms are its relative preference for dopamine D1 or D3 receptors, its relative affinity for serotonin 5HT-2 or 5HT-3 receptors, and/or its enhancement of GABA activity. Clearly the numbers of competing hypotheses demonstrate the varied pharmacology and a lack of exact neurochemical mechanisms underlying schizophrenia and EPS.

Clozapine is 95% absorbed following oral administration and is detected in the blood one half hour after ingestion. Peak serum concentrations occurred at 2 hours. The mean half-life was 12 hours.

Clozapine causes several major side effects and complications. It is more likely than many other antipsychotics to lower the seizure threshold causing a 14% risk of seizures at doses greater than 600 mg per day, necessitating the co-administration of anticonvulsant drugs in some cases. It has also been observed that occasional cataplectic episodes in which a sudden loss of muscle tone during wakefulness often results in a fall. Orthostatic hypotension is perhaps the most serious adverse reaction, accompanied by respiratory depression. Agranulocytosis is the most clinically significant of clozapine's side effects. The approximate incidence rate for agranulocytosis following clozapine use is 0.8%, with a few deaths attributable to this adverse reaction in Europe (Poulsen, Noring, Fog & Gerlach, 1985). There has been one documented death in the United States due to this acute lowering a white blood cells. This problem has been well handled by a special patient management system in which the patient must have weekly monitoring of WBCs before they are provided with their medication for the following week. While this causes some inconvenience and increases the cost of treatment, it is well worth the effort since this medication is prescribed for patients with treatment resistant schizophrenia, 30% of whom realize the significant clinical benefit. Other occasionally troublesome side effects include sedation, weight gain, and hypersalivation.

The clozapine dose is initiated at 25 mg per day and is increased by 25 mg every 2 to 3 days to an effective level. The dose range is 200 to 900 mg per day with a mean of 500 mg per day. Blood levels often help to determine appropriate dosing requirements.

Risperdal (risperidone) is the second "atypical" antipsychotic to be approved in this country. The theorized mechanism of action is blockade of dopamine (D2) and serotonin (5-HT) receptors. The blockade of serotonin (S2) receptors may account for the relative lack of parkinsonian side effects.

Risperidone is well absorbed from the gastrointestinal tract and peak plasma levels are reached in one hour. Therapeutic benefits may be seen in seven days. The half-life of risperidone is thirty hours.

Risperidone appears to be well tolerated in patients taking up to 10 mg per day, with sedation being reported more frequently at higher doses. This drug produces less extrapyramidal symptoms (EPS) than standard antipsychotic drugs. The most common adverse effects reported were agitation, anxiety, insomnia, EPS, headache, nausea, sedation, and tachycardia. Unlike clozapine, risperidone is not associated with agranulocytosis and to date there have been no reported cases of tardive dyskinesia.

Risperidone was released in February 1994, and no specific drug interactions have been reported. Because risperidone is metabolized in the liver by the cytochrome P450 system, the potential exists for interactions with other drugs metabolized in this way (beta-blockers, SSRIs, Tegretol, phenobarbital, and benzodiazepines).

Risperidone should be administered starting with 1 mg po bid in order to minimize potential orthostatic hypotension during the initial titration period. The dose is usually increased by 1 mg bid up to 6 mg per day which is where most patients respond. Non-responders may need up to 16 mg per day. The safety and efficacy of doses greater than 16 mg per day has not been evaluated.

Role of the Occupational Therapist in Medication Management

Occupational therapists have several essential roles in the medical management of clients. As members of the interdisciplinary treatment team, occupational therapists are responsible for monitoring functional status of clients. They are in a position to report to the physician and others what functional impairment the client may have, and to indicate how that changes over time. Since an important goal of medication is to improve function, observations and formal assessment completed by the occupational therapist provide vital information about the effectiveness of the selected medication and its doseage.

In addition, the therapist must know what medication the client is taking, and what its side effects are. For example, several medications cause postural hypotension which can lead to falls. Therapists must be alert to the potential for clients to fall while engaged in activity, and must implement appropriate preventive measures. Other medications cause drowsiness; clients should not use heavy machinery while unduly drowsy. Still other medications may lead to adverse reactions to sunlight; clients should be kept out of the sun while taking such medication.

It is also important to keep in mind that unpleasant side effects can lead to poor compliance on the part of the client. If the therapist has reason to believe that the client is not taking medication as prescribed, this information must be conveyed to the physician. This has become an increasingly important role for non-physicians as treatment is provided much more often in community rather than inpatient settings, putting clients more in charge of their own medication management.

Thus, the therapist must be informed about what kinds of pharmacologic interventions are being undertaken, and report both main effects noted and undue side effects. Therapists should guard against giving medical advice, but should be sure to direct client questions to the physician. In addition, therapists should convey their own concerns about the medication to the physician. Because the physician may not have regular opportunities to observe the client while engaged in activity, such information can be essential to effective medical management.

References

Abou, M. T., & Copper, A. J. (1987). Acute treatment, long-term management and prophylaxis of affective disorders. *Psychiatric Annals, 17,* 301-308.

American Psychiatric Association (1994). *The Diagnostic and Statistical Manual of Mental Disorders* (4th ed.). Washington, DC: Author.

Barton, B. M. & Gitlin, M. J. (1987). Verapamil in treatment resistant mania: An open trial. *Journal of Clinical Pharmacology, 7,* 101-103.

Bassuk, E., & Schoonover, S. (1977). *The practitioner's guide to psychoactive drugs.* New York: Plenum Books.

Busto, V., Sellers, E., Naranjo, C., et al. (1986). Withdrawal reactions after long term therapeutic use of benzodiazepines. *New England Journal of Medicine, 315,* 854-859.

Cade, J. F. J. (1949). Lithium salts in the treatment of psychotic excitement. *Med J Aust, 2,* 349-352.

Calabrese, J. R., Woyshville, M. D., Kimmel, S. E. & Rapport, D. J. (1993). Mixed states and rapid cyclic bipolar disorder and their treatment with divalproex sodium. *Psychiatric Annals, 23*(2), 70-78.

Chiarello, R. J., & Cole, J. (1987). The use of psychostimulants in general psychiatry, a recommendation. *Archives of General Psychiatry, 44,* 286-296.

Christison, G. W., Kirch, D. G., & Wyatt, R. J. (1991). When symptoms persist: Choosing among alternative somatic treatments for schizophrenia. *Schizophrenia Bulletin, 17,* 217-245.

Cole, J., Altesman, R., & Weingarten, C. (1979). Beta-blocking drugs in psychiatry. *McLean Hospital Journal, 4,* 40.

Connors, L.K., & Taylor, E. (1980). Pemoline, methylphednidate, and placebo in children with minimal brain dysfunction. *Archives of General Psychiatry, 37,* 922-930.

Cooper, G. (1988). The safety of fluoxetine—An update. *British Journal of Psychiatry, 153* (suppl. 3), 77-86.

Davis, J. (1985). Antipsychotic drugs. In H. Kaplan & B. Saddock (Eds.), *Comprehensive textbook of psychiatry, IV* (pp. 1481-1537). Baltimore: Williams and Wilkins.

Fang, J. C., Hinrich, J. V., & Ghonheim, M. H. (1987). Diazepam and memory: Evidence for spared memory function. *Pharmacology and Biochemistry of Behavior, 28,* 347-352.

Farde, L. (1989). PET studies of patients treated with antipsychotic drugs. *Psychiatric Annals, 19,* 530-535.

File, S., & Pellow, S. (1987). Behavioral pharmacology of minor tranquilizers. *Pharmacology Therapy, 35,* 265-290.

Glazer, W. H. (1989). An introduction to tardive dyskinesia. *Psychiatric Annals, 19,* 288.

Gold, M., Potash, A. C., & Extein, I. (1984). Laboratory testing and pharmacology. In J.G. Bernstein (Ed.), *Clinical psychopharmacology* (p. 31) Boston: John Wright, PSG, Inc.

Golden, R. N., Devane, C. L., Laizure, S. C., et al. (1988). Buproprion in depression. *Archives of General Psychiatry, 45,* 145-149.

Hackett, T., & Cassem, N. (Eds.) (1978). *Massachusetts General Hospital handbook of general psychiatry.* St. Louis: C.V. Mosby.

Haskell, D., Cole, J., Schneibolk, S., et al. (1986). A survey of diazepam patients. *Psychopharmacology Bulletin, 22,* 434-438.

Hechtman, L., Weiss, G., & Perlman, T. (1984). Young adult outcome of hyperactive children who received long-term stimulant treatment. *Journal of the American Academy of Child Psychiatry, 23,* 261-269.

Hoschl, C., Blahos, J., & Kabes, J. (1986). The use of calcium channel blockers in psychiatry. In C. E. Shagoss, R. C. Josiasson, W. H. Bridger, et al. (Eds.), *Biographical psychiatry 1985* (pp. 330-332). New York: Elsevior Science Publishing.

Janicak, P. G., Davis, J. M., Preskorn, S. H. & Ayd, F. J. (1993). *Principles and practices of psychopharmacology* (pp. 492-495). Baltimore: Williams and Wilkins.

Janicak, P. G., Newman, R. H. & Davis, J. M. (1992). Advances in the treatment of mania and related disorders: A reappraisal. *Psychiatric Annals, 22*(2), 92-103.

Jeavons, P. M. (1982). Sodium valproate and neural tube defects. *Lancet, ii,* 1282-1283.

Jefferson, J. (1989). Cardiovascular effects and toxicity of anxiolytics and antidepressants. *Journal of Clinical Psychiatry, 50,* 365-375.

Joffe, R. J., Post, R. M., Roy-Byrne, P. P., et al (1985). Hematological effects of carbamezapine in patients with affective illness. *American Journal of Psychiatry, 142,* 1196-1199.

Kalinowsky, L. B., Hippius, H., & Helmfried, E. K. (1982). *Biological treatments in psychiatry.* New York: Grune and Stratton, 129.

Kane, J. M. (1989). The current status of neuroleptic therapy. *Journal of Clinical Psychiatry, 50,* 322-328.

Linnoila, M., Erwin, C. W., Brende, A., et al, (1983). Psychomotor effects of diazepam in anxious patients and healthy volunteers. *Journal of Clinical Psychopharmacology, 3,* 88-96.

Loney, J., Kramer, J., & Milich, R. S. (1981). In K. D. Sadow, & J. Loney (Eds.), *Psychosocial aspects of drug treatment for hyperactivity* (pp. 381-415). Boulder, CO: Westview Press.

Lydiard, R. B., Larai, M. T., Ballenger, J. C., et al. (1987). Emergence of depressive symptoms in patients receiving alprazolam for panic disorder. *American Journal of Psychiatry, 144,* 664-665.

Mahta, N. (1983). The chemistry of buproprion. *Journal of Clinical Psychiatry, 44,* 56-59.

McElroy, S. L., Keck, P. E., Pope, H. S., et al. (1991). Correlates of antimanic response to valproate. *Psychopharmacology Bulletin, 27,* 127-133.

Meltzer, H. (1989). Clozapine: Clinical advantage and biologic mechanisms. In S. C. Schults & C. A. Tammingo (Eds.), *Schizophrenia: Scientific process* (pp. 333-340) New York: Oxford University Press.

Montgomery, S. A., Feighner, J. P., Magni, G. (1993). Venlafaxine: A new dimension in antidepressant pharmacotherapy. *J Clinical Psychiatry 54:3,* 119-126.

O'Boyle, C., Barry, H., Fox, E., et al. (1982). Benzodiazepine-induced event amnesia following a stressful surgical procedure. *Psychopharmacology, 9,* 244-247.

Ortiz, A., Dabbagh, M., & Gershon, S. (1984). Lithium clinical use, toxicology, and mode of action. In J. G. Bernstein (Ed.), *Clinical psychopharmacology* (2nd ed., pp. 111-134). Boston: John Wright, PSG.

Par, C. M. B. (1987). Monoamine oxidase inhibitors in the treatment of affective disorders. *Psychiatric Annals, 17,* 309-311.

Pelham, W. E., Bender, M. E., Caddell, J., Booth, S., & Moorer, S. H. (1985). Methylphenidate and children with attention deficit disorder, dose effects on classroom academic and social behavior. *Archives of General Psychiatry, 42,* 948-952.

Post, R. M., George, M. S., Ketter, T. A., Deniloff, K., Leverich, G. S., & Mikalauskas, K. Mechanisms underlying recurrence and cycle acceleration in affect disorders: Implications for long term treatment. In: Montgomery, S., ed. *Psychopharmacology of Depression.* London, England: Oxford University Press.

Poulsen, U. J., Noring, V., Fog, R. & Gerlach, J. (1985). Tolerability and therapeutic effect of clozapine: A retrospective investigation of 216 patients treated with clozapine for up to 12 years. *Acta Psychiat Scand, 71,* 176-185.

Rickels, K., Gordon, P., Sansman, D., et al. (1970). Pemoline and methylphenidate in mildly depressed outpatients. *Clinical Pharmacologic Therapy, 11,* 698-709.

Roose, S., & Glassman, A. (1989). Cardiovascular effects of tricyclic antidepressants in depressed patients with and without heart disease. *Journal of Clinical Psychiatry Monograph, 7,* 1-18.

Schou, M. (1989). Lithium prophylaxis: Myths and realities. *American Journal of Psychiatry, 146,* 573-576.

Schuckit, H. (1988). *Clinical dialogues in psychiatric disorders: Mood disorders. A phamacologic approach.* New York: Science and Medicine.

Schultz, S. C., & Pata, C. N. (1989). Pharmacologic treatment of schizophrenia. *Psychiatric Annals, 19,* 288.

Shader, R. I., & Greenblatt, D. J. (1984). Benzodiazepine overuse-misuse. *Journal of Clinical Psychopharmacology, 4,* 123-124.

Smiley, A. (1987). Effects of minor tranquilizers and antidepressants on psychomotor performance. *Journal of Clinical Psychiatry, 48* (12 suppl.), 22-28.

Sternback, H. (1991). The serotonin syndrome. *American Journal of Psychiatry, 148,* 705-713.

Sussman, N., & Chou, J. (1988). Current issues in benzodiazepine use for anxiety disorders. *Psychiatry Annals, 18,* 139-144.

Tesar, G. E., & Rosenbaum, J. F. (1986). Successful use of clonazepam in patients with treatment resistent panic. *Journal of Nervous and Mental Disorders, 174,* 477-482.

Glossary

Activities of daily living (ADL): The most basic self-care needs, including feeding, hygiene and grooming, toileting, and dressing.

Activity therapies: Therapies in which doing, rather than talking, is the primary mode of intervention.

Affect: "A pattern of observable behaviors that is the expression of a subjectively experienced feeling state (emotion)" (APA, 1987, pg. 391). May be abnormally flat, labile, or inappropriate.

Agraphia: An inability to write, caused by impairment of CNS processing (i.e. not by paralysis).

Anhedonia: An inability to experience pleasure.

Aphasia: A communication deficit which may be *expressive,* i.e., the inability to effectively express a thought, or *receptive,* i.e., the inability to process what is being said. Occurs at the CNS level.

Ataxia: Poor balance and awkward movement which results from CNS processing deficits.

Avolition: Absence of interest or will to undertake activities.

Behaviorism: A theory of behavior and intervention which holds that behavior is learned, that behaviors which are reinforced tend to recur, and those that are not reinforced tend to disappear.

Biofeedback: Provision of visual or auditory cues about physical processes (e.g., heart rate, muscle tension). May allow the individual to gain control of these processes.

Catatonia: Motor abnormality usually characterized by immobility or rigidity, in which no organic base has been identified.

Codependence: A condition in which substance dependence is subtly supported by the codependent who meets some need through the continued dependence of the individual.

Cognitive therapy: An approach to intervention which holds that emotional disturbance is the result of faulty belief systems.

Compulsion: Repetitive, purposeful behavior undertaken to diminish obsessive thoughts. Usually recognized as not genuinely helpful, but feels out of control to the individual.

Confabulation: Fabrication of facts which the individual can't remember. The individual is not aware he or she is fabricating, thus is not intentionally lying.

Defense mechanisms: Patterns of thinking or behavior which are mediated at an unconscious level to provide psychic protection to an individual, e.g., projection, denial, etc.

Delusion: A fixed, firmly held belief system which is not in keeping with external reality.

Desensitization: A technique employed by behaviorists to diminish fear and anxiety related to a stimulus, usually by pairing the stimulus with an incompatible response (e.g., relaxation).

Double depression: A diagnosis of major depressive episode superimposed on a diagnosis of dysthymia.

Dual diagnosis: Presence of more than one DSM diagnosis at the same time, most often a combination of a substance use disorder and some other condition, but may include any situation in which comorbidity exists.

Dyssomnia: Sleep disorder.

Echolalia: Repetitive verbalization which does not fit the situation.

Echopraxia: Repetitive movement which does not fit the situation.

Educational approaches: Interventions which make use of factual learning/teaching to change behaviors.

Ego: A concept developed by Freud, to describe that portion of the personality which mediates between wishes (id) and conscience (superego).

Enuresis: Inability to control urine, usually bed-wetting.

Environmental approaches: Interventions based on changing the environment, e.g., changing support systems, modifying job, home, etc.

Environmental press: The demands of the environment for particular levels of performance by the individual.

Extinction: A behavioral approach to discouraging a particular behavior by ignoring it and reinforcing other more acceptable behaviors.

Family therapy: Intervention into the entire family system, based on the theory that individual psychological difficulties are symptomatic of family disorder.

Flight of ideas: Rapid continuous speech with rapid, unclear shifts from subject to subject.

Flooding: A behavioral technique in which the individual is inundated with an unpleasant stimulus on the theory that this will overwhelm and exhaust any anxiety response.

Group therapy: Any intervention directed toward groups of individuals rather than an individual alone.

Habilitation: Enabling for the first time, as in the case of someone with mental retardation who never acquired a particular skill.

Hallucination: A sensory experience which does not match external reality.

Hyperactivity: Extreme activity, distractibility.

Hypersomnia: Excessive sleeping.

Instrumental activities of daily living (IADL): Self-care activities which are higher order than ADL; includes cooking, shopping, budgeting, home repair, etc.

Loose associations: Thoughts shift with little or no apparent logic.

Mainstreaming: The idea that individuals should, as much as possible, be in the least restrictive environment. Most often applies to educational settings, and having retarded children and others with dysfunction placed in regular classrooms where possible.

Metaanalysis: A type of research in which previous research studies are examined to determine outcome trends.

Milieu therapy: Treatment in which the environment is designed to provide specific levels of press and feedback.

Nervios: A Hispanic idiom for "nerves," used to describe a variety of psychological symptoms in individuals of those cultural groups.

Neurotic: An analytic concept which reflects psychodynamic conflicts that cause an individual difficulty. The individual remains in contact with reality.

Neurotransmitters: Chemical substances which convey new impulses at the synapses (gaps between nerve cells).

Obsession: An irresistible thought pattern, usually anxiety provoking, which intrudes on normal thought processes.

Panic attack: A state of extreme anxiety, usually including sweating, shortness of breath, chest pains and fear. May come on unpredictably or as a result of a particular stimulus.

Paranoia: A thought pattern which reflects a belief that others are persecuting or attempting to harm one, in the absence of a realistic basis for such fears.

Parasomnia: Abnormal sleep behavior, including sleepwalking and bruxing (grinding the teeth).

Perserveration: An inability to shift from thought to thought, persistence of an idea even when the subject changes.

Phobia: Fear of a particular stimulus, e.g., heights, snakes. The stimulus provokes both anxiety and avoidance of the stimulus.

Pica: Compulsive eating of nonnutritive substances like dirt.

Polydrug abuse: Abuse of several psychoactive drugs (e.g., alcohol and cocaine).

Prodromal: A preliminary phase of an illness which warns of upcoming major/primary symptoms.

Psychoanalysis: A verbal therapy based on analytic theories of intrapsychic conflict.

Psychodynamic: Any therapy which examines intrapsychic conflicts.

Psychotic: A psychological state characterized by hallucinations and delusions, i.e., a loss of contact with reality.

Psychotropic medications: Drugs which act to relieve psychological symptoms.

Rational emotive therapy: A form of cognitive therapy. Intervention is designed to provide clients with cognitive understanding and control of emotions.

Reality orientation: A therapeutic intervention often used with demented patients. Includes both group techniques to remind the patient of facts, and patterned environment which provides memory cues.

Reality therapy: A form of therapy designed to provide individual with experience of reasonable consequences of actions.

Rehabilitation: Helping individuals regain skills and abilities which have been lost as a result of illness or disorder.

Reinforcement: A desired outcome of behavior. In behavior therapy, reinforcement is provided to encourage specific activities.

Relaxation: A technique which increases relaxation, including biofeedback, systematic relaxation exercises.

Reliability: The predictability of an outcome, regardless of observer. In diagnosis, refers to the probability that several therapists will apply the same label to a given individual.

Rumination: Repetitive chewing of food regurgitated after ingestion.

Self-concept: The view one has of oneself.

Self-esteem: The value one places on the attributes which comprise one's self-concept.

Self-help: Various methods by which individuals attempt to remedy their difficulties without making use of formal care providers. Examples include Alcoholics Anonymous and several organizations of former mental patients.

Sensory stimulation: A therapeutic intervention which makes use of patterned sensory input.

Sensory integration: The ability of the CNS to process sensory information, also refers to a therapeutic intervention which uses strong kinesthetic and proprioceptive stimulation to attempt to better organize the CNS.

Sensory-motor: Therapeutic interventions which make use of both motor and sensory input in an effort to better organize the CNS.

Sheltered living: Living arrangements such as group homes which provide structure and supervision for individuals who do not require institutionalization but are not fully capable of independent living.

Social skills training: A cognitive/behavioral approach to teaching skills basic to social interaction.

Standard error: The possible range in which a person's "true" score on a test might fall; a number which recognizes the amount by which a score might vary on different days or in different situations.

Superego: An analytic concept which equates roughly to the conscience.

Systematic desensitization: A behavioral procedure which uses relaxation paired with an anxiety provoking stimulus in an attempt to reduce the anxiety response.

Tachycardia: Racing heartbeat.

Teratogenic: Substances which harm the developing fetus, causing birth defects.

Therapeutic community - A structured inpatient environment which is designed to provide rehabilitative experience.

Thought form: The pattern or flow of ideas; the way in which thoughts take form.

Token economy: A structured inpatient environment in which behavioral principles are employed. Some form of token is used for reinforcement/reward of desired behaviors.

Verbal therapies: Any therapy in which talk/discussion is the primary mode of intervention.

Waxy rigidity: A symptom of catatonia in which an individual will assume any position in which he or she is placed, and remain there until moved again.

Zar: A term used in some African and Middle Eastern cultures to suggest possession by spirits.

Appendix A
DSM-IV Classification

NOS = Not Otherwise Specified.

An X appearing in a diagnostic code indicates that a specific code number is required.

An ellipsis (...) is used in the names of certain disorders to indicate that the name of a specific mental disorder or general medical condition should be inserted when recòrding the name (e.g., 293.0 Delirium Due to Hypothyroidism).

Numbers in parentheses are page numbers.

If criteria are currently met, one of the following severity specifiers may be noted after the diagnosis:

Mild
Moderate
Severe

If criteria are no longer met, one of the following specifiers may be noted:

In Partial Remission
In Full Remission
Prior History

Disorders Usually First Diagnosed in Infancy, Childhood, or Adolescence (37)

MENTAL RETARDATION (39)
Note: These are coded on Axis II.

317	Mild Mental Retardation (41)
318.0	Moderate Mental Retardation (41)
318.1	Severe Mental Retardation (41)
318.2	Profound Mental Retardation (41)
319	Mental Retardation, Severity Unspecified(42)

LEARNING DISORDERS (46)

315.00	Reading Disorder (48)
315.1	Mathematics Disorder (50)
315.2	Disorder of Written Expression (51)
315.9	Learning Disorder NOS (53)

MOTOR SKILLS DISORDER

315.4	Developmental Coordination Disorder (53)

COMMUNICATION DISORDERS (55)

315.31	Expressive Language Disorder (55)
315.31	Mixed Receptive-Expressive Language Disorder (58)
315.39	Phonological Disorder (61)
307.0	Stuttering (63)
307.9	Communication Disorder NOS (65)

PERVASIVE DEVELOPMENTAL DISORDERS (65)

299.00 Autistic Disorder (66)

299.80 Rett's Disorder (71)

299.10 Childhood Disintegrative Disorder (73)

299.80 Asperger's Disorder (75)

299.80 Pervasive Developmental Disorder NOS (77)

ATTENTION-DEFICIT AND DISRUPTIVE BEHAVIOR DISORDERS (78)

314.xx Attention-Deficit/Hyperactivity Disorder (78)

.01   Combined Type

.00   Predominantly Inattentive Type

.01   Predominantly Hyperactive-Impulsive Type

314.9 Attention-Deficit/Hyperactivity Disorder NOS (85)

312.8 Conduct Disorder (85)

Specify type: Childhood-Onset Type/ Adolescent-Onset Type

313.81 Oppositional Defiant Disorder (91)

312.9 Disruptive Behavior Disorder NOS (94)

FEEDING AND EATING DISORDERS OF INFANCY OR EARLY CHILDHOOD (94)

307.52 Pica (95)

307.53 Rumination Disorder (96)

307.59 Feeding Disorder of Infancy or Early Childhood (98)

TIC DISORDERS (100)

307.23 Tourette's Disorder (101)

307.22 Chronic Motor or Vocal Tic Disorder (103)

307.21 Transient Tic Disorder (104)

Specify if: Single Episode/Recurrent

307.20 Tic Disorder NOS (105)

ELIMINATION DISORDERS (106)

-----.-- Encopresis (106)

787.6 With Constipation and Overflow Incontinence

307.7 Without Constipation and Overflow Incontinence

307.6 Enuresis (Not Due to a General Medical Condition) (108)

Specify type: Nocturnal Only/Diurnal Only/ Nocturnal and Diurnal

OTHER DISORDERS OF INFANCY, CHILDHOOD, OR ADOLESCENCE

309.21 Separation Anxiety Disorder (110)

Specify if: Early Onset

313.23 Selective Mutism (114)

313.89 Reactive Attachment Disorder of Infancy or Early Childhood (116)

Specify type: Inhibited Type/Disinhibited Type

307.3 Stereotypic Movement Disorder (118)

Specify if: With Self-Injurious Behavior

313.9 Disorder of Infancy, Childhood, or Adolescence NOS (121)

Delirium, Dementia, and Amnestic and Other Cognitive Disorders (123)

DELIRIUM (124)

293.0 Delirium Due to...*[Indicate the General Medical Condition] (127)*

-----.-- Substance Intoxication Delirium (129) *(refer to*

Substance-Related Disorders for substance-specific codes)

-----.-- Substance Withdrawal Delirium (129) (*refer to Substance-Related Disorders for substance-specific codes*)

-----.-- Delirium Due to Multiple Etiologies (*code each of the specific etiologies*) (132)

780.09 Delirium NOS (133)

DEMENTIA (133)

290.xx Dementia of the Alzheimer's Type, With Early Onset (*also code*

331.0 Alzheimer's disease on Axis III) (139)

  .10 Uncomplicated
  .11 With Delirium
  .12 With Delusions
  .13 With Depressed Mood
  Specify if: With Behavioral Disturbance

290.xx Dementia of the Alzheimer's Type, With Late Onset (*also code 331.0 Alzheimer's disease on Axis III*) (139)

  .0 Uncomplicated
  .3 With Delirium
  .20 With Delusions
  .21 With Depressed Mood
  Specify if: With Behavioral Disturbance

290.xx Vascular Dementia (143)

  .40 Uncomplicated
  .41 With Delirium
  .42 With Delusions
  .43 With Depressed Mood
  Specify if: With Behavioral Disturbance

294.9 Dementia Due to HIV Disease (*also code 043.1 HIV infection affecting central nervous system*

on Axis III) (148)

294.1 Dementia Due to Parkinson's Disease (*also code 332.0 Parkinson's disease on Axis III*) (148)

294.1 Dementia Due to Huntington's Disease (*also code 333.4 Huntington's disease on Axis III*) (149)

290.10 Dementia Due to Pick's Disease (*also code 331.1 Pick's disease on Axis III*) (149)

290.10 Dementia Due to Creutzfeldt-Jakob Disease (*also code 046.1 Creutzfeldt-Jakob disease on Axis III*) (150)

294.1 Dementia Due to...[*Indicate the General Medical Condition not listed above*] (*also code the general medical condition on Axis III*) (151)

-----.-- Substance-Induced Persisting Dementia (*refer to Substance-Related Disorders for substance-specific codes*) (152)

-----.-- Dementia Due to Multiple Etiologies (*code each of the specific etiologies*) (154)

294.8 Dementia NOS (155)

AMNESTIC DISORDERS (156)

294.0 Amnestic Disorder Due to... [Indicate the General Medical Condition] (158)

294.1 Dementia Due to Head Trauma (*also code 854.00 head injury on Axis III*) (148)
  Specify if: Transient/Chronic

-----.-- Substance-Induced Persisting Amnestic Disorder (*refer to Substance-Related Disorders for substance-specific codes*) (161)

294.8   Amnestic Disorder NOS (163)

OTHER COGNITIVE DISORDERS (163)

294.9   Cognitive Disorder NOS (163)

Mental Disorders Due to a General Medical Condition Not Elsewhere Classified (165)

293.89   Catatonic Disorder Due to... [*Indicate the General Medical Condition*] (169)

310.1   Personality Change Due to... [*Indicate the General Medical Condition*] (171)
         Specify type: Labile Type/Disinhibited Type/Aggressive Type/Apathetic Type/Paranoid Type/Other Type/Combined Type/Unspecified Type

293.9   Mental Disorder NOS Due to.. [*Indicate the General Medical Condition*] (174)

Substance-Related Disorders (175)

The following specifiers may be applied to Substance Dependence:
With Physiological Dependence/Without Physiological Dependence

Early Full Remission/Early Partial Remission/Sustained Full Remission/Sustained Partial Remission On Agonist Therapy/In a Controlled Environment

The following specifiers apply to Substance-Induced Disorders as noted:
With Onset During Intoxication/With Onset During Withdrawal

ALCOHOL-RELATED DISORDERS (194)

Alcohol Use Disorders

303.90   Alcohol Dependence (195)
305.00   Alcohol Abuse (196)

Alcohol-Induced Disorders

303.00   Alcohol Intoxication (196)
291.8   Alcohol Withdrawal (197)
         Specify if: With Perceptual Disturbances
291.0   Alcohol Intoxication Delirium (129)
291.0   Alcohol Withdrawal Delirium (129)
291.2   Alcohol-Induced Persisting Dementia (152)
291.1   Alcohol-Induced Persisting Amnestic Disorder (161)
291.x   Alcohol-Induced Psychotic Disorder (310)
    .5   With Delusions
    .3   With Hallucinations
291.8   Alcohol-Induced Mood Disorder (370)
291.8   Alcohol-Induced Anxiety Disorder (439)
291.8   Alcohol-Induced Sexual Dysfunction (519)
291.8   Alcohol-Induced Sleep Disorder (601)
291.9   Alcohol-Related Disorder NOS (204)

AMPHETAMINE (OR AMPHETAMINE-LIKE)-RELATED DISORDERS (204)

Amphetamine Use Disorders

304.40   Amphetamine Dependence (206)
305.70   Amphetamine Abuse (206)

Amphetamine-Induced Disorders

292.89 Amphetamine Intoxication (207)
   Specify if: With Perceptual Disturbances

292.0   Amphetamine Withdrawal (208)

292.81 Amphetamine Intoxication Delirium (129)

292.xx Amphetamine-Induced Psychotic Disorder (310)

   .11   With Delusions

   .12   With Hallucinations

292.84 Amphetamine-Induced Mood Disorder, (370)

292.89 Amphetamine-Induced Anxiety Disorder (439)

292.89 Amphetamine-Induced Sexual Dysfunction (519)

292.89 Amphetamine-Induced Sleep Disorder (601)

292.9   Amphetamine-Related Disorder NOS (211)

CAFFEINE-RELATED DISORDERS (212)

Caffeine-Induced Disorders

305.90 Caffeine Intoxication (212)

292.89 Caffeine-Induced Anxiety Disorder (439)

292.89 Caffeine-Induced Sleep Disorder (601)

292.9   Caffeine-Related Disorder NOS (215)

CANNABIS-RELATED DISORDERS (215)

Cannabis Use Disorders

304.30 Cannabis Dependence (216)

305.20 Cannabis Abuse (217)

Cannabis-Induced Disorders

292.89 Cannabis Intoxication (217)
   Specify if: With Perceptual Disturbances

292.81 Cannabis Intoxication Delirium (129)

292.xx Cannabis-Induced Psychotic Disorder (310)

   .11   With Delusions

   .12   With Hallucinations

292.89 Cannabis-Induced Anxiety Disorder (439)

292.9   Cannabis-Related Disorder NOS (221)

COCAINE-RELATED DISORDERS (221)

Cocaine Use Disorders

304.20 Cocaine Dependence (222)

305.60 Cocaine Abuse (223)

Cocaine-Induced Disorders

292.89 Cocaine Intoxication (223)
   Specify if: With Perceptual Disturbances

292.0   Cocaine Withdrawal (225)

292.81 Cocaine Intoxication Delirium (129)

292.xx Cocaine-Induced Psychotic Disorder (310)

   .11   With Delusions

   .12   With Hallucinations

292.84 Cocaine-Induced Mood Disorder (370)

292.89 Cocaine-Induced Anxiety Disorder (439)

292.89 Cocaine-Induced Sexual Dysfunction (519)

292.89 Cocaine-Induced Sleep Disorder (601)

292.9   Cocaine-Related Disorder NOS (229)

HALLUCINOGEN-RELATED DISORDERS (229)

Hallucinogen Use Disorders
304.50 Hallucinogen Dependence (230)
305.30 Hallucinogen Abuse (231)

Hallucinogen-Induced Disorders
292.89 Hallucinogen Intoxication (232)
292.89 Hallucinogen Persisting Perception Disorder (Flashbacks) (233)
292.81 Hallucinogen Intoxication Delirium (129)
292.xx Hallucinogen-Induced Psychotic Disorder (310)
   .11   With Delusions
   .12   With Hallucinations
292.84 Hallucinogen-Induced Mood Disorder (370)
292.89 Hallucinogen-Induced Anxiety Disorder (439)
292.9   Hallucinogen-Related Disorder NOS (236)

INHALANT-RELATED DISORDERS (236)

Inhalant Use Disorders
304.60 Inhalant Dependence (238)
305.90 Inhalant Abuse (238)

Inhalant-Induced Disorders
292.89 Inhalant Intoxication (239)
292.81 Inhalant Intoxication Delirium (129)
292.82 Inhalant-Induced Persisting Dementia (152)
292.xx Inhalant-Induced Psychotic Disorder (310)
   .11   With Delusions
   .12   With Hallucinations

292.84 Inhalant-Induced Mood Disorder (370)
292.89 Inhalant-Induced Anxiety Disorder (439)
292.9   Inhalant-Related Disorder NOS (242)

NICOTINE-RELATED DISORDERS (242)

Nicotine Use Disorder
305.10 Nicotine Dependencea (243)

Nicotine-Induced Disorder
292.0   Nicotine Withdrawal (244)
292.9   Nicotine-Related Disorder NOS (247)

OPIOID-RELATED DISORDERS (247)

Opioid Use Disorders
304.00 Opioid Dependence (248)
305.50 Opioid Abuse (249)

Opioid-Induced Disorders
292.89 Opioid Intoxication (249)
           Specify if: With Perceptual Disturbances
292.0   Opioid Withdrawal (250)
292.81 Opioid Intoxication Delirium (129)
292.xx Opioid-Induced Psychotic Disorder (310)
   .11   With Delusions
   .12   With Hallucinations
292.84 Opioid-Induced Mood Disorder (370)
292.89 Opioid-Induced Sexual Dysfunction (519)
292.89 Opioid-Induced Sleep Disorder (601)
292.9   Opioid-Related Disorder NOS (255)

PHENCYCLIDINE (OR PHENCYCLIDINE-LIKE)-RELATED DISORDERS (255)

Phencyclidine Use Disorders

304.90 Phencyclidine Dependence (256)

305.90 Phencyclidine Abuse (257)

Phencyclidine-Induced Disorders

292.89 Phencyclidine Intoxication (257)
Specify if: With Perceptual Disturbances

292.81 Phencyclidine Intoxication Delirium (129)

292.xx Phencyclidine-Induced Psychotic Disorder (310)

.11 With Delusions

.12 With Hallucinations

292.84 Phencyclidine-Induced Mood Disorder (370)

292.89 Phencyclidine-Induced Anxiety Disorder (439)

292.9 Phencyclidine-Related Disorder NOS (261)

SEDATIVE-, HYPNOTIC-, OR ANXIOLYTIC-RELATED DISORDERS (261)

Sedative, Hypnotic, or Anxiolytic Use Disorders

304.10 Sedative, Hypnotic, or Anxiolytic Dependence (262)

305.40 Sedative, Hypnotic, or Anxiolytic Abuse (263)

Sedative-, Hypnotic-, or Anxiolytic-Induced Disorders

292.89 Sedative, Hypnotic, or Anxiolytic Intoxication(263)

292.0 Sedative, Hypnotic, or Anxiolytic Withdrawal (264)
Specify if: With Perceptual Disturbances

292.81 Sedative, Hypnotic, or Anxiolytic Intoxication Delirium (129)

292.81 Sedative, Hypnotic, or Anxiolytic Withdrawal Delirium (129)

292.82 Sedative-, Hypnotic, or Anxiolytic-Induced Persisting Dementia (152)

292.83 Sedative-, Hypnotic-, or Anxiolytic-Induced Persisting Amnestic Disorder (161)

292.xx Sedative-, Hypnotic-, or Anxiolytic-Induced Psychotic Disorder (310)

.11 With Delusions

.12 With Hallucinations

292.84 Sedative-, Hypnotic-, or Anxiolytic-Induced Mood Disorder (370)

292.89 Sedative-, Hypnotic-, or Anxiolytic-Induced Anxiety Disorder (439)

292.89 Sedative-, Hypnotic-, or Anxiolytic-Induced Sexual Dysfunction (519)

292.89 Sedative-, Hypnotic-, or Anxiolytic-Induced Sleep Disorder (601)

292.9 Sedative-, Hypnotic-, or Anxiolytic-Related Disorder NOS (269)

POLYSUBSTANCE-RELATED DISORDER

304.80 Polysubstance Dependence (270)

OTHER (OR UNKNOWN) SUBSTANCE-RELATED DISORDERS (270)

Other (or Unknown) Substance Use Disorders

304.90 Other (or Unknown)Substance Dependencea (176)

305.90 Other (or Unknown) Substance Abuse (182)

Other (or Unknown) Substance-Induced Disorders

292.89 Other (or Unknown) Substance Intoxication (183)
Specify if: With Perceptual Disturbances

292.0 Other (or Unknown) Substance-Withdrawal (184)
Specify if: With Perceptual Disturbances

292.81 Other (or Unknown) Substance-Induced Delirium 9129)

292.82 Other (or Unknown) Substance-Induced Persisting Dementia (152)

292.83 Other (or Unknown) Substance-Induced Persisting Amnestic Disorder (161)

292.xx Other (or Unknown) Substance-Induced Psychotic Disorder (310)

.11 With Delusions

.12 With Hallucinations

292.84 Other (or Unknown) Substance-Induced Mood Disorder (370)

292.89 Other (or Unknown) Substance-Induced Anxiety Disorder (439)

292.89 Other (or Unknown) Substance-Induced Sexual Dysfunction (519)

292.89 Other (or Unknown) Substance-Induced Sleep Disorder (601)

292.9 Other (or Unknown) Substance-Related Disorder NOS (272)

Schizophrenia and Other Psychotic Disorders (273)

295.xx Schizophrenia (274)
The following Classification of Longitudinal Course applies to all subtypes of Schizophrenia:
Episodic With Interepisode Residual Symptoms (*specify if:* With Prominent Negative Symptoms)/ Episodic With No Interepisode Residual Symptoms/Continuous (*specify if:* With Prominent Negative Symptoms)

Single Episode In Partial Remission (*specify if:* With Prominent Negative Symptoms)/Single Episode In Full Remission

Other or Unspecified Pattern

.30 Paranoid Type (287)

.10 Disorganized Type (287)

.20 Catatonic Type (288)

.90 Undifferentiated Type (289)

.60 Residual Type (289)

295.40 Schizophreniform Disorder (290)
Specify if: Without Good Prognostic Features/ With Good Prognostic Features

295.70 Schizoaffective Disorder (292)
Specify type: Bipolar Type/Depressive Type

297.1 Delusional Disorder (296)
Specify type: Erotomanic Type/Grandiose Type/Jealous Type/Persecutory Type/ Somatic Type/Mixed Type/ Unspecified Type

298.8 Brief Psychotic Disorder (302)
Specify if: With Marked Stressor(s)/ Without Marked Stressor(s)/With Postpartum Onset

297.3 Shared Psychotic Disorder (305)

293.xx Psychotic Disorder Due to... [*Indicated the General Medical Condition*] (306)

.81 With Delusions

.82 With Hallucinations

-----.-- Substance-Induced Psychotic Disorder (*refer to Substance-Related Disorders for substance-specific codes*) (310)
Specify if: With Onset During Intoxication/ With Onset During Withdrawal

298.9 Psychotic Disorder NOS (315)

Mood Disorders (317)

Code current state of Major Depressive Disorder or Bipolar I Disorder in fifth digit:

1 = Mild
2 = Moderate
3 = Severe Without Psychotic Features
4 = Severe With Psychotic Features
   Specify: Mood-Congruent Psychotic Features/ Mood-Incongruent Psychotic Features
5 = In Partial Remission
6 = In Full Remission
0 = Unspecified

The following specifiers apply (for current or most recent episode) to Mood Disorders as noted:

Severity/Psychotic/Remission Specifiers/Chronic/With Catatonic Features/ With Melancholic Features/With Atypical Features/ With Postpartum Onset

The following specifiers apply to Mood Disorders as noted:

With or Without Full Interepisode Recovery/ With Seasonal Pattern/iWith Rapid Cycling

DEPRESSIVE DISORDERS

296.xx Major Depressive Disorder, (339)
   .2x   Single Episode
   .3x   Recurrent
300.4   Dysthymic Disorder (345)
   Specify if: Early Onset/Late Onset
   Specify: With Atypical Features
311   Depressive Disorder NOS (350)

BIPOLAR DISORDERS

296.xx Bipolar I Disorder, (350)
   .0x   Single Manic Episodea
      Specify if: Mixed
   .40   Most Recent Episode Hypomanic
   .4x   Most Recent Episode Manic

   .6x   Most Recent Episode Mixed
   .5x   Most Recent Episode Depressed
   .7   Most Recent Episode Unspecified
296.89 Bipolar II Disordera,b,c,d,e,f,g,h,i (359)
   Specify (current or most recent episode): Hypomanic/Depressed
301.13 Cyclothymic Disorder (363)
296.80 Bipolar Disorder NOS (366)
293.83 Mood Disorder Due to...*[Indicate the General Medical Condition]* (366)
   Specify type: With Depressive Features/ With Major Depressive-Like Episode/ With Manic Features/With Mixed Features
-----/-- Substance-Induced Mood Disorder (*refer to Substance-Related Disorders for substance-specific codes*) (370)
   Specify type: With Depressive Features/ With Manic Features/With Mixed Features
   Specify if: With Onset During Intoxication/ With Onset During Withdrawal
296.90 Mood Disorder NOS (375)

Anxiety Disorders (393)

300.01 Panic Disorder Without Agoraphobia (397)
300.21 Panic Disorder With Agoraphobia (397)
300.22 Agoraphobia Without History of Panic Disorder (403)
300.29 Specific Phobia (405)
   Specify type: Animal Type/Natural Environment Type/Blood-Injection-Injury Type/ Situational Type/Other Type
300.23 Social Phobia (411)
   Specify if: Generalized

300.3   Obsessive-Compulsive Disorder (417)
Specify if: With Poor Insight

309.81 Posttraumatic Stress Disorder (424)
Specify if: Acute/Chronic
Specify if: With Delayed Onset

308.3   Acute Stress Disorder (429)

300.02 Generalized Anxiety Disorder (432)

293.89 Anxiety Disorder Due to...[Indicate the General Medical Condition] (436)
Specify if: With Generalized Anxiety/ With Panic Attacks/With Obsessive-Compulsive Symptoms

-----.-- Substance-Induced Anxiety Disorder (*refer to Substance-Related Disorders for substance-specific codes*) (439)
Specify if: With Generalized Anxiety/ With Panic Attacks/With Obsessive-Compulsive Symptoms/With Phobic Symptoms/With Phobic Symptoms
Specify if: With Onset During Intoxication/ With Onset During Withdrawal

300.00 Anxiety Disorder NOS (444)

Somatoform Disorders (445)

300.81 Somatization Disorder (446)

300.81 Undifferentiated Somatoform Disorder (450)

300.11 Conversion Disorder (452)
Specify type: With Motor Symptom or Deficit/With Sensory Symptom or Deficit/ With Seizures or Convulsions/With Mixed Presentation

307.xx Pain Disorder (458)
.80   Associated With Psychological Factors
.89   Associated With Both Psychological Factors and a General Medical Condition
Specify if: Acute/Chronic

300.7   Hypochondriasis (462)
Specify if: With Poor Insight

300.7   Body Dysmorphic Disorder (466)

300.81 Somatoform Disorder NOS (468)

Factitious Disorders (471)

300.xx Factitious Disorder (471)
.16   With Predominantly Psychological Signs and Symptoms
.19   With Predominantly Physical Signs and Symptoms
.19   With Combined Psychological and Physical Signs and Symptoms

300.19 Factitious Disorder NOS (475)

Dissociative Disorders (477)

300.12 Dissociative Amnesia (478)

300.13 Dissociative Fugue (481)

300.14 Dissociative Identity Disorder (484)

300.6   Depersonalization Disorder (488)

300.15 Dissociative Disorder NOS (490)

Sexual and Gender Identity Disorders (493)

SEXUAL DYSFUNCTIONS (493)
The following specifiers apply to all primary Sexual Dysfunctions:
Lifelong Type/Acquired Type Generalized Type/ Situational Type Due to Psychological Factors/ Due to Combined Factors

302.9   Sexual Disorder NOS (538)

Eating Disorders (539)

307.1   Anorexia Nervosa (539)
Specify type: Restricting Type; Binge-Eating/ Purging Type
307.51 Bulimia Nervosa (545)
Specify type: Purging Type/Nonpurging Type
307.50 Eating Disorder NOS (550)

Sleep Disorders (551)

PRIMARY SLEEP DISORDERS (553)
Dyssomnias (553)
307.42 Primary Insomnia (553)
307.44 Primary Hypersomnia (557)
Specify if: Recurrent
347   Narcolepsy (562)
780.59 Breathing-Related Sleep Disorder (567)
307.45 Circadian Rhythm Sleep Disorder (573)
Specify type: Delayed Sleep Phase Type/ Jet Lag Type/Shift Work Type/ Unspecified Type
307.47 Dyssomnia NOS (579)

Parasomnias (579)
307.47 Nightmare Disorder (580)
307.46 Sleep Terror Disorder (583)
307.46 Sleepwalking Disorder (587)
307.47 Parasomnia NOS (592)

SLEEP DISORDERS RELATED TO ANOTHER MENTAL DISORDER (592)
307.42 Insomnia Related to...[*Indicate the Axis I or Axis II Disorder*] (592)

307.44 Hypersomnia Related to... [*Indicate the Axis I or Axis II Disorder*] (592)

OTHER SLEEP DISORDERS
780.xx Sleep Disorder Due to...[*Indicate the General Medical Condition*] (597)
   .52   Insomnia Type
   .54   Hypersomnia Type
   .59   Parasomnia Type
   .59   Mixed Type
-----.-- Substance-Induced Sleep Disorder (*refer to Substance-Related Disorders for substance-specific codes*) (601)
Specify type: Insomnia Type/Hypersomnia Type/Parasomnia Type/Mixed Type
Specify if: With Onset During Intoxication/With Onset During Withdrawal

Impulse-Control Disorders Not Elsewhere Classified (609)

312.34 Intermittent Explosive Disorder (609)
312.32 Kleptomania (612)
312.33 Pyromania (614)
312.31 Pathological Gambling (615)
312.39 Trichotillomania (618)
312.30 Impulse-Control Disorder NOS (621)

Adjustment Disorders (623)

309.xx Adjustment Disorder (623)
   .0   With Depressed Mood
   .24   With Anxiety
   .28   With Mixed Anxiety and

Depressed Mood
.3   With Disturbance of Conduct
.4   With Mixed Disturbance of
Emotions and Conduct
.9   Unspecified
Specify if: Acute/Chronic

Personality Disorders (629)

Note: These are coded on Axis II.

301.0   Paranoid Personality Disorder (634)

301.20 Schizoid Personality Disorder (638)

301.22 Schizotypal Personality Disorder (641)

301.7   Antisocial Personality Disorder (645)

301.83 Borderline Personality Disorder (650)

301.50 Histrionic Personality Disorder (655)

301.81 Narcissistic Personality Disorder (658)

301.82 Avoidant Personality Disorder (662)

301.6   Dependent Personality Disorder (665)

301.4   Obsessive-Compulsive Personality Disorder (669)

301.9   Personality Disorder NOS (673)

Other Conditions That May Be a Focus of Clinical Attention (675)

PSYCHOLOGICAL FACTORS AFFECTING MEDICAL CONDITION (675)

316   ...[Specified Psychological Factor] Affecting...[*Indicate the General Medical Condition*] (675)
Choose name based on nature of factors:
Mental Disorder Affecting Medical Condition
Psychological Symptoms Affecting Medical Condition
Personality Traits or Coping Style Affecting Medical Condition
Maladaptive Health Behaviors Affecting Medical Condition
Stress-Related Physiological Response Affecting Medical Condition
Other or Unspecified Psychological Factors Affecting Medical Condition

MEDICATION-INDUCED MOVEMENT DISORDERS (678)

332.1   Neuroleptic-Induced Parkinsonism (679)

333.92 Neuroleptic Malignant Syndrome (679)

333.7   Neuroleptic-Induced Acute Dystonia (679)

333.99 Neuroleptic-Induced Acute Akathisia (679)

333.82 Neuroleptic-Induced Tardive Dyskinesia (679)

333.1   Medication-Induced Postural Tremor (680)

333.90 Medication-Induced Movement Disorder NOS (680)

OTHER MEDICATION-INDUCED DISORDER

995.2   Adverse Effects of Medication NOS (680)

RELATIONAL PROBLEMS (680)

V61.9   Relational Problem Related to a Mental Disorder or General Medical Condition (681)

V61.20   Parent-Child Relational Problem (681)

V61.1   Partner Relational Problem (681)

V61.8   Sibling Relational Problem (681)

V62.81   Relational Problem NOS (681)

PROBLEMS RELATED TO ABUSE OR NEGLECT (682)

V61.21   Physical Abuse of Child (682) (*code 995.5 if focus of attention is on victim*)

V61.21   Sexual Abuse of child (682) (*code 995.5 if focus of attention is on victim*)

V61.21   Neglect of Child (682) (*code 995.5 if focus of attention is on victim*)

V61.1   Physical Abuse of Adult (682) (*code 995.81 if focus of attention is on victim*)

V61.1   Sexual Abuse of Adult (682) (*code 995.81 if focus of attention is on victim*)

ADDITIONAL CONDITIONS THAT MAY BE A FOCUS OF CLINICAL ATTENTION (683)

V15.81   Noncompliance With Treatment (683)

V65.2   Malingering (683)

V71.01   Adult Antisocial Behavior (683)

V71.02   Child or Adolescent Antisocial Behavior (684)

V62.89   Borderline Intellectual Functioning (684)
         Note: This is coded on Axis II

780.9   Age-Related Cognitive Decline (684)

V62.82   Bereavement (684)

V62.3   Academic Problem (685)

V62.2   Occupational Problem (685)

313.82   Identity Problem (685)

V62.89   Religious or Spiritual Problem (685)

V62.4   Acculturation Problem (685)

V62.89   Phase of Life Problem (685)

Additional Codes

300.9   Unspecified Mental Disorder (nonpsychotic) (687)

V71.09   No Diagnosis or Condition on Axis I (687)

799.9   Diagnosis or Condition Deferred on Axis I (687)

V71.09   No Diagnosis on Axis II (687)

799.9   Diagnosis Deferred on Axis II (687)

Multiaxial System

Axis I   Clinical Disorders
          Other Conditions That May Be a Focus of Clinical Attention

Axis II   Personality Disorders
          Mental Retardation

Axis III General Medical Conditions

Axis IV   Psychosocial and Environmental Problems

Axis V   Global Assessment of Functioning

Appendix B

Uniform Terminology
For Reporting Occupational
Therapy Services,
Third Edition

This is an official document of The American Occupational Therapy Association. This document is intended to provide a generic outline of the domain of concern of occupational therapy and is designed to create common terminology for the profession and to capture the essence of occupational therapy succinctly for others.

It is recognized that the phenomena that constitute the profession's domain of concern can be categorized, and labeled, in a number of different ways. This document is not meant to limit those in the field, formulating theories or frames of reference, who may wish to combine or refine particular constructs. It is also not meant to limit those who would like to conceptualize the profession's domain of concern in a different manner.

Introduction

The first edition of *Uniform Terminology* was approved and published in 1979 (AOTA, 1979). In 1989, the *Uniform Terminology for Occupational Therapy— Second Edition* (AOTA, 1989) was approved and published. The second document presented an organized structure for understanding the areas of practice for the profession of occupational therapy. The document outlined two domains. **PERFORMANCE AREAS** (activities of daily living [ADL], work and productive activities, and play or leisure) include activities that the occupational therapy practitioner[1] emphasizes when determining functional abilities. **PERFORMANCE**

COMPONENTS (sensorimotor, cognitive, psychosocial, and psychological aspects) are the elements of performance that occupational therapists assess and, when needed, in which they intervene for improved performance.

This third edition has been further expanded to reflect current practice and to incorporate contextual aspects of performance. *Performance Areas, Performance Components,* and *Performance Contexts* are the parameters of occupational therapy's domain of concern. *Performance areas* are broad categories of human activity that are typically part of daily life. They are activities of daily living, work and productive activities, and play or leisure activities. *Performance components* are fundamental human abilities that—to varying degrees and in differing combinations—are required for successful engagement in performance areas.

These components are sensorimotor, cognitive, and psychosocial and psychological. *Performance contexts* are situations or factors that influence an individual's engagement in desired and/or required performance areas. Performance contexts consist of *temporal* aspects (chronological, developmental, life cycle, and disability status); and *environmental* aspects (physical, social, and cultural). There is an interactive relationship among performance areas, performance components, and performance contexts. Function in performance areas is the ultimate concern of occupational therapy, with performance components considered as they relate to participation in performance areas. Performance areas and performance components are always viewed within performance contexts. Performance contexts are taken into consideration when determining function and dysfunction relative to performance areas and performance components, and in planning intervention. For example, the occupational therapist does not evaluate strength (a performance component) in isolation. Strength is considered as it affects necessary or desired tasks (performance areas). If the individual is interested in homemaking, the occupational therapy practitioner would consider the interaction of strength with homemaking tasks. Strengthening could be addressed through kitchen activities, such as cooking and putting groceries away. In some cases, the practitioner would employ an adaptive approach and recommend that the family switch from heavy stoneware to lighter-weight dishes, or use lighter-weight pots on the stove to enable the individual to make dinner safely without becoming fatigued or compromising safety.

Occupational therapy assessment involves examining performance areas, performance components, and performance contexts. Intervention may be directed toward elements of performance areas (e.g., dressing, vocational exploration), performance components (e.g., endurance, problem solving), or the environmental aspects of performance contexts. In the last case, the physical and/or social environment may be altered or augmented to improve and/or maintain function. After identifying the performance areas the individual wishes or needs to address, the occupational therapist assesses the features of the environments in which the talks will be performed. If an individual's job requires cooking in a restaurant as opposed to leisure cooking at home, the occupational therapy practitioner faces several challenges to enable the individual's success in different environments. Therefore, the third critical aspect of performance is the performance context, the features of the environment that affect the person's ability to engage in functional activities.

This document categorizes specific activities in each of the performance areas (ADL, work and productive activities, play or leisure). This categorization is based on what is considered "typical," and is not meant to imply that a particular individual characterizes personal activities in the same manner as someone else. Occupational therapy practitioners embrace individual differences, and so would document the unique pattern of the individual being served, rather than forcing the "typical" pattern on him or her and family. For example, because of experience or culture, a particular individual might think of home management as an ADL task rather than "work and productive activities" (current listing). Socialization might be considered part of play or leisure activity instead of its current listing as part of "activities of daily living," because of life experience or cultural heritage.

Examples in Practice

Uniform Terminology—Third Edition, defines occupational therapy's domain of concern, which includes performance areas, performance components, and performance contexts. While this document may be used by occupational therapy practitioners in a number of different areas (e.g., practice, documentation, charge systems, education, program development, marketing, research, disability classifications, and regulations), it focuses on the use of uniform terminology in practice. This document is not intended to define specific occupational therapy interventions. Examples of how performance areas, performance components, and performance contexts translate into practice are provided below.

- An individual who is injured on the job may have the potential to return to work and productive activities, which is a performance area. In order to achieve the outcome of returning to work and productive activities, the individual may need to address specific performance components such as strength, endurance, soft tissue integrity, time management, and the physical features of performance contexts, like structures and objects in his or her environment. The occupational therapy practitioner, in collaboration with the individual and other members of the vocational team, uses planned interventions to achieve the desired outcome. These interventions may include activities such as an exercise program, body mechanics instruction, and job site modifications, all of which may be provided in a work-hardening program.
- An elderly individual recovering from a cerebral vascular accident may wish to

live in a community setting, which combines the performance areas of ADL with work and productive activities. In order to achieve the outcome of community living, the individual may need to address specific performance components, such as muscle tone, gross motor coordination, postural control, and self-management. It is also necessary to consider the sociocultural and physical features of performance contexts, such as support available from other persons, and adaptations of structures and objects within the environment. The occupational therapy practitioner, in cooperation with the team, utilizes planned interventions to achieve the desired outcome. Interventions may include neuromuscular facilitation, practice of object manipulation, and instruction in the use of adaptive equipment and home safety equipment. The practitioner and individual also pursue the selection and training of a personal assistant to ensure the completion of ADL tasks. These interventions may be provided in a comprehensive inpatient rehabilitation unit.

- A child with learning disabilities is required to perform educational activities within a public school setting. Engaging in educational activities is considered the performance area of work and productive activities for this child. To achieve the educational outcome of efficient and effective completion of written classroom work, the child may need to address specific performance components. These include sensory processing, perceptual skills, postural control, motor skills, and the physical features of performance contexts, such as objects (e.g., desk, chair) in the environment. In cooperation with the team, occupational therapy interventions may include activities like adapting the student's seating in the classroom to improve postural control and stability, and practicing motor control and coordination. This program could be developed by an occupational therapist and supported by school district personnel.

- The parents of an infant with cerebral palsy may ask to facilitate the child's involvement in the performance areas of activities of daily living and play. Subsequent to assessment, the therapist identifies specific performance components, such as sensory awareness and neuromuscular control. The practitioner also addresses the physical and cultural features of performance contexts. In collaboration with the parents, occupational therapy interventions may include activities such as seating and positioning for play, neuromuscular facilitation techniques to enable eating, facilitating parent skills in caring for and playing with their infant, and modifying the play space for accessibility. These interventions may be provided in a home-based occupational therapy program.

- An adult with schizophrenia may need and want to live independently in the community, which represents the performance areas of activities of daily living, work and productive activities, and leisure activities. The specific performance categories may be medication routine, functional mobility, home management, vocational exploration, play or leisure performance, and social interaction. In order to achieve the outcome of living independently, the individual may need to address specific performance components such as topographical orientation, memory, categorization, problem solving, interests, social conduct, time management, and sociocultural features of performance contexts, such as social factors (e.g., influence of family and friends) and roles. The occupational therapy practitioner, in cooperation with the team, utilizes planned interventions to achieve the desired outcome. Interventions may include activities such as training in the use of public transportation, instruction in budgeting skills, selection of and participation in social activities, and instruction in social conduct. These interventions may be provided in a community-based mental health program.

- An individual with a history of substance abuse may need to re-establish family roles and responsibilities, which represent the performance areas of activities of daily living, work and productive activities, and leisure activities. In order to achieve the outcome of family participation, the individual may need to address the performance components of roles, values, social conduct, self-expression, coping skills, self-control, and the sociocultural features of performance contexts, such as custom, behavior, rules, and rituals. The occupational therapy practitioner, in cooperation with the team, utilizes planned intervention to achieve the desired outcomes. Interventions may include roles and values exercises, instruction in stress management techniques, identification of family roles and activities, and support to develop family leisure routines. These interventions may be provided in an inpatient acute care unit.

Person-Activity-Environment Fit

Person-activity-environment fit refers to the match among skills and abilities of the individual; the demands of the activity; and the characteristics of the physical, social, and cultural environments. It is the interaction among the performance areas, performance components, and performance contexts that is important and determines the success of the performance. When occupational therapy practitioners provide services, they attend to all of these aspects of performance and the interaction among them. They also attend to each individual's unique personal history. The personal history includes one's skills and abilities (performance components), the past performance of specific life tasks (performance areas), and experience within particular environments (performance contexts). In addition to personal history, anticipated life tasks and role demands influence performance.

When considering the person-activity-environment fit, variables such as novelty, importance, motivation, activity tolerance, and quality are salient. Situations range from those that are completely familiar, to those that are novel and have never been experienced. Both the novelty and familiarity within a situation contribute to the overall task performance. In each situation, there is an optimal level of novelty that engages the individual sufficiently and provides enough information to perform the task. When too little novelty is present, the individual may miss cues and opportunities to perform. When too much novelty is present, the individual may become confused and distracted, inhibiting effective task performance.

Humans determine that some stimuli and situations are more meaningful than others. Individuals perform tasks they deem important. It is critical to identify what the individual wants or needs to do when planning interventions.

The level of motivation an individual demonstrates to perform a particular task is determined by both internal and external factors. An individual's biobehavioral state (e.g., amount of rest, arousal, tension) contributes to the potential to be responsive. The features of the social and physical environments (e.g., persons in the room, noise level) provide information that is either adequate or inadequate to produce a motivated state.

Activity tolerance is the individual's ability to sustain a purposeful activity over time. Individuals must not only select, initiate, and terminate activities, but they must also attend to a task for the needed length of time to complete the task and accomplish their goals.

The quality of performance is measured by standards generated by both the individual and others in the social and cultural environments in which the performance occurs. Quality is a continuum of expectations set within particular activities and contexts.

I. Performance Areas
  A. Activities of Daily Living
      1. Grooming
      2. Oral Hygiene
      3. Bathing/Showering
      4. Toilet Hygiene
      5. Personal Device Care
      6. Dressing
      7. Feeding and Eating
      8. Medication Routine
      9. Health Maintenance
     10. Socialization
     11. Functional Communication
     12. Functional Mobility
     13. Community Mobility
     14. Emergency Response
     15. Sexual Expression

B. Work and Productive Activities
  1. Home Management
     a. Clothing Care
     b. Cleaning
     c. Meal Preparation/Cleanup
     d. Shopping
     e. Money Management
     f. Household Maintenance
     g. Safety Procedures
  2. Care of Others
  3. Educational Activities
  4. Vocational Activities
     a. Vocational Exploration
     b. Job Acquisition
     c. Work or Job Performance
     d. Retirement Planning
     e. Volunteer Participation
C. Play or Leisure Activities
  1. Play or Leisure Exploration
  2. Play or Leisure Performance

II. Performance Components
A. Sensorimotor Component
  1. Sensory
     a. Sensory Awareness
     b. Sensory Processing
        (1) Tactile
        (2) Proprioceptive
        (3) Vestibular
        (4) Visual
        (5) Auditory
        (6) Gustatory
        (7) Olfactory
     c. Perceptual Processing
        (1) Stereognosis
        (2) Kinesthesia
        (3) Pain Response
        (4) Body Scheme
        (5) Right-Left Discrimination
        (6) Form Constancy
        (7) Position in Space

(8) Visual-Closure
(9) Figure Ground
(10) Depth Perception
(11) Spatial Relations
(12) Topographical Orientation
2. Neuromusculoskeletal
a. Reflex
b. Range of Motion
c. Muscle Tone
d. Strength
e. Endurance
f. Postural Control
g. Postural Alignment
h. Soft Tissue Integrity
3. Motor
a. Gross Coordination
b. Crossing the Midline
c. Laterality
d. Bilateral Integration
e. Motor Control
f. Praxis
g. Fine Motor Coordination/Dexterity
h. Visual-Motor Integration
i. Oral-Motor Control
B. Cognitive Integration and Cognitive Components
1. Level of Arousal
2. Orientation
3. Recognition
4. Attention Span
5. Initiation of Activity
6. Termination of Activity
7. Memory
8. Sequencing
9. Categorization
10. Concept Formation
11. Spatial Operations
12. Problem Solving
13. Learning
14. Generalization

C. Psychosocial Skills and Psychological Components
1. Psychological
   a. Values
   b. Interests
   c. Self-Concept
2. Social
   a. Role Performance
   b. Social Conduct
   c. Interpersonal skills
   d. Self-Expression
3. Self-Management
   a. Coping Skills
   b. Time Management
   c. Self-Control

III. Performance Contexts
A. Temporal Aspects
1. Chronological
2. Developmental
3. Life Cycle
4. Disability Status
B. Environment
1. Physical
2. Social
3. Cultural

Uniform Terminology for Occupational Therapy—Third Edition

"Occupational Therapy" is the use of purposeful activity or interventions to promote health and achieve functional outcomes. "Achieving functional outcomes" means to develop, improve, or restore the highest possible level of independence of any individual who is limited by a physical injury or illness, a dysfunctional condition, a cognitive impairment, a psychosocial dysfunction, a mental illness, a developmental or learning disability, or an adverse environmental condition. Assessment means the use of skilled observation or evaluation by the administration and interpretation of standardized or nonstandardized tests and measurements to identify areas for occupational therapy services.

Occupational therapy services include, but are not limited to:

1. The assessment, treatment, and education of or consultation with the

individual, family, or other persons;

2. Interventions directed toward developing, improving, or restoring daily living skills, work readiness or work performance, play skills or leisure capacities, or enhancing educational performances skills; or

3. Providing for the development, improvement, or restoration of sensorimotor, oral-motor, perceptual or neuromuscular functioning; or emotional, motivational, cognitive, or psychosocial components of performance.

These services may require assessment of the need for and use of interventions such as the design, development, adaptation, application, or training in the use of assistive technology devices; the design, fabrication, or application of rehabilitative technology such as selected orthotic devices; training in the use of assistive technology, orthotic or prosthetic devices; the application of physical agent modalities as an adjunct to or in preparation for purposeful activity; the use of ergonomic principles; the adaptation of environments and processes to enhance functional performance; or the promotion of health and wellness (AOTA, 1993, p. 1117).

I. Performance Areas
Throughout this document, activities have been described as if individuals performed the tasks themselves. Occupational therapy also recognizes that individuals arrange for tasks to be done through others. The profession views independence as the ability to self-determine activity performance, regardless of who actually performs the activity.

A. *Activities of Daily Living*—Self-maintenance tasks.

1. *Grooming*—Obtaining and using supplies; removing body hair (use of razors, tweezers, lotions, etc.); applying and removing cosmetics; washing, drying, combing, styling, and brushing hair; caring for nails (hands and feet), caring for skin, ears, and eyes; and applying deodorant.

2. *Oral Hygiene*—Obtaining and using supplies; cleaning mouth; brushing and flossing teeth; or removing, cleaning and re-inserting dental orthotics and prosthetics.

3. *Bathing/Showering*—Obtaining and using supplies; soaping, rinsing, and drying all body parts; maintaining bathing position; transferring to and from bathing positions.

4. *Toilet Hygiene*—Obtaining and using supplies; clothing management; maintaining toileting position; transferring to and from toileting position; cleaning body; and caring for menstrual and continence needs (including catheters, colostomies, and suppository management).

5. *Personal Device Care*—Cleaning and maintaining personal care items, such as hearing aids, contact lenses, glasses, orthotics, prosthetics, adaptive equipment, and contraceptive and sexual devices.

6. *Dressing*—Selecting clothing and accessories appropriate for the time of day, weather, and occasion; obtaining clothing from storage area; dressing and undressing in a sequential fashion; fastening and adjusting clothing and shoes; and applying and removing personal devices, prostheses, or orthoses.

7. *Feeding and Eating*—Setting up food; selecting and using appropriate utensils and tableware; bringing food or drink to mouth; sucking, masticating, coughing, and swallowing; and management of alternative methods or nourishment.

8. *Medication Routine*—Obtaining medication, opening and closing containers, following prescribed schedules, taking correct quantities, reporting problems and adverse effects, and administering correct quantities using prescribed methods.

9. *Health Maintenance*—Developing and maintaining routines for illness prevention and wellness promotion, such as physical fitness, nutrition, and decreasing health risk behaviors.

10. *Socialization*—Accessing opportunities and interacting with other people in appropriate contextual and cultural ways to meet emotional and physical needs.

11. *Functional Communication*—Using equipment or systems to send and receive information, such as writing equipment, telephones, typewriters, communication boards, call lights, emergency systems, Braille writers, telecommunication devices for the deaf, and augmentative communication systems.

12. *Functional Mobility*—Moving from one position or place to another, such as in-bed mobility, wheelchair mobility, transfers (wheelchair, bed, car, tub/shower, toilet, chair, floor); performing functional ambulation and transporting objects.

13. *Community Mobility*—Moving self in the community and using public or private transportation, such as driving, or accessing buses, taxi cabs, or other public transportation systems.

14. *Emergency Response*—Recognizing sudden, unexpected hazardous situations, and initiating action to reduce the threat to health and safety.

15. *Sexual Expression*—Engaging in desired sexual activities.

B. *Work and Productive Activities*—Purposeful activities for self-development, social contribution, and livelihood.

1. *Home Management*—Obtaining and maintaining personal and household possessions and environment.

   a. *Clothing Care*—Obtaining and using supplies; sorting, laundering (hand, machine, and dry clean); folding; ironing; storing; and mending.

   b. *Cleaning*—Obtaining and using supplies; picking up; putting away;

vacuuming; sweeping and mopping floors; dusting; polishing; scrubbing; washing windows; cleaning mirrors; making beds; and removing trash and recyclables.

 c. *Meal Preparation and Cleanup*—Planning nutritious meals; preparing and serving food; opening and closing containers, cabinets, and drawers; using kitchen utensils and appliances; cleaning up and storing food safely.

 d. *Shopping*—Preparing shopping lists (grocery and other); selecting and purchasing items; selecting method of payment; and completing money transactions.

 e. *Money Management*—Budgeting, paying bills, and using bank systems.

 f. *Household Maintenance*—Maintaining home, yard, garden appliances, vehicles, and household items.

 g. *Safety Procedures*—Knowing and performing preventive and emergency procedures to maintain a safe environment and prevent injuries.

2. *Care of Others*—Providing for children, spouse, parents, pets or others, such as the physical care, nurturing, communicating, and using age-appropriate activities.

3. *Educational Activities*—Participating in a learning environment through school, community, or work-sponsored activities, such as exploring educational interests, attending to instruction, managing assignments, and contributing to group experiences.

4. *Vocational Activities*—Participating in work-related activities.

 a. *Vocational Exploration*—Determining aptitudes, developing interests and skills, and selecting appropriate vocational pursuits.

 b. *Job Acquisition*—Identifying and selecting work opportunities, and completing application and interview processes.

 c. *Work or Job Performance*—Performing job tasks in a timely and effective manner; incorporating necessary work behaviors.

 d. *Retirement Planning*—Determining aptitudes, developing interests and skills, and identifying appropriate avocational pursuits.

 e. *Volunteer Participation*—Performing unpaid activities for the benefit of selected individuals, groups, or causes.

C. *Play or Leisure Activities*—Intrinsically motivating activities for amusement, relaxation, spontaneous enjoyment, or self-expression.

1. *Play or Leisure Exploration*—Identifying interests, skills, opportunities, and appropriate play or leisure activities.

2. *Play or Leisure Performance*—Planning and participating in play or leisure activities; maintaining a balance of play or leisure activities with work and productive activities, and activities of daily living; obtaining, utilizing, and

maintaining equipment and supplies.

II. Performance Components

A. *Sensorimotor Component*—The ability to receive input, process information, and produce output.

1. *Sensory*

a. *Sensory Awareness*—Receiving and differentiating sensory stimuli.

b. *Sensory Processing*—Interpreting sensory stimuli.

(1) *Tactile*—Interpreting light touch, pressure, temperature, pain, and vibration through skin contact/receptors.

(2) *Pro-prioceptive*—Interpreting stimuli originating in muscles, joints, and other internal tissues to give information about the position of one body part in relation to another.

(3) *Vestibular*—Interpreting stimuli from the inner ear receptors regarding head position and movement.

(4) *Visual*—Interpreting stimuli through the eyes, including peripheral vision and acuity, awareness of color and pattern.

(5) *Auditory*—Interpreting and localizing sounds, and discriminating background sounds.

(6) *Gustatory*—Interpreting tastes.

(7) *Olfactory*—Interpreting odors.

c. *Perceptual Processing*—Organizing sensory input into meaningful patterns.

(1) *Stereognosis*—Identifying objects through proprioception, cognition, and the sense of touch.

(2) *Kinesthesia*—Identifying the excursion and direction of joint movement.

(3) *Pain Response*—Interpreting noxious stimuli.

(4) *Body Scheme*—Acquiring an internal awareness of the body and the relationship of body parts to each other.

(5) *Right-Left Discrimination*—Differentiating one side of the body from the other.

(6) *Form Constancy*—Recognizing forms and objects as the same in various environments, positions, and sizes.

(7) *Position in Space*—Determining the spatial relationship of figures and objects to self or other forms and objects.

(8) *Visual-Closure*—Identifying forms or objects from incomplete presentations.

(9) *Figure Ground*—Differentiating between foreground and background forms and objects.

(10) *Depth Perception*—Determining the relative distance between ob-

jects, figures, or landmarks and the observer, and changes in planes of surfaces.

(11) *Spatial Relations*—Determining the position of objects relative to each other.

(12) *Topographical Orientation*—Determining the location of objects and settings and the route to the location.

2. *Neuromusculoskeletal*

a. *Reflex*—Eliciting an involuntary muscle response by sensory input.

b. *Range of Motion*—Moving body parts through an arc.

c. *Muscle Tone*—Demonstrating a degree of tension or resistance in a muscle at rest and in response to stretch.

d. *Strength*—Demonstrating a degree of muscle power when movement is resisted, as with objects or gravity.

e. *Endurance*—Sustaining cardiac, pulmonary, and musculoskeletal exertion over time.

f. *Postural Control*—Using righting and equilibrium adjustments to maintain balance during functional movements.

g. *Postural Alignment*—Maintaining biomechanical integrity among body parts.

h. *Soft Tissue Integrity*—Maintaining anatomical and physiological condition of interstitial tissue and skin.

3. *Motor*

a. *Gross Coordination*—Using large muscle groups for controlled, goal-directed movements.

b. *Crossing the Midline*—Moving limbs and eyes across the midsagittal plane of the body.

c. *Laterality*—Using a preferred unilateral body part for activities requiring a high level of skill.

d. *Bilateral Integration*—Coordinating both body sides during activity.

e. *Motor Control*—Using the body in functional and versatile movement patterns.

f. *Praxis*—Conceiving and planning a new motor act in response to an environmental demand.

g. *Fine Coordination/Dexterity*—Using small muscle groups for controlled movements, particularly in object manipulation.

h. *Visual-Motor Integration*—Coordinating the interaction of information from the eyes with body movement during activity.

i. *Oral-Motor Control*—Coordinating oropharyngeal musculature for controlled movements.

B. *Cognitive Integration and Cognitive Components*
1. *Level of Arousal*—Demonstrating alertness and responsiveness to environmental stimuli.
2. *Orientation*—Identifying person, place, time, and situation.
3. *Recognition*—Identifying familiar faces, objects, and other previously presented materials.
4. *Attention Span*—Focusing on a task over time.
5. *Initiation of Activity*—Starting a physical or mental activity.
6. *Termination of Activity*—Stopping an activity at an appropriate time.
7. *Memory*—Recalling information after brief or long periods of time.
8. *Sequencing*—Placing information, concepts, and actions in order.
9. *Categorization*—Identifying similarities of and differences among pieces of environmental information.
10. *Concept Formation*—Organizing a variety of information to form thoughts and ideas.
11. *Spatial Operations*—Mentally manipulating the position of objects in various relationships.
12. *Problem Solving*—Recognizing a problem, defining a problem, identifying alternative plans, selecting a plan, organizing steps in a plan, implementing a plan, and evaluating the outcome.
13. *Learning*—Acquiring new concepts and behaviors.
14. *Generalization*—Applying previously learned concepts and behaviors to a variety of new situations.
C. *Psychosocial Skills and Psychological Components*—The ability to interact in society and to process emotions.
1. *Psychological*
   a. *Values*—Identifying ideas or beliefs that are important to self and others.
   b. *Interests*—Identifying mental or physical activities that create pleasure and maintain attention.
   c. *Self-Concept*—Developing the value of the physical, emotional, and sexual self.
2. *Social*
   a. *Role Performance*—Identifying, maintaining, and balancing functions one assumes or acquires in society (e.g., worker, student, parent, friend, religious participant).
   b. *Social Conduct*—Interacting using manners, personal space, eye contact, gestures, active listening, and self-expression appropriate to one's environment.
   c. *Interpersonal Skills*—Using verbal and nonverbal communication to interact in a variety of settings.

      d. *Self-Expression*—Using a variety of styles and skills to express thoughts, feelings, and needs.

3. *Self-Management*

      a. *Coping Skills*—Identifying and managing stress and related reactors.

      b. *Time Management*—Planning and participating in a balance of self-care, work, leisure, and rest activities to promote satisfaction and health.

      c. *Self-Control*—Modifying one's own behavior in response to environmental needs, demands, constraints, personal aspirations, and feedback from others.

III. Performance Contexts

Assessment of function in performance areas is greatly influenced by the contexts in which the individual must perform. Occupational therapy practitioners consider performance contexts when determining feasibility and appropriateness of interventions. Occupational therapy practitioners may choose interventions based on an understanding of contexts, or may choose interventions directly aimed at altering the contexts to improve performance.

    A. *Temporal Aspects*

      1. *Chronological*—Individual's age.

      2. *Developmental*—Stage or phase of maturation.

      3. *Life Cycle*—Place in important life phases, such as career cycle, parenting cycle, or educational process.

      4. *Disability Status*—Place in continuum of disability, such as acuteness of injury, chronicity of disability, or terminal nature of illness.

    B. *Environment*

      1. *Physical*—Nonhuman aspects of contexts. Includes the accessibility to and performance within environments having natural terrain, plants, animals, buildings, furniture, objects, tools, or devices.

      2. *Social*—Availability and expectations of significant individuals, such as spouse, friends, and caregivers. Also includes larger social groups which are influential in establishing norms, role expectations, and social routines.

      3. *Cultural*—Customs, beliefs, activity patterns, behavior standards, and expectations accepted by the society of which the individual is a member. Includes political aspects, such as laws that affect access to resources and affirm personal rights. Also includes opportunities for education, employment, and economic support.

References

American Occupational Therapy Association. (1979). *Occupational therapy output reporting system and uniform terminology for reporting occupational therapy services.* Rockville, MD: Author.

American Occupational Therapy Association. (1989). Uniform terminology for occupational therapy—

Second edition. *American Journal of Occupational Therapy, 43,* 808-815.
American Occupational Therapy Association. (1993). Definition of occupational therapy practice for state regulation (Policy 5.3.1). *American Journal of Occupational Therapy, 47,* 1117-1121.

Authors:
The Terminology Task Force:
  Winifred Dunn, PhD, OTR, FAOTA—Chairperson
  Mary Foto, OTR, FAOTA
  Jim Hinojosa, PhD, OTR, FAOTA
  Barbara A. Boyt Schell, PhD, OTR/L, FAOTA
  Linda Kohlman Thomson, MOT, OTR, OT(C), FAOTA
  Sarah D. Hertfelder, MEd, MOT, OTR/L—Staff Liaison

for The Commission on Practice
Jim Hinojosa, PhD, OTR, FAOTA—Chairperson

Adopted by the Representative Assembly 7/94

NOTE: This document replaces the following documents, all of which were rescinded by the 1994 Representative Assembly:

Occupational Therapy Product Output Reporting System (1979)
Uniform Terminology for Reporting Occupational Therapy Services—First Edition (1979)
Uniform Occupational Therapy Evaluation Checklist (1981)
Uniform Terminology for Occupational Therapy—Second Edition (1989)

Uniform Terminology—Third Edition:
Application to Practice

Introduction

This document was developed to help occupational therapists apply *Uniform Terminology, Third Edition* to practice. The original grid format (Dunn, 1988) enabled occupational therapy practitioners to systematically identify deficit and strength areas of an individual and to select appropriate activities to address these areas in occupational therapy intervention (Dunn & McGourty, 1990). For the third edition, the profession is highlighting "Contexts" as another critical aspect of performance. A second grid provides therapy practitioners with a mechanism to consider the contextual features of performance in activities of daily living (ADL), work and productive activity, and play/leisure. "Performance Areas" and "Performance Components" (Figure A) focus on the individual. These features are embedded in the "Performance Contexts" (Figure B).

On the original grid (Dunn, 1988), the horizontal axis contains the Performance Areas of Activities of Daily Living, Work and Productive Activities, and Play or Leisure Activities (see Figure A). These Performance Areas are the functional outcomes occupational therapy addresses. The vertical axis contains the Performance Components, including Sensorimotor Components, Cognitive Components, and Psychosocial Components. The Performance Components are the skills and abilities that an individual uses to engage in the Performance Areas. During an occupational therapy assessment, the occupational therapy practitioner determines an individual's abilities and limitations in the Performance Components and how they affect the individual's functional outcomes in the Performance Areas.

Figure A—Uniform Terminology Grid
(Performance Areas and Performance Components)
Performance Areas

I. Performance Components
    A. Sensorimotor Component
        1. Sensory
            a. Sensory Awareness
            b. Sensory Processing
                (1) Tactile
                (2) Pro-prioceptive
                (3) Vestibular
                (4) Visual
                (5) Auditory
                (6) Gustatory
                (7) Olfactory
            c. Perceptual Processing
                (1) Stereognosis
                (2) Kinesthesia
                (3) Pain Response
                (4) Body Scheme
                (5) Right-Left Discrimination
                (6) Form Constancy
                (7) Position in Space
                (8) Visual-Closure
                (9) Figure Ground
                (10) Depth Perception

(11) Spatial Relations
(12) Topographical Orientation
2. Neuromusculoskeletal
  a. Reflex
  b. Range of Motion
  c. Muscle Tone
  d. Strength
  e. Endurance
  f. Postural Control
  g. Postural Alignment
  h. Soft Tissue Integrity
3. Motor
  a. Gross Coordination
  b. Crossing the Midline
  c. Laterality
  d. Bilateral Integration
  e. Motor Control
  f. Praxis
  g. Fine Coordination/Dexterity
  h. Visual-Motor Integration
  i. Oral-Motor Control
B. Cognitive Integration and Cognitive Components
  1. Level of Arousal
  2. Orientation
  3. Recognition
  4. Attention Span
  5. Initiation of Activity
  6. Termination of Activity
  7. Memory
  8. Sequencing
  9. Categorization
  10. Concept Formation
  11. Spatial Operations
  12. Problem Solving
  13. Learning
  14. Generalization
C. Psychosocial Skills and Psychological Components
  1. Psychological
    a. Values
    b. Interests

        c. Self-Concept
    2. Social
        a. Role Performance
        b. Social Conduct
        c. Interpersonal Skills
        d. Self-Expression
    3. Self-Management
        a. Coping Skills
        b. Time Management
        c. Self-Control

SPECIAL NOTE: The first application document (Dunn & McGourty, 1989) describes how to use the original *Uniform Terminology* grid with a variety of individuals. It is quite useful to introduce these concepts. However, the third edition of *Uniform Terminology* contains some changes in the Performance Areas and Performance Components lists. Be sure to check for the terminology currently approved in the third edition before applying this information in current practice environments.

With the addition of Performance Contexts into *Uniform Terminology*, occupational therapy practitioners must consider how to interface what the individual wants to do (i.e., performance areas) with the contextual features that may support or block performance. Figure B illustrates the interaction of Performance Areas and Performance Contexts as a model for therapists' planning.

Figure B—Uniform Terminology Grid
(Performance Areas and Performance Contexts)
Performance Areas

I. Performance Contexts
    A. Temporal Aspects
        1. Chronological
        2. Developmental
        3. Life Cycle
        4. Disability Status
    B. Environment
        1. Physical
        2. Social
        3. Cultural

The grid in Figure B can be used to analyze the contexts of performance for a particular individual. For example, when working with a toddler with a developmental disability who needs to learn to eat, the occupational therapy practitioner would consider all the Performance Contexts features as they might impact on this toddler's ability to master eating. Unlike the grid in Figure A, in which the occupational therapy practitioner selects *both* Performance Areas (i.e., what the individual wants or needs to do) and the Performance Component (i.e., a person's strengths and needs), in this grid (Figure B) the occupational therapy practitioner only selects the Performance Area. After the Performance Area is identified through collaboration with the individual and significant others, the occupational therapy practitioner considers **all** Performance Context features as they might impact on performance of the selected task.

Intervention Planning

Intervention planning occurs both within the general domain of concern of occupational therapy (i.e., uniform terminology) and by considering the profession's theoretical frames of reference that offer insights about how to approach the problem. In Figure A, the occupational therapy practitioner considers the Performance Areas that are of interest to the individual and the individual's strengths and concerns within the Performance Components. The intervention strategies would emerge from the cells on the grid that are placed at the intersection of the Performance Areas and the targeted Performance Components (strength and/or concern). For example, if a child needed to improve sensory processing and fine coordination for oral hygiene and grooming, an occupational therapy practitioner might select a sensory integrative frame of reference to create intervention strategies, such as adding textures to handles and teaching the child sand and bean digging games. Dunn and McGourty (1989) discuss this in more detail.

When using Figure B, the occupational therapy practitioner considers the Performance Contexts features in relation to the desired Performance Area. The occupational therapy practitioner would analyze the individual's temporal, physical, social, and cultural contexts to determine the relevance of particular interventions. For example, if the child mentioned above was a member of a family in which having messy hands from sand play was unacceptable, the occupational therapy practitioner would consider alternate strategies that are more compatible with their lifestyle. For example, perhaps the family would be more interested in developing puppet play. This would still provide the child with opportunities to experience the textures of various puppets and the hand movements required to manipulate the puppets in play context, without adding the messiness of sand. When occupational therapy practitioners consider contexts, interventions become more relevant and applicable to individual's lives.

Case Example 1

Sophie, a 75-year-old lady who was widowed 3 years ago, is recovering from a cerebral vascular accident and has been transferred from an acute care unit to an inpatient medical rehabilitation unit. Prior to her admission, she was living in a small house in an isolated location and has no family living nearby. She was driving independently and frequently ran errands for her friends. She is adamant in her goal to return to her home after discharge. All of her friends are quite elderly and are not able to provide many resources for support.

Sophie and the team collaborated to identify her goals. Sophie decided that she wanted to be able to meet her daily needs with little or no assistance. Almost all of the Performance Areas are critical in order to achieve the outcome of community living in her own home. Being able to cook all of her meals, bathe independently, and have alternative transportation available is necessary. Because of their significant impact on the patient's function in the Performance Areas, some of the Performance Components that may need to be addressed are figure ground, muscle tone, postural control, fine coordination, memory, and self-management.

In the selection of occupational therapy interventions, it is critical to analyze the elements of Performance Contexts for the individual. The physical and social elements of her home environment do not support returning home without modifications to her home and additional social supports being established. Railings must be added to the front steps, provision of and instruction in the use of a tub seat, and instruction in the use of specialized transportation may need to occur. If this same individual had been living in an apartment in a retirement community prior to her CVA, the contexts of performance would support a return home with fewer environmental modifications being needed. Being independent in cooking might not be necessary due to meals being provided, and the bathroom might already be accessible and safe. If the individual had friends and family available, the social support network might already be established to assist with shopping and transportation needs. The occupational therapy interventions would be different due to the contexts in which the individual will be performing. Interventions must be selected with the impact of the Performance Contexts as an essential element.

Case Example 2

Malcolm is a 9-year-old boy who has a learning disability which causes him to have a variety of problems in school. His teachers complain that he is difficult to manage in the classroom. Some of the Performance Components that may need to be addressed are his self-control such as interrupting, difficulty sitting during instruction, and difficulty with peer relations. Other children avoid him on the playground, because he doesn't follow rules, doesn't play fair, and tends to anger quickly when confronted. The performance component impairment with concept formation is reflected in his sloppy and disorganized classroom assignments.

The critical elements of the Performance Contexts are the temporal aspect of age-appropriateness of his behavior and the social environment aspect of his immature socialization. The significant cultural and temporal aspects of his family are that they place a high premium on athletic prowess.

The occupational therapy practitioner intervenes in several ways to address his behavior in the school environment. The occupational therapy practitioner focuses on structuring the classroom environment and facilitating consistent behavioral expectations for Malcolm by educational personnel. She also consults with the teachers to develop ways to structure activities which will support his ability to relate to other children in a positive way.

In contrast, another child with similar learning disabilities, but who is 12 years old and in the 7th grade might have different concerns. Elements of the Performance Contexts are the temporal aspect of the age-appropriateness of his behavior; and the social environment context of school where "bullying" behavior is unacceptable and in which completing assignments is expected. In addressing the cultural Performance Contexts the occupational therapy practitioner recognizes from meeting the parents that they have only average expectation for academic performance but value athletic accomplishments.

Since teachers at his school consider completion of home assignments to be part of average performance, the occupational therapy practitioner works with the child and parents on time management and reinforcement strategies to meet this expectation. After consultation with the coach, she works with the father to create activities to improve his athletic abilities. When occupational therapy practitioners consider family values as part of the contexts of performance, different intervention priorities may emerge.

Authors:

The Terminology Task Force:
  Winifred Dunn, PhD, OTR, FAOTA—Chairperson
  Mary Foto, OTR, FAOTA
  Jim Hinojosa, PhD, OTR, FAOTA
  Barbara A. Boyt Schell, PhD, OTR/L, FAOTA
  Linda Kohlman Thomson, MOT, OTR, OT(C), FAOTA
  Sarah D. Hertfelder, MEd, MOT, OTR/L—Staff Liaison

for The Commission on Practice—1994

Jim Hinojosa, PhD, OTR, FAOTA—Chairperson

NOTE: This document replaces the 1989 *Application of Uniform Terminology to Practice* that accompanied the *Uniform Terminology for Occupational Therapy—Second Edition.*

I. Performance Areas	II. Performance Components	III. Performance Contexts
A. Activities of Daily Living	A. Sensorimotor Component	A. Temporal Aspects
1. Grooming	1. Sensory	1. Chronological
2. Oral Hygiene	a. Sensory Awareness	2. Developmental
3. Bathing/Showering	b. Sensory Processing	3. Life Cycle
4. Toilet Hygiene	(1) Tactile	4. Disability Status
5. Personal Device Care	(2) Proprioceptive	B. Environmental Aspects
6. Dressing	(3) Vestibular	1. Physical
7. Feeding and Eating	(4) Visual	2. Social
8. Medication Routine	(5) Auditory	3. Cultural
9. Health Maintenance	(6) Gustatory	
10. Socialization	(7) Olfactory	
11. Functional Communication	c. Perceptual Processing	
12. Functional Mobility	(1) Stereognosis	
13. Community Mobility	(2) Kinesthesia	
14. Emergency Response	(3) Pain Response	
15. Sexual Expression	(4) Body Scheme	
B. Work and Productive Activities	(5) Right-Left Discrimination	
1. Home Management	(6) Form Constancy	
a. Clothing Care	(7) Position in Space	
b. Cleaning	(8) Visual-Closure	
c. Meal Preparation/Cleanup	(9) Figure Ground	
d. Shopping	(10) Depth Perception	
e. Money Management	(11) Spatial Relations	
f. Household Maintenance	(12) Topographical Orientation	
g. Safety Procedures	2. Neuromusculoskeletal	
2. Care of Others	a. Reflex	
3. Educational Activities	b. Range of Motion	
4. Vocational Activities	c. Muscle Tone	
a. Vocational Exploration	d. Strength	
b. Job Acquisition	e. Endurance	
c. Work or Job Performance	f. Postural Control	
d. Retirement Planning	g. Postural Alignment	
e. Volunteer Participation	h. Soft Tissue Integrity	
C. Play or Leisure Activities	3. Motor	
1. Play or Leisure Exploration	a. Gross Coordination	
2. Play or Leisure Performance	b. Crossing the Midline	
	c. Laterality	
	d. Bilateral Integration	
	e. Motor control	
	f. Praxis	
	g. Fine Coordination/Dexterity	
	h. Visual-Motor Integration	
	i. Oral-Motor Control	
	B. Cognitive Integration and Cognitive Components	
	1. Level of Arousal	
	2. Orientation	
	3. Recognition	
	4. Attention Span	
	5. Initiation of Activity	
	6. Termination of Activity	
	7. Memory	
	8. Sequencing	
	9. Categorization	
	10. Concept Formation	
	11. Spatial Operations	
	12. Problem Solving	
	13. Learning	
	14. Generalization	
	C. Psychosocial Skills and Psychological Components	
	1. Psychological	
	a. Values	
	b. Interests	
	c. Self-Concept	
	2. Social	
	a. Role Performance	
	b. Social Conduct	
	c. Interpersonal Skills	
	d. Self-Expression	
	3. Self-Management	
	a. Coping Skills	
	b. Time Management	
	c. Self-Control	

Index